MUTAGENESIS

Advances in Modern Toxicology

Editor
Myron A. Mehlman

Advances in Modern Toxicology

VOLUME 5

MUTAGENESIS

EDITED BY

W. GARY FLAMM
NATIONAL CANCER INSTITUTE

MYRON A. MEHLMAN
MEDICAL DEPARTMENT
MOBIL OIL CORPORATION

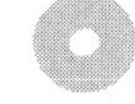

HEMISPHERE
PUBLISHING CORPORATION

Washington   London

A HALSTED PRESS BOOK

JOHN WILEY & SONS
New York   London   Sydney   Toronto

Hemisphere Publishing Corporation
1025 Vermont Ave., N.W., Washington, D.C. 20005

Distributed solely by Halsted Press, a Division of John Wiley & Sons, Inc., New York.

1 2 3 4 5 6 7 8 9 0   D O D O   7 8 3 2 1 0 9 8

Library of Congress Cataloging in Publication Data
Main entry under title:

Mutagenesis.

    (Advances in modern toxicology: v. 5)
    Includes index.
    I. Chemical mutagenesis. I. Flamm, W. G., date.
II. Mehlman, Myron A. III. Series.
QH465.C5M87   575.2'92   77-26342
ISBN 0-470-99393-6

CONTENTS

PREFACE

Research in the area of chemical mutagenesis has been carried out for about three decades now. One could say it has passed through a number of phases: a period of surprising discovery, one of gradual illumination, a period of developing dogma, and finally a period of reflection. During the early years of research, the justifications for undertaking such work probably varied inversely with the number of researchers involved. As it became generally recognized that chemical mutagens were sufficiently common and ubiquitous as to pose a threat to exposed human populations, the reasons for undertaking research in the area became fewer and researchers more numerous.

Today we are witnessing the creation of new laws and the promulgations of new regulatory requirements under existing laws that are likely to change forever the face of chemical mutagenesis. It bears remembering that efforts to develop toxicologically sound mutagenic test systems began only about ten years ago. In 'the course of that period certain tests came into favor and fell from favor; some may again return to favor. During this ten-year period of reasonably intense activity, a number of texts and volumes have been written on the subject in general and the test methods specifically. This monograph is in part born of the belief that regulatory test requirements are imminent and that an effort must be made to provide better understanding of the public health issues, needs, and requirements.

The introductory section attempts to explain the relationship between mutagenic test systems and the diseases of genetic origin that occur in human populations, as well as the need to develop guidelines for determining maximum permissible levels of chemical mutagens. In passing, it is noted that mutagens share with carcinogens a one-hit mechanism for the production of their respective biological effects. Nevertheless, mutagens may prove far more tractable in terms of assessing and quantifying risk given the fact that much is known regarding their mechanism of action, the target molecule, and, of course, the target tissue. It should also be pointed out that the main purpose of this volume is to address mutagenesis in terms of genetic disease burden—in other words, the risk to future generations.

The section on modifying factors makes evident the need to consider a variety of biochemical, metabolic, and molecular aspects of the problem that can enhance, inhibit, or be totally responsible for the mechanism and events of mutagenesis. Because there appears to be a reasonably good analogy between carcinogenesis and mutagenesis regarding the impact of nutrition and because considerably more is known about nutrition and carcinogenesis, most of the chapter dealing with this subject has addressed carcinogenesis.

The section on test methods is not intended to be comprehensive in any sense. Instead, tests were selected because they were at opposite poles in terms of the type of mutation measured and the method of measurement in order to illustrate test system methodology. Rather than repeat material contained in many other volumes on this subject, the emphasis here is on defining current and future needs and discussing the types of tests that at fledgling stages of development hold considerable promise. Implicit in this approach is the belief that the field of chemical/environmental mutagenesis is a dynamic one that will require the development and reassessment of many tests and experience many changes.

The next section deals with chemical mutagens per se, their sources, and the nature and character of human exposure to them. This subject is divided into naturally occurring and synthetic mutagens. The final section discusses information systems on chemical environmental mutagens and provides the reader with a guide to the use and accessibility of the Environmental Mutagen Information Center. It is hoped that this monograph, having taken a some-what different approach from other volumes on the subject, will prove to be of special interest to those involved in the toxicological assessment and public health considerations attending chemical mutagens.

Part 1

INTRODUCTION

CHAPTER 1

GENETIC DISEASES IN HUMANS VERSUS MUTAGENICITY TEST SYSTEMS

W. Gary Flamm
Division of Cancer Cause and Prevention
National Cancer Institute
Bethesda, Maryland

INTRODUCTION

An attempt will be made in this chapter to outline briefly the major categories of human diseases that are of genetic origin, and to describe the types of available experimental systems with the capability of detecting and measuring the genetic events responsible for the diseases in each category. For the sake of simplicity, the body of knowledge regarding diseases of genetic origin will be divided into the four main categories.

CATEGORIES OF GENETIC DISEASES

The first and perhaps best defined category in terms of disease incidence consists of chromosomal mutations (Shaw, 1972). It should be recognized that even here new genetic disorders are continually being discovered, largely because of the development and application of new chromosome banding techniques in cytogenetics. The classic and most frequently encountered chromosomal mutations in humans are mongolism, Klinefelter's syndrome, and Turner's syndrome. Mongoloid idiocy, or Down's syndrome as it is known medically, is a chromosomal mutation involving chromosome 21. This mutation can arise through a variety of genetic events, the most common being nondisjunction (by far the most frequent) and translocation occurring in the germinal cells of either the mother or the father.

The seriousness and morbidity of mongolism are common knowledge, but it should be mentioned here that the incidence of the disease among live births has been estimated to be approximately 0.2% in the United States (McKusick, 1968, 1970). Assuming 3–4 million births in the United States 6,000–8,000 mongoloid children are born each year in this country alone. It should also be pointed out that mongolism is the most frequent single definable entity causing severe mental deficiency.

No attempt will be made to describe the other genetic disorders attributable to chromosomal mutations, except to state that collectively they occur with a frequency slightly greater than that for mongolism—approximately 0.3% (McKusick, 1968, 1970). It is emphasized and should be noted that the great majority of these chromosomal mutations are new, having arisen in the germ cells of either the mother or the father of the mutant progeny.

This category of genetic diseases can be summarized by stating that 1 of every 200 live births, or 15,000–20,000 newborns per year, are affected by chromosomal mutation, and that the majority of such mutations are new, having arisen in the germ cells that transmitted them.

Now, the question is what types of animal systems are available for detecting and measuring the genetic events responsible for these kinds of chromosomal mutations. There are two major methods. However, both are still under development, in the sense that efforts are being made to define the protocols that are best or at least adequate for performing these tests. The two methods that have been used in mammals—or, more particularly, in mice—for measuring genetic events that give rise to Down's, Klinefelter's, and Turner's syndromes and other chromosomal diseases are the X-chromosome loss method, which is being perfected at Oak Ridge National Laboratory by Dr. William Russell, and the indirect heritable translocation test, which is also under study at Oak Ridge and at several other laboratories in the United States and Europe (Generoso et al., 1977).

The details of these tests are described elsewhere (Flamm and Mehlman, 1978). For this chapter it need only be stated that either the female or the male is treated with the suspect compound for an appropriate period of time, after which the animals are mated and the progeny are examined by a variety of methods to see whether they are mutants. In the case of the heritable translocation test, the males from treated fathers are mated to virgin females; should their reproductive performance prove to be affected in a specific way, they are set aside as possible presumptive translocation heterozygotes. Whether they are mutant translocation heterozygotes can be determined definitively by a cytogenetic-cytological investigation of meiotic chromosomes at the time of pairing. Because the translocation occurred in the germ line of the treated male, all of the cells of the male offspring should contain the translocation, and, as the germ cells of the male offspring attempt to pass through the meiotic phase of spermatogenesis, failure of homologous chromosomes to pair as they should proves that a translocation has occurred.

In the X-chromosome loss test, female mice are treated and their female progeny examined for the existence of an XO phenotype based on the use of a morphologic marker on the X-chromosome.

There are, of course, a number of other approaches by which chromosomal aberrations may be detected and measured. These methods include *in vitro* techniques utilizing somatic cells in tissue culture and *in vivo* procedures where cells from either the bone marrow or lymphocytes of treated animals are examined for chromosomal aberrations. These end points are neither explicit nor readily interpretable in that the assessment is one of chromosome damage (usually chromosome breaks and gaps) and cell death, and not necessarily of heritable or transmissible effects. Despite the fact that muta-geneticists have used chromosome and chromatid breaks and gaps for a number of years to identify substances suspected of being chromosomal mutagens, it is not likely that all agents that have the capability of breaking chromosomes will always and necessarily have the capability of producing heritable effects in germinal cells.

It is probably fair to state that when the relevance of chromosomal breaks as induced by a specific chemical substance has been established, chromosomal breaks can be used as a very effective research tool. But one should remain skeptical of accepting a substance as a mutagen only on the basis of experiments that show that the chemical can produce chromosomal breaks when cells are treated *in vitro*. The evidence in support of that view is inadequate at present, and, indeed, it is possible that future research will show that certain of the assay systems used for measuring chromosomal breaks are not always relevant to mutagenesis.

The next category of human genetic diseases comprises those occurring through mutations of single genes that are dominant. Dominant mutation means that anyone carrying the mutant gene will express the mutant trait. It also implies that 50% of the children of such individuals will express the mutant trait. For these genes, the mutant trait usually involves structural anomalies and physical malformations, as opposed to functional alterations. However, among approximately 1,000 dominant mutations known to occur in human populations, there are certain exceptions to this rule.

For instance, nine forms of cancer are known to occur through mutations of dominant genes. These are single, autosomal genes. These cancers are collectively referred to as hereditary neoplasms (Fraumeni, 1973). The best studied of these nine is bilateral retinoblastoma, which has an incidence of 1 in 20,000 births. This incidence translates into approximately 200 cases per year. Because of the high mortality once associated with bilateral retinoblastoma, virtually all cases in the past have undoubtedly been new mutations.

The most common of the hereditary neoplasms is probably polyposis coli, with a frequency of about 1 in 8,000, or approximately 500 cases per year (Fraumeni, 1973). This disease is characterized by numerous polyps of the rectum and colon, which invariably progress into carcinomas with advancing age.

The other seven hereditary neoplasms are also rare. Their collective incidence is probably no more than 1 per 5,000, or less than 1,000 cases per year (Fraumeni, 1973).

The total disease burden attributable to mutations of dominant genes, including hereditary neoplasms, is of the same order of magnitude as that for chromosomal mutations—and the two categories taken together would represent an incidence of approximately 1%. It should be remembered, however, that many dominant gene mutations result in structural anomalies, which we would classify not as diseases but as disorders. And while they may not come to clinical attention, they nevertheless constitute a real departure from the norm, and certainly impact on an individual's quality of life. The figure of 1%, therefore, is highly conservative and may be looked on as an underestimate. In the interest of saving space, I shall describe the third category of mutations in humans before discussing the types of laboratory test systems that are useful in measuring the genetic events responsible for dominant gene mutations.

This third category of mutations consists of the recessive mutations, and for these to be expressed both genes of a homologous chromosomal pair, composed of one chromosome from the mother and one from the father, must be similarly affected. Thus, it is possible to carry a defective gene without ever expressing the corresponding defect or trait. Mating to an individual carrying the same defect can result in two phenotypically normal parents producing children with the disease corresponding to that particular recessive mutation. Sickle-cell anemia is an excellent example of such a mutation. Two individuals can carry the sickling trait, but unless their maternal and paternal hemoglobin genes are of the sickle-cell mutant type, these individuals themselves will appear essentially normal. Should they have children, however, their offspring have a 25% chance of inheriting two sickle-cell mutant genes, in which case they would express the recessive disease of sickle-cell anemia.

Unlike the first two categories, recessive gene mutations are cryptic and can remain dormant through many generations, until a single mating occurs in which both homologous mutant genes are present in the offspring. It is at this time that the mutant gene reveals its character and expresses its full effect on the affected individual.

Another means by which recessive genes can acquire expression is through a second mutation. Indeed, it should be recognized that there is a high degree of heterozygocity in human populations. That is, perhaps as much as several percent of the total recessive genes present in the human genome are already in a mutant form or at least deviate from the norm in a significant way. Assuming this to be the case, then a reasonably high percentage of mutations is likely to occur at a gene where either the maternal or the paternal complement is already mutant. This, then, would lead to the expression of the disease characterized by the recessive mutation.

There are over 1,000 known genetic disorders that have the genetic properties of a recessive mutation. Many of these, such as phenylketonuria, alkaptonuria, galactosemia, and homocystinuria, are well known to any student of biochemistry. Indeed, surveys have revealed that at any given time 5-6% of the patients in the pediatric wards of major metropolitan hospitals are suffering from diseases caused by single-gene defects that can be defined genetically as recessive mutations (Childs et al., 1972).

There are, unquestionably, a variety of genetic events responsible for this myriad of mutations in humans. At the molecular level, many are known to be base-pair substitutions, but there is every likelihood that these mutations occur by a variety of other molecular mechanisms as well, such as frameshifts, interstitial deletions, terminal deletions, and others (Drake, 1970).

In any case, both dominant and recessive mutations are classified as gene mutations, and the only methods thought to be useful for detecting and measuring these kinds of mutations are methods that measure heritable effects. Bacteria can be used for this and will measure a variety of mutational events, including base-pair substitutions and frameshifts. *Neurospora* is useful for measuring inter- and intragenic deletions and gene conversions as well as point mutations. Indeed, I could proceed to name any number of test systems that have the capability of detecting genetic events of importance to humans, but little would be accomplished in so doing. Each system has its own advantages and disadvantages, and clearly the major challenge is to provide adequately for the kind of metabolic transformations or activations expected to occur in humans. Once this has been done and it has been found that a substance is genetically active, the task of assessing potency remains.

This apparently is best approached by combining genetic investigations with pharmacokinetic studies, and it is my view that mammalian cells in tissue culture may prove highly useful in providing the necessary genetic evidence with respect to potential and potency, while intact animals will need to be used to address all relevant pharmacokinetic aspects. After all, we know the target organ is essentially the gonads and the target molecule is essentially DNA. Indeed, because of this knowledge, the prospects for conducting meaningful studies that quantify the genetic risk attributable to specific levels of exposure seem excellent.

The final category of genetic diseases includes such common disorders as diabetes, epilepsy, schizophrenia, and essential hypertension—all of which are believed to have a strong genetic component because of their recurrence in families. These conditions are presumably transmitted as multiple-gene disorders and are poorly understood in genetic terms. Indeed, it is not by any means clear that the incidence of these diseases would increase with increases in mutation rate. At the present state of understanding, it cannot be argued that any of the current mutagenicity methods would necessarily be relevant to this group of familial diseases.

CONCLUSION

To assess the potential dangers of environmental mutagens, one must first understand the mutation process, including the nature and origins of mutation and the ways in which mutations are likely to be produced by various agents that impinge on humans. One must also have some understanding of the mechanism of inheritance and the role of mutation in disease and evolutionary processes.

REFERENCES

Childs, B., Miller, S.M. and Bearn, A., 1972. Gene mutation as a cause of human disease. In *Mutagenic effects of environmental contaminants*, eds. H. E. Sutton and M. I. Harris, pp. 3–14. New York: Academic Press.

Drake, J. W. 1970. *The molecular basis of mutation*. San Francisco: Holden-Day.

Flamm, W. G. and Mehlman, M., eds. 1978. *Advances in modern toxicology*, vol. 5 *Mutagenesis*. Washington, D.C.: Hemisphere.

Fraumeni, J. F. 1973. Genetic factors. In *Cancer medicine*, eds. J. Holland and E. Frei, pp. 7–15. Philadelphia: Lea and Febiger.

Generoso, W., Cain, K. T. and Huff, W. 1978. Inducibility by chemical mutagens of heritable translocations in male and female germ cells of mice. In *Advances in modern toxicology*, vol. 5 *Mutagenesis*, eds. W. G. Flamm and M. Mehlman, pp. 109–129. Washington, D.C.: Hemisphere.

McKusick, V. A. 1968. *Mendelian inheritance in man*, 2nd ed. Baltimore: Johns Hopkins.

McKusick, V. A. 1970. *Annu. Rev. Genet.* 4: 1.

Shaw, M. W. 1972. Chromosome mutations in man. In *Mutagenic effects of environmental contaminants*, eds. H. E. Sutton and M. I. Harris, pp. 81–97. New York: Academic Press.

CHAPTER 2

SOME GUIDELINES FOR DETERMINING MAXIMUM PERMISSIBLE LEVELS OF CHEMICAL MUTAGENS

John W. Drake
Department of Microbiology
University of Illinois
Urbana, Illinois

INTRODUCTION

Some Aspects of Mutation in Humans

Although individual cases of mutation in humans may appear to be very rare events, the aggregate deleterious effects of spontaneous mutation are distressingly common. It is instructive to consider the incidence of mutation in comparison with two specific dangerous diseases, poliomyelitis and cancer. The former was relatively rare even before the introduction of vaccines, seriously affecting no more than 1 individual in 10,000 even in most epidemic years. Just as in the case of many human mutations, however, poliomyelitis most dramatically affects the very young, and was deemed worthy of a massive attempt at eradication. Cancer, on the other hand, will arise in nearly one-fourth of the population, and will prove fatal to a large proportion of its victims; because of this high incidence, it, too, is deemed worthy of massive attack. It is an unfortunate fact that the gross human mutation rate is much nearer to the rate of cancer than it is to the rate of poliomyelitis.

There are a variety of ways of estimating the total human spontaneous mutation rate, none of them alone being very satisfactory but all of them pointing to the same general value. Estimates of the average mutation rate per individual human gene per sexual generation range from about 10^{-4} (Neel, 1973) to about 10^{-7} (Stevenson and Kerr, 1967), and estimates of the total number of human genes range from 10^4 to 10^5. The product of the means of these two ranges is $(10^{-4} \times 10^{-7})^{0.5} \times (10^4 \times 10^5)^{0.5} = 0.1$, suggesting that 10% of all human gametes harbor a newly arisen mutation. Similarly, the BEIR report (Advisory Committee on the Biological Effects of Ionizing Radiations, 1972) estimated the incidence of human genetic disease at 6%. Each of these figures, however, probably seriously underestimates the true value, since neither includes diseases determined by several genes acting in concert, or relatively mild diseases that may in the aggregate produce a vast amount of human suffering.

Comprehensive estimates of the total rate of appearance of deleterious mutations have been obtained thus far in only one higher eukaryote, *Drosophila melanogaster* (Mukai et al., 1972). The types of mutations scored in these fruit fly experiments excluded many that are routinely observed in humans, such as dominant and visible mutations. On the other hand, the exceedingly sensitive scoring system employed readily detected mutations that reduced fruit fly viability by only a very few percent (at least under the rather luxurious living conditions provided the flies) and, as a result, detected by far the largest class of mutations. The mutation rate estimated in these experiments was ≥ 0.43 per haploid genome per sexual generation. Since there are no indications either that the mutation rate per gene is substantially lower in humans than in the fruit fly or that the number of human genes is smaller than the number of fruit fly genes, 43% is a reasonable lower limit for the spontaneous rate of deleterious mutation in humans.

If the human spontaneous mutation rate per gamete is ≥ 0.43, then the rate per zygote is ≥ 0.86, and almost everyone appears to harbor approximately one newly (and harmfully) mutated gene. Furthermore, the majority of these mutations are probably only mildly deleterious and are therefore subject to only weak selection. As a result, the average individual is apt to carry not only a newly mutated gene, but also several mutated genes inherited from relatively recent ancestors. It is not very clear at present how this relatively large burden of mutations is tolerated, but one answer to this question may lie in a tendency for the typical genetic death (that is, failure to reproduce, for whatever reason) to subtract a greater than average number of defective genes from the gene pool. This is particularly apt to happen if typically rather mildly deleterious mutations interact synergistically, rather than simply additively, as they accumulate in individuals.

The principal mechanism that enables a diploid species to carry an average of several deleterious genes per individual, a genetic burden that might well be lethal several times over in a haploid species, is the recessiveness of many mutations. When two versions (alleles) of a gene coexist in a common cell, as is nearly always the case for the higher eukaryotes, and when the resulting phenotype is determined exclusively by only one of these two alleles, then that allele is said to be dominant and its counterpart to be recessive. Fully recessive and fully dominant alleles are favorite objects of study by geneticists because they make superior laboratory tools compared with (codominant) alleles with intermediate degrees of expression, and, probably because of this partiality, geneticists sometimes do not adequately stress the fact that completely recessive or dominant alleles occur infrequently. The typical newly arisen mutant allele is neither fully recessive nor fully dominant, but is somewhere in between, usually closer to the recessive than to the dominant end of the spectrum. The typical deleterious mutant allele that has persisted for a number of generations within a population, however, is much more recessive than is the typical newly arisen mutant allele, an obvious result of the culling action of natural selection. It appears that the average environmentally induced mutation is not going to be very different in character from the average truly spontaneous mutation. Therefore, the lack of complete recessiveness of most newly arisen mutant alleles implies that the expression of induced genetic damage is not, as is sometimes assumed, largely postponed until that distant time when the progeny of defective genes once again find themselves in a double dose in a single individual. On the contrary, some considerable fraction of whatever damage we may do to our germ cells will be visited directly on our own children.

While gene defects are often expressed at least in part in the very next generation, an only moderately increased mutation rate is unlikely to be recognized by the populace at large without expert assistance. Obvious birth defects are of mixed origin, some being determined genetically and others by quite different causes, and even a specific type of birth defect may sometimes be determined genetically and at other times by nongenetic causes. The numbers of birth defects that are almost exclusively of genetic origin, that are attributable to new mutations not present in either parent, and that are readily recognized at or near birth by the layman (or even by the physician) are quite small. The collective deleterious effects of mutations producing only mild disease, or producing only a fraction of the incidence of a specific illness, are likely to be far greater than illnesses attributable to well-defined defects detectable at or shortly after birth. Only a small fraction of the total damage resulting from mutation is therefore likely to impinge on the awareness of the average individual. The total cost to society may be very large, however, whether measured in terms of dollars diverted to medical care, in terms of lost human-days of employment, or, more subjectively, in terms of total human suffering.

Geneticists concerned with the problems of environmental mutagenesis tend to focus primarily on damage to the gene pool, damage that can be passed on to future generations. Other types of genetic damage, such as mutations in somatic cells (somatic mutations) or mutations so severe in their effects that the zygote dies very early in development (such as dominant lethal mutations), are of relatively little consequence to future generations. A somatic mutation may be of considerable consequence, however, to the individual who harbors the affected cell, particularly if the mutation occurs early enough in development to affect a large fraction of somatic tissue, or if the mutant cell propagates more rapidly than does a normal cell. There is little reason to believe that germ line mutation rates are substantially different from somatic cell mutation rates, or that the types of mutations that arise are very different in the two types of cells. Environmental mutagenesis will therefore affect not only future generations, but our own as well. Somatic mutation is also of considerable immediate practical importance because screening for environmental mutagens is frequently conducted with cells that are reproducing mitotically rather than meiotically.

One unnecessarily noisy ghost needs laying while we are still surveying general aspects of mutation in humans—namely, the recurrent idea that rare advantageous mutations would somehow significantly balance the majority of deleterious mutations artificially induced by environmental mutagenesis. The defect in this idea is not that some mutations are not advantageous: new mutations undoubtedly continue to contribute to the process of Darwinian evolution in all species. The already great genetic variability of natural populations, however, including the probability that virtually all possible (single) base-pair substitutions arise repeatedly in such populations over relatively short times, strongly suggests that spontaneous mutation alone is quite sufficient to produce large numbers of potentially advantageous mutations. For instance, the spontaneous mutation rate per base pair per sexual generation is unlikely to be less than 10^{-9} in humans (Drake, 1969, 1974), so that this value times the present total human population (now about 4×10^9) already exceeds unity. Furthermore, the clear evidence that mutation rates themselves evolve (Drake, 1974) implies that the spontaneous mutation rate may already be optimal. It is therefore difficult to argue that an artificially induced general decrease in average human health can be justified by the generation of rare advantageous mutations when the latter already appear to exist in sufficient numbers. [Certain experiments involving radiation-induced mutations in fruit fly populations seem to hint at net beneficial effects; see, for instance, Maruyama and Crow (1975). These effects, however, are irrelevant to our concerns about environmental mutagenesis. They may well be of doubtful statistical significance when they do occur (Pandey, 1975); they are specifically observed in highly inbred lines, which are already relatively deficient in natural genetic variability; and even then they are probably restricted in their occurrence to those relatively few generations during which the test populations are most rapidly adapting to a novel environment.]

The claim is sometimes made that modern medicine, as well as an artificially increased human mutation rate, will contribute to future genetic ill health by permitting the reproduction of genetically defective individuals who would, in previous centuries, have experienced genetic death. Although this may be true of a few specific diseases, I have never encountered a quantitative attempt to generalize this concept to the average human disease (which is, after all, very mild, particularly during the genetically crucial first three decades of life). I strongly suspect that medicine has as yet made little quantitatively significant progress in enhancing the transmission of defective genes, although selection in favor of resistance to bacterial disease may have been slightly relaxed. Increased standards of living, on the other hand, may indeed produce just such a relaxation of selection against a wide variety of defective genes. Among the factors that ought to be considered most closely in this context are excessive thermoregulation of living and working areas and excessive distribution of devices to decrease physical exertion.

Absolute versus Flexible Limits

Let us suppose that reliable methods have been developed and applied to the screening of potential environmental mutagens, and that mutagenicity is detected from time to time either in compounds already present in the environment or in compounds newly considered for distribution. Let us also suppose that a consensus also exists to the effect that unrestricted distribution of environmental mutagens should not be allowed. What limits, then, should be applied? Two general strategies are available. (Both, however, would presumably ban the distribution of any mutagenic agent whose benefits were nil or highly ephemeral, or of any mutagenic agent for which a nonmutagenic equivalent were readily available.)

The first strategy involves establishing absolute limits of exposure, including limits on all mutagens summed, limits on individual agents, limits for the protection of the total population, and limits for the protection of special groups of individuals at higher than average risk. Within this general framework, more specific and more restrictive prohibitions may also be constructed, for instance against a mutagen whose dispersion cannot be adequately monitored. In strategies of this type even highly beneficial compounds may be banned when, for instance, they cause the absolute limit on total artificial environmental mutagens to be approached. In the extreme case, the absolute limit would consist of a total ban on any compound for which any mutagenicity is detected in any accepted test system.

The second strategy is to deal with each particular environmental mutagen as it is detected, without reference to any ceiling on total mutagenic exposure either to the total population or to particular individuals. The distribution of a mutagen would be permitted only to the extent that its intended applications produced benefits that outweighed the total genetic damage summed over all affected generations. This strategy assumes that methods can actually be developed to quantitate both the benefits and the damages in ways that will allow meaningful comparisons to be made.

Each of these strategies has favorable and unfavorable aspects, which depend to a large degree on the extent to which a particular society tolerates unrestricted discussion of important issues and on the extent to which that society's economic and political institutions have evolved public responsibility. A strong argument in support of absolute and inflexible bans is the possibility that selfish economic forces might bring great pressures to bear on a flexible system, so that it would occasionally bend sufficiently to allow the distribution of mutagens that were not well balanced (by the algebra of the flexible system itself) by corresponding benefits. A further argument against flexible bans is that the risk-benefit calculations that would have to be performed would need to take into account the damage done to all future generations;

together with all the other immense difficulties that arise in calculating comprehensive risk/benefit ratios, this requirement would tend to make the resulting decisions unconvincing. An argument against absolute and inflexible bans is that they do not allow us to deal effectively with unanticipated situations whose characteristics are poorly described by contemporary criteria; should, for instance, an agent that virtually abolishes dental decay but that also increases the human mutation rate by 15% be distributed?

I will assume in further discussion that attempts will increasingly be made to establish absolute limits, although attempts to develop the science of risk-benefit measurement might eventually evolve quite different approaches to the problem of limiting environmental mutagens.

GUIDELINES FOR ADOPTING ABSOLUTE LIMITS

Characteristics of the Mutational Response

A number of aspects of the mutational response, both in humans and in numerous other species, are very relevant to the task in hand. Perhaps the most important is the matter of thresholds, particularly since the presence or absence of thresholds for a large proportion of mutagenic agents would quickly sharpen the question of whether a total ban on the distribution of even a weak mutagen would be reasonable. The widespread occurrence of DNA repair systems (including systems already identified or strongly implied in human cells) does suggest that sufficiently small doses of a mutagen might be virtually completely nonmutagenic. Experimentally, however, thresholds can only be inferred with confidence from dose-response curves well populated with accurate experimental points at low doses. As far as I am aware, such curves, whether or not they are linear, have never revealed a convincing example of a threshold mutagenic effect. If thresholds do exist, therefore, they are sufficiently small to be undetectable by the genetic technology applied thus far, and they are widely considered, at least by geneticists, not to exist at all. This opinion is reinforced by the observation that all repair systems studied to date allow a certain (if rather variable) fraction of premutational lesions to escape repair. It would be most reassuring if mutagenic thresholds did actually exist at the rather low levels of exposure that we hope will turn out to be characteristic of most environmental mutagens. In the absence of convincing data to this effect, however, it would be foolish to risk assuming the existence of any thresholds.

What, then, is the actual shape of the dose-response curve of the typical mutagen, particularly at low doses? Unfortunately, dose-dependency curves show enough variability to make broad generalizations difficult. Whereas even deletions may be induced directly proportionally to dose in some systems, even point mutations may be induced proportionally to the square or some higher power of the dose in other systems. Since measurements of induced mutation rates will offer relatively little predictive value in the absence of dose-response data, we can assume that dose dependencies will probably be measured in several different test systems for all potentially important environmental mutagens. The problem will always remain, however, of how to interpolate between zero dose and the smallest experimental dose for which an accurate measure of the mutagenic response is available. The best way to proceed under these circumstances seems to be to interpolate linearly, regardless of the shape of the dose-response curve at high doses. Since higher-power dose-response curves do sometimes change to linear curves at low doses, it will certainly not be safe to assume that a higher-power dose-response relationship will be maintained all the way to zero dose. (As far as I know, however, dose-response curves that are convex at low doses have never been observed in studies of mutagenesis, so that underestimation of the mutagenic hazard from this cause is unlikely.)

Both the magnitude of the mutational response and the shape of the dose-response curve sometimes depend on the dose rate—that is, on the time over which a given dose is administered. Dose rate effects generally consist of increased mutagenicity at higher dose rates, and can be large. Whenever a potentially important environmental mutagen is comprehensively investigated, therefore, tests should be included to detect dose rate effects.

Perhaps the next most important aspect of the mutational response, and one about which much less can be stated with confidence, is the extent and nature of interactions among mutagens, including interactions between mutagens and their nonmutagenic synergists. There is already considerable literature demonstrating the existence of such interactions, which turn out to be very diverse and difficult to categorize. Certain acridines, for instance, may be mutagenic during meiosis but antimutagenic during mitosis, and may either reduce or enhance the action of other mutagens, depending on the nature of the second mutagen and the conditions of exposure. Most interaction tests are conducted with relatively large doses of both agents, compared with the exposures that might often occur in nature. Unlike the question of single-mutagen thresholds, however, there are no very compelling experiments known to me to indicate just where synergistic interactions will occur, or whether they will continue to occur at low levels of exposure. The logistic problems involved in mass screening for interactions among even moderate numbers of environmental mutagens, to say nothing of nonmutagenic agents that might be synergists, are discouragingly huge, and little systematic screening of this type is likely to occur in the near future. In the absence of specific information, there is little recourse other than to assume that all mutagenic agents act additively. However, in the case of some potentially important environmental mutagens already studied, this assumption would have proved to be too optimistic (Couch and Friedman, 1975). It should also be borne in mind that the collective action of numerous weak mutagens might be more than additive simply because of dose rate effects.

The final aspect of the mutational response to be considered in this section is its generality: To what extent can we expect different screening systems to respond uniformly to a given agent? Were we assured that all systems would, in fact, respond uniformly—they do not, of course—our task would be much easier, since the relatively very expensive, tedious, and insensitive intact animal systems could be entirely replaced by the inexpensive, rapid, and highly sensitive microbial systems. The rather dogmatic assertion is sometimes made that all genes are composed of DNA and that mutagenesis in any one system implies mutagenesis in all (so that failure to detect mutagenesis in some systems, but not others, implies incompetence, at least on the part of the test organism itself). This is excessively naive. First, all mutagens may not (probably do not) act directly on DNA; some instead may affect the enzymes of DNA replication and repair, which will certainly differ in at least minor ways among organisms. Second, a probably rather large fraction of potential mutagens require specific metabolic activation; similarly, some mutagens are undoubtedly subject to metabolic inactivation. One hardly expects the relevant enzymatic activities to be ubiquitous, either among organisms or among tissues. Third, barriers may exist between the blood or other tissues and the germ cells, and may either prevent or promote the access of the mutagen to the critical cells; and these barriers too are likely to be highly organism-specific. An additional complicating factor arises from the high degree of genetic polymorphism now recognized to be characteristic of most genes in most species: instead of possessing only a single wild-type allele, most genes exist in an array of wild-type alleles, some (but not necessarily all) expressing functional differences. It is therefore necessary to remember that any test system that employs a highly inbred line, or even the immediate progeny from crosses between two such lines, expresses far less genetic diversity than does a normal population and may therefore produce atypical and misleading results.

What, then, are we to do about the variable responses that we anticipate will occur, and that have indeed already been observed, among diverse test systems? Since it is unthinkable to contemplate using humans as test organisms to detect mutagenicity, we will always have to extrapolate from other test systems. Because of the very diversity that we already know to exist, however, any positive mutagenic result must be taken very seriously; even if observed in bacteria, for instance, but not in cultured human cells, it is still quite possible that an important fraction of humans will indeed produce a mutagenic response when challenged with the compound in question. The same principle also extends to tests conducted with other microorganisms, with fruit flies, or even with plants. Only when but a single test system is positive out of many, when the battery of test systems includes several mammalian components, and when there is some reasonable explanation for the anomalous response that predicts that it will be absent in humans, will we be justified in classifying the compound as probably safe.

How Much Time Do We Have?

If environmental mutagenesis began to increase the human mutation rate today, how long would we have to act? First of all, under present conditions as large an increase as 100% over the spontaneous background could easily go undetected for many years, and it could require a decade or more to unequivocally prove that it occurred. Current proposals to monitor a considerable fraction of newborns for a variety of well-defined mutational events could result, within not too many years, in the ability to detect perhaps a 50% increase in the human mutation rate within an interval as short as 1 yr (Neel et al., 1973). The usefulness of such a screening program, however, would be limited by its ability to generate information about the cause of any detected increase (Crow, 1971). Since this type of screening would be likely only to identify a crisis without providing the data to resolve it, and would also be very expensive, I continue to assume that the detection of a powerful environmental mutagen that has slipped past at least a cursory screening system would require the better part of a generation.

Even upon the identification of such a mutagen, its immediate withdrawal from circulation might not very rapidly decrease its environmental concentration. Some long-lived agricultural chemicals require years or decades to decay, and some organic heavy metal complexes may require centuries. Furthermore, even the disappearance of the mutagen from the environment would leave a residue of already mutated germ cells, which would persist for approximately one more generation. Finally, natural selection would require many more generations to eliminate the majority of the deleterious genes created by our hypothetical genetic catastrophe.

Many thousands of chemicals are already environmentally distributed, and many hundreds are sufficiently widely distributed to find their way into the average human body in at least milligram quantities per generation. Given the diversity of such chemicals and the lack of mutagenicity testing in the past, it is highly unlikely that none are mutagenic for humans, or that, for those that are mutagenic, 1 mg per person per generation is innocuous. (While it is inappropriate even to begin to list specific suspect chemicals here, such information is in fact available, for instance in the pages of *Mutation Research* and from the data banks of the Environmental Mutagen Information Center.) Testing should therefore begin immediately.

Choosing Absolute Limits

Here I ask the reader to imagine being a member of a group of respected but technologically and philosophically heterogeneous colleagues dedicated to the prevention of harm to the populace at large. Suppose this group is to be charged with constructing protective rules (of the absolute type) that are enforceable, susceptible to general consensus, and logically consistent. How, then, can such rules actually be devised? A crucial first consideration is that we do not, in fact, possess a sound quantitative basis for the design of the rules we seek for the particular case of environmental mutagenesis. If we do not initially abjure all possible exposure to even the weakest of environmental mutagens, however, we will immediately have removed ourselves from the simplistic to the quantitative realm of decision making. In the absence of suitable data, any such decision will be largely arbitrary. There may, however, be a few side roads leading partly away from this impasse.

The first is an appeal to higher (or simply to previous) authority. Other groups have dealt with similarly intractable problems. They have generated inoffensive answers; these have accumulated acceptance and therefore comprise a useful reference base. This is a traditional human approach to the solution of complex problems where the critical data are insufficient, or where the data are available but the inferences are difficult to formulate rigorously.

The second is an attempt to equate the particular problem with other, unrelated problems that have already been resolved on a societal (although not necessarily scientific) basis. The fascination of moving water tempts us to build houses on alluvial river banks, despite the experience of centuries, and we collectively pay the price for such behavior in a fairly open-eyed manner, just as we implicitly accept the price of breathing noxious air in order to inhabit city centers. Thus, to the extent that we directly perceive the benefits and risks involved, rules can fairly readily be devised by simple comparisons with more familiar situations. An example might be to equate the acceptable number of genetically defective newborn individuals with the number of persons killed in automobile accidents in an identical period of time.

Unfortunately, this second method is grossly inadequate for establishing maximum permissible environmental levels of mutagenic agents. The key to the application of this method is perception by the afflicted population, and while we probably readily perceive the claimed benefits of, for instance, cosmetics or agricultural chemicals, we certainly do not as a society perceive mutagenic hazards. Compared with cancer and infectious diseases, mutation is both relatively esoteric and poorly understood. We are also concerned with a hazard that may be visited more harshly on our descendants than on ourselves.

The side roads clearly fail to lead us directly to our desired rules. As a result, it seems inescapable that any rules devised to limit the distribution of environmental mutagens will have to be at least somewhat arbitrary for the present.

COMMITTEE 17 RECOMMENDATIONS

History of Committee 17

A fascinating debate has developed over the past several years concerning how best to test for mutagenicity, the optimal order in which to apply these tests and select compounds for testing, and the applications of the resulting data. In only one case, however, has a highly specific set of exposure limits been recommended—namely, in the report of Committee 17 of the (American branch of the) Environmental Mutagen Society (Drake et al., 1975).

The Environmental Mutagen Society is an incorporated nonprofit society dedicated to the avoidance of environmental mutagenesis. It is composed of a majority of geneticists and a substantial minority of toxicologists, industrial safety specialists, and members of government regulatory and/or health agencies with responsibilities in this general area. (Since the founding of the original Environmental Mutagen Society in North America, European, Japanese, and Indian Environmental Mutagen Societies have come into existence.) Committee 17 was created by action of the Environmental Mutagen Society Council during their meeting of October 17, 1972, wherein a vigorous discussion developed around the question of whether the society should support an extension of the concept of the Delaney Amendment to environmental mutagens. (The Delaney Amendment totally bans the addition to foods of any carcinogenic agent, and at the time there were signs of possible Senate action with respect to the mutagenicity problem.) The committee was charged with reviewing this general problem, the enabling resolution being very briefly described in item 17 of the official minutes. (The title of the committee was adopted by the author, who was also to become the committee chairman, as a precise but neutral label, in order to avoid any predetermination of the scope of the committee's duties. Both the enabling resolution and the discussion that preceded it were, in fact, quite vague in a number of directions, and it was necessary to begin the deliberations of the committee by self-definition of its tasks. In any event, however, and despite its controversial nature, the Committee 17 report was approved by the Environmental Mutagen Society Executive Board.)

Committee 17 had neither the time nor the budget (nor, in fact, an assignment by the Environmental Mutagen Society Council) to compile a detailed description and critique of contemporary testing systems. (These are, in any case, all in a state of rapid evolution.) Instead, the committee was more concerned with describing the fundamental nature of the environmental mutagenic hazard, the nature of the information that would be needed to cope with the hazard, and the question of how to apply this information when it became available. Probably the two most controversial problems attacked were how to extrapolate induced mutation rates from test systems to humans, and how to design rules to limit human exposures to mutagens. It is the result of the latter inquiry by Committee 17 that will be discussed here.

Recommended Limits

The committee's deliberations quickly revealed a consensus in favor of a system of absolute limits to be placed on environmental mutagens, but with little sympathy for an absolute ban along the lines of the Delaney Amendment. The question of how to choose recommended exposure limits then quickly narrowed to the quantitative aspects of the problem. For instance, general agreement rapidly developed that a level of environmental mutagenesis sufficient to double the "spontaneous" mutation rate would be quire intolerable by almost all criteria, even though geneticists are uncertain about the magnitude of the spontaneous mutation rate in humans in the hypothetical absence of even natural environmental mutagens. At the other extreme, a discussion about the extent to which such environmental mutagens of natural origin—such as aflatoxins, ionizing and near-ultraviolet radiation, components of natural smog, and natural nitrites and nitrates—already impinge on the human gene pool generated a consensus that a limit as low as a 1% artificially induced increase over the spontaneous background would be unrealistic, and quite possibly totally unattainable in practice. Within this wide range, however, from 1 to 100% over the spontaneous background, it was remarkably difficult to formulate logical guidelines for a choice of limits.

At this point the deliberations of a preceding group with somewhat similar concerns and outlooks became very influential (Advisory Committee on the Biological Effects of Ionizing Radiations, 1972). Chapter V of the BEIR report was concerned with genetic effects of ionizing radiation. In it, the total incidence of genetic disease was estimated to be about 6%, although, as noted previously, this is likely to be a considerable underestimate because it includes neither diseases of complex (multigenic) etiology nor diseases of individually mild effect. The BEIR report endorsed a previously recommended limit of exposure to artificial ionizing radiation that it was estimated would correspond to an induced increase of some 2.5–25% over the spontaneous mutation rate, the range of values reflecting uncertainties about the radiation rate-doubling dose (the dose required to induce as many mutations per generation as arise spontaneously). The members of Committee 17 agreed that this was a reasonable range within which to set limits, but also decided that it was unreasonable to allow so much damage by a single type of environmental mutagen. It was felt instead that the limit should apply to the sum of all environmental mutagens of artificial origin. (Note that if medically administered radiations are omitted from consideration, as was the case in the BEIR report recommendations, the current average exposure to ionizing radiations of artificial origin amounts to less than 3% of the limit endorsed by the BEIR report, while natural radiation equals 53% of this limit, and medically administered radiations equal 18–35% of the limit.)

The Committee 17 members considered two ways in which to endorse quantitatively similar limits. The first approach was to accept the same limits (expressed in specific units of radiation exposure) as recommended by the BEIR report, namely 5 rem per generation (per sexual generation, that is, or per the first 30 yr of life), or 170 mrem/yr. [A rem (rad equivalent man) expresses the amount of radiation damage to human tissue per incident rad. It takes into account the nature of the target tissue, the type of damage in question, and the nature of the radiation itself. A rad (radiation absorbed dose) is 100 ergs absorbed per gram of material.] The effective application of this limit, however, requires that we determine the relative mutagenicity of chemicals compared to ionizing radiations. Chemical mutagenicity must therefore be expressed in units equivalent to the rem. The choice of the committee was the REC, or rem equivalent chemical: if a certain chemical exposure induces the same number of mutants in a test system as does 1 rem of ionizing radiation, then the chemical exposure corresponds to 1 REC. At present there are certain drawbacks to the REC, both as defined and as applied. First, it is not always immediately clear how to calculate the number of rads that correspond to 1 rem in subhuman mutagenicity test systems, and the calculations can quickly become complex. It may therefore become necessary to redefine the REC as the rad equivalent chemical. Second, the ratio of chemical- to radiation-induced mutagenicity may vary with the test system and with the type of genetic damage (nondisjunction, deletions, point mutations, and so on). It may therefore become necessary to specify ways to average or weigh different REC values obtained with the same chemical in different systems.

The second approach of the committee, one that recognized that major difficulties might arise in the practical application of the REC, was based on the human spontaneous mutation rate. Implicit in this approach was the assumption that this rate will be measured more accurately in the future than it has been to date, and that such measurements will reveal the baseline spontaneous rate independently of perturbations already introduced by known or unknown environmental mutagens of natural or artificial origin. If progress toward this end is too slow, however, an acceptable substitute might be an average somatic mutation rate measured at several different loci in cultured human cells. The committee recommended adoption of a limit consisting approximately of the mean of the uncertainty range (2.5–25%) of the values that resulted when the BEIR report translated radiation doses into mutagenic equivalents. Specifically, the Committee 17 report recommended that the total dose of environmental mutagens of artificial origin, including radiations but excluding medically administered mutagens (see below), be limited to that which would produce an average increase in the human mutation rate of 12.5%.

It is implicit in both methods of limiting total REC exposure that the relevant time span for summing exposures is the reproductive life-span. This is usually taken to be the first 30 yr of life, but changing population and family structures might significantly increase the average reproductive life-span. If the total reproductive life-span exposure were to approach the maximum permissible level, therefore, it would then become necessary to decrease the total allowable annual mutagenic exposure to some value less than, for instance, 170 mREC.

It is a common experience with hazards that some individuals are, by the nature of their occupations or personal habits, more highly exposed than others. Committee 17 also endorsed the principle, previously supported by the BEIR report, that maximum permissible doses to such individuals still within their reproductive life-span should be limited to 10 times the exposure limit for the average member of the population.

Committee 17 made no recommendations whatsoever concerning exposure to environmental mutagens of individuals who are beyond their reproductive life-span, or who, for whatever reasons, have a very low probability of reproducing. Such individuals are genetically deceased, however alive and vigorous they may be in other ways. The direct relevance of environmental mutagens to such persons is probably limited to the carcinogenic properties of mutagens.

The committee discussions soon led to a novel problem, not specifically encountered by groups previously concerned with radiation-induced genetic hazards: the potentially very large number of qualitatively different chemical mutagens. The problem is somewhat akin to, but quantitatively much more difficult than, that of pooling the radiation hazards from fallout, nuclear power plants, medicine, laboratories of diverse types, and the mining and manufacturing of sources of radiations. It is quite possible that a rather large number of chemical mutagens might compete for space within the limited universe defined by the overall recommended limits, and also that a small number of compounds of relatively great mutagenicity (but presumably with important benefits in some other context) might dominate the limited mutagenic space. The committee therefore recommended that no single mutagenic agent should be allowed to exceed 10% of the total mutagenic budget. Even if some compound produced a substantial benefit, its distribution should not be allowed to grow beyond the point where it exceeded this limit (0.5 REC per 30 yr, or 17 mREC/yr).

The limits recommended by Committee 17 were designed for a reasonably civilized and stable world. It is possible that even if these limits obtain widespread acceptance, they will still come into grave conflict with some of the pressures now building in the world. For instance, should a strongly mutagenic herbicide or pesticide be used, even on an emergency basis, to avert the possibility of famine, particularly if the persons to be saved from famine were a population distinct from those who would be exposed to the mutagen? Should a major industry suffer large-scale economic dislocation, with propagating effects throughout the general economy, if and when it was found to be responsible for the dissemination of a dangerous mutagen, particularly one for which no safe substitute is readily available? Questions of this type are difficult enough to answer when only the extant population is affected, but become even more challenging when it is primarily the health of unborn generations that is at risk. My own belief is that we should be prepared to accept very considerable short-term deprivations in order to avoid any substantial possibility of major long-term damage to the human gene pool. This is, however, by no means an area in which one can assume the consensus even of an informed public.

Problem of Medical Sources

The BEIR report specifically excluded from its exposure limits radiations of medical (including dental) origin. The Committee 17 report did likewise for medically administered chamicals, but very clearly left open the possibility that this exemption might be withdrawn in the future. It is notable that medically administered ionizing radiations alone would consume some 18–35% of the entire mutagenic budget at present, and if medical drugs were equally hazardous then the problem would obviously become very severe. It would be well worthwhile to attempt to determine whether the therapeutic effects of such treatments (especially of radiations, where the necessary data may be more readily available) exceed the integrated deleterious effects, including both mutagenesis and carcinogenesis. It would probably also be wise to consider that, while mutagenicity screening programs may soon begin to limit and perhaps even to reduce whatever genetic damage is being done by licit drugs, genetically significant doses of medically administered radiations may tend to increase both because of an expansion of the financial base supporting medical care and because of increasing pressures (via malpractice suits) on the medical profession to employ more diagnostic irradiation. However, just as legal pressures on the automotive industry are forcing technological advances that reduce air pollution, legal pressures might well be applied both on the medical profession itself and on the underlying bio-engineering industries to limit ionizing radiation exposures.

My feeling is that the medical profession ought to be the first (and certainly not the last) to exhibit concern for genetic damage by limiting as much as possible all medical applications of mutagenic agents. The great resistance only a few decades ago within the medical profession to the idea that X-irradiation was dangerous should certainly not serve as a precedent. Some questions that seem ripe for reexamination are whether chest X-ray programs really turn a profit when balanced against their possible genetic and carcinogenic effects, whether current dental irradiation technology ensures virtually zero gonadal doses in actual practice, and whether all of the commonly administered antibiotics are free of mutagenicity.

CORRELATIVE GUIDELINES

Measuring Exposure

Establishing maximum levels of exposure is a futile exercise unless exposure itself can be measured. Compared with the already difficult problems encountered in measuring environmental radiation levels, measuring environmental levels of chemical mutagens is likely to be extremely difficult. The kinds of information that will be needed to determine human environmental exposures to mutagenic compounds were also considered in the Committee 17 report. Briefly, it will be necessary to monitor total production levels, distribution patterns, persistence in the environment, and metabolic disposition within the human body.

Production or importation figures should be easily obtainable from primary manufacturers or importers, if necessary with a little prodding from regulatory agencies. Distribution patterns may be much more difficult to ascertain, however, since fairly detailed information may be required, and the kind of information needed by the geneticist or regulatory agency may not coincide with the kind of information of routine interest to, and already gathered by, manufacturers and their primary distributors. Since this kind of information is just as important as are mutagenicity test data themselves, and since it is more and more the responsibility of manufacturers to provide the latter information, Committee 17 recommended that manufacturers be required to provide the former as well.

Measuring average human exposure also involves measuring the persistence of the mutagenic agent in the environment—as of agricultural chemicals in the soil, rivers, and lakes, for instance—and in the human body itself. Particular attention should be given to the situation where a weak mutagen exhibits great persistence, so that its integrated effects over years or decades would become relatively massive. Again assigning primary responsibility for data collection to the entity that stands to make a profit, Committee 17 recommended that the needed data be provided by the manufacturers.

Many (probably most) environmental mutagens are relatively innocuous until metabolically converted to an active form, either within the human body or by some intermediate organism. The efficiency of conversion needs to be determined for the typical route by which the compound enters the body, if quantitative risk extrapolation is to be maximally feasible from subhuman test systems. Ideally, it would also be advisable to determine the concentration of the active form of the mutagen not only in, for instance, the blood, but also in the germ cells themselves. I suspect that data of this type are going to be very difficult to obtain, but they should still be sought, perhaps by indirect methods.

Choosing Testing Strategies

Many more chemicals are already manufactured and distributed, and are being introduced yearly, than can be run through the available mutagen screening systems in the near future. Furthermore, only a tiny fraction of these compounds can be tested in the more involved mammalian screening systems unless and until a rather large effort is made to create suitable testing facilities and to train personnel. On the other hand, some of the more simple microbial testing systems can be applied to large numbers (hundreds to thousands) of compounds essentially immediately. What, then, are the guidelines for deciding which chemicals are to be tested first?

Two of the most compelling guidelines are directly suggested by the nature of the problem itself: priority should be assigned to a chemical to the extent that it is actually present in the environment, and to the extent that it is chemically related to known mutagens. The extent to which a compound is significantly present in the environment can be assessed in two ways—namely, by its gross production level and distribution pattern, and by the extent to which it arrives in the immediate neighborhood of the human body (as in the case of cosmetics and food additives, for instance).

Even the very large number of potentially suspect compounds already in distribution could, without unreasonable or excessive effort, be tested in the rapid microbial screening systems within only a few years, and if only a relatively small fraction of these compounds exhibited mutagenicity, they could then be subjected to much more elaborate testing in higher organisms. (A passing grade obtained in the preliminary examination would not, however, constitute a certificate of graduation to safe status, and retesting with other systems should continue at later times.) Similarly, the rapid screening systems could be profitably applied early in the development of new compounds, along with the most preliminary tests for the desirable activity being sought, and mutagenically active (and, by inference, carcinogenic) compounds could be rapidly eliminated from serious consideration before substantial further investments were made in their development.

Committee 17 recommended, however, that no new compound should be introduced into the environment until it had passed not only the simple tests, but also the best available mammalian tests.

Note added in proof: Much has occurred since this paper was prepared, including conceptual, systems, and legislative advances; hence the sometimes rather dated material included.

REFERENCES

Advisory Committee on the Biological Effects of Ionizing Radiations. 1972. *The effects on populations of exposure to low levels of ionizing radiation.* Washington, D.C.: National Academy of Sciences-National Research Council.

Couch, D. B. and Friedman, M. A. 1975. *Mutat. Res.* 31: 109.

Crow, J. F. 1971. In *Chemical mutagens. Principles and methods for their detection*, ed. A. Hollaender, vol. 2, pp. 591–605. New York: Plenum.

Drake, J. W. 1969. *Nature (Lond.)* 221: 1132.

Drake, J. W. 1974. *Symp. Soc. Gen. Microbiol.* 24: 41.

Drake, J. W., Abrahamson, S., Crow, J. F., Hollaender, A., Lederberg, S., Legator, M. S., Neel, J. V., Shaw, M. W. , Sutton, H. E., von Borstel, R. C., Zimmering, S., de Serres, F. J. and Flamm, W. G. 1975. *Science* 187: 503.

Maruyama, T. and Crow, J. F. 1975. *Mutat. Res.* 27: 241.
Mukai, T., Chigusa, S. I., Mettler, L. E. and Crow, J. F. 1972. *Genetics* 72: 335.
Neel, J. V. 1973. *Proc. Natl. Acad. Sci. U.S.A.* 70: 3311.
Neel, J. V., Tiffany, T. O. and Anderson, N. G. 1973. In *Chemical mutagens. Principles and methods for their detection*, ed. A. Hollaender, vol. 3, pp. 105–150. New York: Plenum.
Pandey, J. 1975. *Mutat. Res.* 27: 249.
Stevenson, A. C. and Kerr, C. B. 1967. *Mutat. Res.* 4: 339.

Part 2

MODIFYING INFLUENCES

DNA REPAIR AS IT RELATES TO MUTAGENESIS AND GENE EXPRESSION IN MAMMALIAN CELLS AND TISSUES

Michael W. Lieberman

Environmental Mutagenesis Branch
National Institute of Environmental Health Sciences
National Institutes of Health
Research Triangle Park, North Carolina

INTRODUCTION

One of the most exciting developments in eukaryotic molecular biology over the past decade has been the discovery of processes competent to repair a wide variety of physical and chemical insults to the genome. Many laboratories are presently involved in trying to understand the molecular mechanisms involved in eukaryotic repair processes. Another area of importance is the analysis of the pathophysiologic significance of repair. In terms of impact on human health, it is the cellular consequences of molecular events that must be focused on; however, this task is inherently much more difficult than understanding molecular mechanisms because of the complexity of the events that must be analyzed. It is with this thought that this chapter has been written, and it is hoped that it will serve to relate data at the molecular level to problems that are generally thought of as cellular. Repair of specific types of damage, adequacy of restoration of the damaged area, and functional consequences of repair are dealt with. In addition, the usefulness of repair synthesis as a screen for genetically active agents in the environment is analyzed. Little space has been given to the analysis of molecular mechanisms per se since there is already much awareness of the importance of this area.

Dr. Lieberman's present address is Department of Pathology, Washington University School of Medicine, St. Louis, Missouri 63110.

TYPES OF DNA REPAIR

It is now widely appreciated that several different types of DNA repair occur in mammalian cells. These have been reviewed elsewhere and will not be reviewed in detail here (Beers et al., 1972; Cleaver, 1973, 1974; Regan and Setlow, 1974; Sutherland et al., 1974; Hanawalt and Setlow, 1975; Lehmann et al., 1975; Lieberman, 1976a). Excision repair (long patch repair) and rejoining of single-strand breaks (short patch repair) are the most extensively studied repair processes in mammalian cells. More work is beginning to appear on postreplication repair and efforts to identify recombinational events in mammalian cells (see Hanawalt and Setlow, 1975). Although initial efforts to identify photoreactivation in placental mammals were unsuccessful, Sutherland's group has identified an enzyme from some cell types of placental mammals that will photoreactivate pyrimidine dimers. With the exception of the photoreactivation process, there have been few generally accepted purifications and isolations of enzymes involved in repair. Consequently, a detailed molecular analysis of repair processes is not available; however, a great number of ingenious experiments with cultured cells have begun to supply some information on how these processes work. Although, in general, there is at least a superficial resemblance between prokaryotic and eukaryotic repair processes, too little is known to allow an intimate comparison (e.g., see Lieberman, 1976a).

INTRAGENOMAL DISTRIBUTION OF DNA REPAIR SYNTHESES

Studies of the removal of thymine dimers and of bound carcinogens and mutagens have usually found incomplete removal of damaged sites (e.g., Roberts et al., 1971; Witschi et al., 1971; Lieberman and Dipple, 1972; Slor, 1973; Cleaver, 1974; Takebe et al., 1974; Lieberman et al., 1976; see also Table 1). Typically, 30–70% of damage is removed in the course of these experiments. While this observation may have a variety of explanations, including selective excision of particular types of damage (see below), toxicity of these agents, and saturation of repair mechanisms, one intriguing possibility is that certain sites in the genome are more repairable than others. It is now known that removal of damage from the prokaryotic genome is usually more extensive than that from mammalian genomes (e.g., Lieberman and Dipple, 1972; Venitt and Tarmy, 1972; Slor, 1973; Ikenaga, et al., 1975) and that the organizations of the two types of genomes are apparently very different (Graham et al., 1974; R. Kornberg, 1974; A. Kornberg, 1974; Sollner-Webb and Felsenfeld, 1975).

Two studies (Meltz and Painter, 1973; Lieberman and Poirier, 1974a) concerned the distribution of repair synthesis following UV radiation, *N*-acetoxy-2-acetylaminofluorine (NA-AAF), and 7-bromomethylbenz[*a*]an-

TABLE 1 Disappearance of Bound Carcinogen *In Vivo*

Organ	Species	Carcinogen	Approximate time to reach maximum binding (hr)	Approximate $t_{1/2}$	Reference
Skin	Mouse	β-Propiolactone	12	12	Boutwell et al., 1969
Skin	Mouse	7-Bromomethyl-12-methylbenz[a]anthracene	6–12	12–18	Rayman and Dipple, 1973
Skin	Mouse	7-Bromomethylbenz[a]-anthracene	100	24 hr	Rayman and Dipple, 1973
Mammary gland	Rat	Dimethylbenz[a]anthracene	24	6–13 days	Janss et al., 1972
Liver	Rat	N-Hydroxyacetylamino-fluorene	1	12 hr	Szafarz and Weisburger, 1969
Liver	Rat	N-Hydroxyacetylamino-fluorene	$\leqslant 16$	2–6 days	Witschi et al., 1971
Liver	Rat	N-Hydroxyacetylamino-fluorene	$\leqslant 18$	3–7 days (product 1) Not removed (product 2)	Kriek, 1972
Liver	Rat	Dimethylnitrosamine	$\leqslant 5$	5–15 hr (O^6-methylguanine) 35–45 hr (other products)	O'Connor et al., 1973
Liver	Rat	Dimethylnitrosamine	$\leqslant 5$	3 days (N^7-methylguanine)	Capps et al., 1973
Liver	Rat (10-day-old)	Ethylnitrosourea	1–4	64 hr (N^7-ethylguanine) 36 hr (O^6-ethylguanine) 12 hr (N^3-ethyladenine)	Goth and Rajewsky, 1974
Brain	Rat (10-day-old)	Ethylnitrosourea	1–4	89 hr (N^7-ethylguanine) 229 hr (O^6-ethylguanine) 12 hr (N^3-ethyladenine)	Goth and Rajewsky, 1974

thracene (7BrMeBA) (all agents that induce large patch repair) among DNA sequences of varying degrees of repetitiveness in HeLa cells and confluent diploid fibroblasts. They found that highly repetitive sequences, moderately repetitive sequences, and "unique sequences" (the C_0t 10,000 fraction) were all repaired to about the same extent. In a similar study, Lieberman and Poirier (1974b) found that mouse satellite DNA, a highly repetitive, nontranscribed set of sequences, was repaired to about the same extent as the rest of the genome (main-band DNA). The implication of these findings is that a great variety of sequences are repairable in the mammalian genome and that at least one set of sequences that does not code for a specific protein is repairable. These observations suggest—but, of course, do not conclusively demonstrate—that the informational content of an individual sequence is not a factor in determining whether that sequence will be repaired.

A number of studies indicate that the organization of chromatin within the nucleus is of importance in determining which lesions are repairable. Wilkins and Hart (1974) found that pyrimidine dimers were removed more slowly from DNA complexed to protein than from naked DNA; they concluded that nuclear proteins masked some sites and prevented or retarded repair in these regions. In another study, the intranuclear distribution of DNA repair synthesis was examined after damage with UV radiation and three chemical carcinogens (Harris et al., 1974). This group found less repair synthesis in DNA located near the nuclear membrane and presumed to be heterochromatic by ultrastructural criteria. In addition, the distribution of repair synthesis in the inner core (representing euchromatic DNA) was found to be clustered (nonrandom). Although the authors were unable to analyze the distribution of damage with their methodology, their data suggest that repair synthesis is not uniformly distributed throughout the nucleus. Another group (Berliner et al., 1975) suggested that there is more repair in the peripheral region of the nucleus of UV-irradiated human lymphocytes. Although this peripheral region contains much heterochromatin, the authors suggested that it is not only heterochromatin but also peripherally located euchromatin that shows more repair. A pre- liminary report (Ramanathan et al., 1975) suggests that nuclease-accessible sites (Sollner-Webb and Felsenfeld, 1975) are more readily damaged by the carcinogen dimethylnitrosamine and that this damage is more readily removed than damage at nuclease-insensitive sites. Preliminary data of Tlsty, Smerdon, and Lieberman (unpublished) suggest that nuclease-sensitive sites are repaired more readily than resistant sites in human diploid fibroblasts damaged with NA-AAF or UV radiation. Thus, at present there is no general agreement on the basis for any selectivity of excision repair processes, but it appears that the selectivity is not based simply on sequence repetitiveness or transcriba- bility. The precise nature of this selectivity will have to await further elucidation of chromatin structure. In this regard, it is of interest that mammalian cells do not repair UV radiation damage to mitochondrial DNA (Clayton et al., 1974).

ACCURACY OF REPAIR SYNTHESIS

A major consideration in the evaluation of the role of repair synthesis in eukaryotic cells is the accuracy of the repair process. If repair is truly error free, then restoration of nucleotide sequence may mean full restoration of function (however, see below). On the other hand, misrepair could result in the introduction of different types of errors, preservation of the same type of errors, or even a net increase in the amount of damage (for a review of this subject as it relates to mammalian cells, see Lieberman, 1976a). It is important to emphasize here that, except for some information on the excision repair system, we know very little about the error-proneness of repair processes (however, see Maher et al., 1976).

Repair synthesis associated with excision repair has been evaluated both biochemically and genetically. A study utilizing such techniques as pyrimidine isostich profiles, S_1 nuclease digestion studies, and thermal elution chromatography suggested that most nucleotides are inserted in a template-directed fashion (i.e., accurately) (Lieberman and Poirier, 1974c; Lieberman, 1976a). This contention is supported by the observation that all four nucleosides are substrates for repair synthesis after damage with two chemical carcinogens (Lieberman and Poirier, 1973). Establishment of the incorporation of all four nucleosides is of importance, since they would all be required for an accurate filling of the large gap left by a repair nuclease. As has been pointed out previously (Lieberman, 1976a), all such biochemical studies have an inherent limitation in that they are insensitive to very low levels of infidelity ($< 1\%$) while most mutational phenomena (one manifestation of inaccurate repair) occur at much lower frequencies. The major advantage of chemical studies is that they provide a biochemical basis for the genetic analysis of the error-proneness of the repair process.

Recently, Maher and her associates have examined induced mutation frequencies at the hypoxanthine-guanine phosphoribosyltransferase (HGPRT) locus in a series of normal and excision repair-deficient human fibroblasts [xeroderma pigmentosum (XP) cells] (Maher and Wessel, 1975; Maher et al., 1976). In general, they found that the induced mutation frequency is higher in xeroderma cells; the most repair-deficient of these also have the highest induced mutation frequencies. They examined the effects of both UV radiation and chemical carcinogens. These data agree with the biochemical studies mentioned above and suggest that the excision repair system is at least error-correcting and perhaps error free.

The last few years have seen the development of systems to study postreplication repair in mammalian cells. Much interest has developed in this area since in bacteria postreplication repair (or at least recombination repair, which seems to be closely related to postreplication repair) appears to be error prone (Kondo, 1973; Witkin and George, 1973; Witkin, 1975a). To date, there have been no biochemical studies of the accuracy of postreplication repair largely because of technical difficulties in performing the requisite experiments. In this regard, it is of interest that Witkin has suggested that mutagens and carcinogens induce an error-prone repair system in bacteria and may do the same in mammalian cells (Witkin, 1975a, 1975b). Mammalian cells (i.e., thymus) contain a terminal transferase that adds nucleotides to an existing DNA chain without template direction; it is possible that it or related enzymes could be involved in the postreplication repair process and thus provide a biochemical basis for the postulated error-prone repair system.

Lehmann et al. (1975) have demonstrated that XP variants that have normal excision repair are partially deficient in postreplication repair. A recent report suggests that XP variants have lower survival rates than normal strains and higher induced mutation frequencies (Maher et al., 1975). At present the significance of this finding, especially in relation to prokaryotic work, is unclear, but it is hoped that a great deal of interesting work will develop from these discoveries.

BINDING OF CARCINOGENS AND MUTAGENS
TO DNA AND THEIR REMOVAL

In theory, excision repair involves both the removal of damage and the synthesis of a new segment of DNA following this removal. Although repair synthesis (repair replication, unscheduled DNA synthesis) has been relatively easy to demonstrate, removal studies tend to be somewhat more difficult. They require a radioactive carcinogen or mutagen or a sensitive assay for pyrimidine dimers; the latter is difficult to develop, especially for low (and biologically meaningful) levels of damage. Thus, for example, it has been relatively easy to demonstrate repair synthesis in the mouse (e.g., Hart and Setlow, 1974; Lieberman and Poirier, 1974b), but a clear demonstration of dimer removal has depended on careful measurements and low levels of damage (Setlow et al., 1972; Lehmann, 1972). Nevertheless, it is now widely accepted that repair synthesis is indicative of the removal (or at least the spontaneous loss) of some DNA damage. In general, the interesting problems have centered around the rate of loss of adducts, whether loss is enzymatic or spontaneous, and the extent to which there is selectivity in the removal process.

Over the past decade studies have demonstrated the disappearance of bound carcinogen from mammalian organs *in vivo* (Table 1). Often these data have been interpreted in terms of repair processes, but in most instances repair synthesis was not actually measured (however, see Bowden et al., 1975). Thus it is not clear at present that all these cases actually represent repair phenomena. Careful correlative studies of removal, repair synthesis, and ligation in the same tissue at the same time remain to be done. Other problems associated with the analysis of removal of damaged nucleotides *in vivo* include those of carcinogen-induced cell death and normal cell turnover (Boutwell et al., 1969) and the possibility of chemical instability of adducts and spontaneous loss (Kriek, 1972; Goth and Rajewski, 1974). Of particular interest is the finding of Goth and Rajewski (1974) that O^6-ethylguanine, following the administration of ethylnitrosourea, is removed more rapidly from liver than from brain; this finding may be related to the propensity of ethylnitrosourea to produce brain tumors. The authors speculate that the proliferative *potential* of liver may be related to the ability of hepatocytes to remove O^6-ethylguanine. However, Witschi et al. (1971) found no difference in the rate of removal of acetylaminofluorene (AAF) moieties between normal livers and those undergoing regeneration following partial hepatectomy. Capps et al. (1973) made similar observations with respect to the removal of N^7-methylguanine from liver DNA.

Removal studies *in vitro* with mammalian cells have been somewhat easier to do. Ultraviolet irradiation and thymine dimer analysis have resulted in a large amount of data on removal damage as a function of time (e.g., Cleaver, 1974). In addition, simultaneous studies of repair synthesis are facilitated by the ease with which cultured cells may be manipulated. Thus Takebe and co-workers (1974) were able to study the removal of thymine dimers, unscheduled DNA synthesis, and rejoining of single-strand breaks in several normal human cells, XP cells, and rodent lines as well as to assess host cell reactivation. Such a study would be very difficult and time-consuming with whole animals. Roberts et al. (1971) were able to look at repair synthesis and the removal of damage induced by methylating agents from two cell types. Lieberman and Dipple (1972) and Slor (1973) studied the removal of 7BrMeBA from human lymphocytes. Ikenaga et al. (1975) looked at the removal of 4-nitroquinoline-1-oxide (4NQO) adducts from rodent and human DNA. The removal of NA-AAF-induced adducts from the DNA of a variety of normal human cells, XP cells, and rodent cells has been carried out (Lieberman et al., 1976; Amacher and Lieberman, 1977; Amacher et al., 1977). The major conclusions from these *in vitro* studies are: (1) carcinogen may be removed from the genomes of mammalian cells, but removal is rarely complete; (2) XP cells are less competent to remove bound carcinogen than are normal human cells; and (3) removal is often most rapid in the first 12 hr but continues for at least a 2-day period (the longest measured). At present, it is not clear to what extent such factors as level of binding and toxicity of administered agents affect results.

Several studies have focused on rates of removal of different products. In a study of removal of adducts from the DNA of cultured human lymphocytes, Lieberman and Dipple (1972) found that the N^6-adenine derivative of methylbenz[*a*]anthracene was removed about twice as readily as the N^2-guanine derivative. Ikenaga et al. (1975) showed that 4NQO adducts are less readily removed from mammalian DNA than is an unstable adduct that releases 4-aminoquinoline-1-oxide on hydrolysis. (The fact that XP cells differed from normal cells in the rate of removal of this adduct demonstrates that some excision system is operating.) These data and the *in vivo* data of Goth and Rajewsky (1974) and of Kriek (1972) indicate that differential rates of removal of adducts occur in mammalian cells. Work with prokaryotic species has revealed similar phenomena, but the results differ quantitatively and qualitatively from those found in mammalian cells (e.g., Lawley and Orr, 1970; Venitt and Tarmy, 1972; Kirtikar and Goldthwait, 1974; Lawley and Warren, 1975; see also Lieberman, 1976a).

Repair studies have emphasized simple DNA damage, and yet there is evidence that both radiation and chemicals produce DNA-protein cross-links (Grunicke et al., 1973; Han et al., 1975; Metzger and Daune, 1975) and damage to DNA-associated proteins (e.g., Turberville and Craddock, 1971). Whether DNA-protein cross-links are repairable remains an open question. Likewise, we know little about the role of cross-links in mutagenesis or gene expression. No doubt this will be an area of active investigation in the near future.

TISSUE DISTRIBUTION OF REPAIR SYNTHESIS

One important aspect of the relation between repair and neoplasia rests in the distribution of repair synthesis among cell types in the body. One prevalent hypothesis suggests that carcinogens are mutagenic for somatic cells and that the mutations produced lead to neoplasia. To the extent that the somatic mutation theory of neoplasia has merit, repair in somatic cells is of importance. Since some chemotherapeutic agents and ionizing irradiation produce not only DNA damage but also neoplasia, interest in the tissue distribution of repair synthesis goes beyond concern about environmental and industrial carcinogens and mutagens. In this regard, analysis of repair in relation to the types of tumors produced might be of great interest. At present, data are restricted to repair synthesis (unscheduled DNA synthesis, repair replication), the disappearance of labeled carcinogen (see above), and rejoining of strand breaks. No work has been done on photoreactivation, postreplication repair, or recombination repair *in vivo*.

Because of ready accessibility and interest in XP, skin has been studied extensively. It has been demonstrated that UV irradiation of normal human skin followed by intradermal injection of [^{3}H]thymidine resulted in unscheduled DNA synthesis in epidermal cells (basal cells, Malpighian cells, granular cells) as well as in dermal fibroblasts and vascular endothelial cells (J. Epstein et al., 1970; W. Epstein et al., 1971). In contrast, similar treatment of skin from two XP patients showed no unscheduled DNA synthesis, while that from a third patient showed 15–25% of normal repair synthesis. Unscheduled

DNA synthesis in basal epidermal cells from patients with a variety of sun-sensitive or cancer-prone syndromes showed normal or near-normal repair synthesis. In a study of full-thickness "skin" biopsies (including the paniculus carnosus muscle) from rat, mouse, and miniature pig, Lieberman and Forbes (1973) found that both epidermal cells and dermal fibroblasts underwent unscheduled DNA synthesis following UV irradiation and three chemical carcinogens (NA-AAF, 7BrMeBA, and β-propiolactone). Muscle nuclei showed little or no unscheduled DNA synthesis.

Of interest in relation to repair in skin is the recent clinical trial of oral methoxypsoralen and long-wavelength UV irradiation in the treatment of psoriasis (Parrish et al., 1974). This regimen confines damage largely to specific regions of the skin. Presumably, repair is not completely effective in removing the DNA cross-links produced by this treatment or it would probably be ineffective. Nevertheless, the dilemma of therapeutic response versus potential neoplastic risk and the role of repair in titrating these two sequelae are clearly highlighted by this approach.

Circulating human lymphocytes have been examined for unscheduled DNA synthesis, usually following removal and resuspension in cell culture medium. The conclusion from most studies has been that normal lymphocytes undergo unscheduled DNA synthesis in response to ionizing irradiation, UV irradiation, chemical carcinogens, and alkylating agents (Evans and Norman, 1968; Frey-Wettstein et al., 1969; Connor and Norman, 1971; Lieberman et al., 1971). Lymphocytes from most XP patients have reduced or absent unscheduled DNA synthesis after UV radiation, 4NQO, or 7BrMeBA (Burk et al., 1971; Jacobs et al., 1972; Slor, 1973). One report suggests that long-lived lymphocytes (small peripheral blood lymphocytes and lymph node lymphocytes) undergo more unscheduled DNA synthesis in response to UV irradiation than do short-lived lymphocytes (small lymphocytes from thymus) (Frey-Wettstein et al., 1969).

A number of reports have indicated that granulocytes from peripheral blood (usually neutrophils) show much reduced or absent unscheduled DNA synthesis following exposure to ionizing radiation, UV radiation, or chemical carcinogens (Frey-Wettstein et al., 1969; Connor and Norman, 1971; Lieberman et al., 1971). These cells, like small lymphocytes from thymus, are short-lived. It is unlikely, however, that longevity correlates closely with repair. Thus, differentiated muscle that persists for the life of the individual shows reduced repair (Stockdale, 1971; Lieberman and Forbes, 1973), while epithelial granular cells are short-lived, but show repair equal to that of basal cells that persist as dividing stem cells for the life of the individual (J. Epstein et al., 1970; Lieberman and Forbes, 1973).

Several studies indicate that hepatocytes undergo repair synthesis. Exposure of liver biopsies to UV radiation or NA-AAF resulted in unscheduled DNA synthesis when they were placed in culture medium containing [^{3}H]thymidine (Lieberman and Forbes, 1973). Farber's laboratory has adapted the technique of McGrath and Williams (1966) for use *in vivo*: their findings indicate that many agents produce damage to hepatocyte DNA (detected as single-strand breaks in alkaline sucrose gradients) and that this damage is repaired (detected as strand rejoining) (Cox et al., 1973a, 1973b; Damjanov et al., 1973; Stewart et al., 1973; Cox and Irving, 1975). Stich and Kieser (1974) have used trypsinized hepatocyte suspensions to investigate unscheduled DNA synthesis following exposure to dimethylnitrosamine.

Unscheduled DNA synthesis and strand rejoining have also been reported for pulmonary and renal parenchyma (Lieberman and Forbes, 1973; Stich and Kieser, 1974; Cox and Irving, 1975).

Work on the central nervous system has revealed an interesting pattern. Lett et al. (1972) were able to demonstrate strand rejoining in the DNA of canine granular cerebellar neurons following ionizing radiation. Following UV irradiation or NA-AAF, both agents that apparently require endonuclease activity for repair, no unscheduled DNA synthesis was seen in rabbit granular cell neurons, Purkinje cells or cerebellar glial cells; however, the vascular endothelial cells appeared to repair well (Lieberman and Forbes, 1973). Goth and Rajewsky (1974) found that O^6-ethylguanine, which probably requires endonucleolytic action for removal, was eliminated more slowly from brain than N^7-ethylguanine, which is probably lost at least in part by nonenzymatic means; this finding is in contrast to that in liver, in which the O^6 product is removed faster than the N^7 product (Table 1). These authors suggest that analysis of repair by specific cell types would be of interest. One explanation consistent with most of these findings is that neurons and glial cells have low levels of repair endonucleases but are able to repair lesions in which strand breakage occurs subsequent to chemical or physical injury.

For a while it was suspected that normal tissues might be competent to repair damage, but that their hyperplastic or neoplastic derivatives might be deficient in this regard. It was argued that the absence of repair during the early stages of neoplasia would result in a cascade effect on neoplastic progression and perhaps account for the greater sensitivity of some cancers to chemo- and radiotherapy. In general, experimental findings have not supported this speculation. Huang et al. (1972) found that lymphocytes from patients with chronic lymphatic leukemia showed greater unscheduled DNA synthesis and dimer removal following exposure to UV radiation than those from normal donors. Frey-Wettstein et al. (1969) found similar levels of unscheduled DNA synthesis in normal lymphocytes and chronic lymphocytic leukemia lymphocytes. Norman, et al. (1972) were able to demonstrate unscheduled DNA synthesis in trypsinized preparations of human cells from ovarian, endometrial, cervical, breast, colonic, and "mouth" carcinomas following exposure to UV or ionizing radiation. Examination of normal mouse skin, chronically irradiated skin that was histologically normal, hyperplastic mouse skin, and squamous cell carcinomas from mouse skin following exposure to UV irradiation or NA-AAF revealed substantial unscheduled DNA synthesis in cells from all tissues examined (Lieberman and Forbes, 1973). While the results were difficult to quantitate, the authors felt that they indicated that loss of DNA repair capacity was not responsible for neoplastic progression. A more recent quantitative examination of repair in normal liver and hyperplastic nodules demonstrated increased unscheduled DNA synthesis in nodules compared with normal liver; these findings are similar to the results of other studies of repair and neoplastic transformation discussed above (Kitagawa et al., 1975).

In terms of the "genetic toxicology" of the whole animal, the studies cited above will have to be expanded greatly. It would be of great importance to examine a variety of tissues with several agents, not only for the ability to perform the steps necessary for excision repair, but also for the presence of other repair systems. In the future, more emphasis must be placed on the quantitative aspects of repair processes—and especially comparative data from different tissues. Work of this sort in the developing embryo might be especially interesting as a possible explanation for the selective teratologic effects of some agents.

REPAIR AND GENE EXPRESSION

This section deals with the problem of gene expression and related biochemical events. Other topics such as mutagenesis and host cell reactivation, which are related to gene expression in the sense that their functional consequences may be alteration of an "expressed gene," are dealt with subsequently.

Does damage to the genome and its subsequent repair or misrepair result in the expression of unexpressed cellular potential or the repression of expressed properties? For eukaryotes this question is especially important, since the regulation and organization of the eukaryotic genome appears to be much more complex than that of the prokaryotic genome (for a recent review of this subject, see Lewin, 1974). One may consider briefly three types of events that could bring about altered gene expression in conjunction with accurate restoration of the sequence of the DNA: (1) alterations in chromatin structure, (2) alterations in nuclear proteins, and (3) modification of DNA bases.

In the mammal, DNA is organized and packaged in chromatin, and, while it is still not clear what the significance of these arrangements is in terms of gene expression, current work with *Drosophila* suggests the importance of chromosomal structure in gene expression in eukaryotes (e.g., Glover et al., 1975). Even transient alteration of these relationships could result in activation of repressed genetic material. Consider, for instance, a single-strand break produced either by ionizing radiation or by an endonuclease in response to damage. Among other things, this break may have the effect of isolating a particular gene from neighboring sequences. This isolation might be evanescent or prolonged and could result in turning the transcription of the gene product on or off. The effect might be a direct one (i.e., the result of simple strand scission) or an indirect one (strand scission might result in alteration of protein-DNA interaction). In addition to simple strand scission, gaps produced during excision or postreplication repair might be present for a considerable length of time before closing (Lehmann et al., 1975) and might have similar regulatory effects. Thus, even though repair might subsequently result in accurate restoration of the genome, its transient effects might be of great importance. Although it is not clear that any of these events or others like them would lead to an alteration of gene expression, investigation in this area would be of interest.

DNA, histones, nonhistone proteins, and small amounts of RNA form a complex structure known as chromatin. Although recently some exciting advances have been made in our understanding of this structure, at present only the most general features of how proteins and nucleic acids are associated in chromatin are known (e.g., Clark and Felsenfeld, 1974; R. Kornberg, 1974; Noll et al., 1975). Since it is generally felt that DNA-nuclear protein interactions and the type and extent of posttranscriptional modification of these proteins (phosphorylation, acetylation, and methylation) are, at least in part, responsible for alterations in gene expression, any alterations that the repair process itself produces might be of interest. At present, any possible relationship remains largely unexplored. However, in collaboration with Stein's laboratory, we have recently begun to explore one aspect of this problem. We have looked for the accumulation of newly synthesized histones and acidic nuclear proteins during the repair process (Stein et al., 1976). The rationale behind these experiments was that certain agents (UV radiation, NA-AAF) result in the replacement of about 100 nucleotides (equivalent to 10 turns of the double helix). Removal of a piece of DNA this large could disturb relationships between DNA and nuclear protein. If these proteins were actually dissociated from the DNA, their replacement might involve synthesis of new proteins. Within the limits of the sensitivity of our experiments, we could not detect any accumulation of new nuclear proteins. There are several possible interpretations of this finding: (1) a more sensitive assay for the detection of newly synthesized nuclear proteins may be needed; (2) DNA-protein relations are undisturbed during repair; (3) if there is dissociation of DNA and proteins during repair, the old proteins are reutilized during reassociation; or (4) repair does not stimulate the synthesis of new proteins but may result in posttranscriptional modification of existing protein.

Finally, repair processes could affect the modification of nucleic acids. The only known naturally occurring alteration in mammalian DNA is the methylation of cytosine moieties. Usually about 2–5% of the cytosine is methylated. Little is known about the distribution of 5-methylcytosine in DNA, and nothing is known about its function. During DNA replication, methylation of cytosine occurs soon after synthesis of the DNA strand. At present it is not known whether methylation occurs at all after repair synthesis or, if it does, how long the lag is. Conceivably, unmethylated regions of DNA might be important in altering gene expression directly or indirectly by altering chromatin structure.

Most of the discussion above has concerned ways in which repair might alter the organization of nuclear material and thus effect changes in gene expression. To date, no one has looked specifically at the question of gene expression. There are relatively few good markers to use and, in order to analyze this process, individual cells and not cell populations must be analyzed. Conceptually, the demonstration of any alteration in gene expression resulting from repair processes would be of great importance, since it would establish that the restoration of DNA sequence and hence of genetic information does not inevitably result in the complete restoration of cellular function.

INHIBITORS OF REPAIR

Much effort has gone into the search for compounds that would specifically inhibit DNA repair. Undoubtedly much of this effort derived from the successful use of other relatively specific inhibitors such as puromycin, cycloheximide, hydroxyurea, cytosine arabinoside, and actinomycin D to understand cell function. In addition, there has been the implicit assumption that DNA damage is somehow related to neoplasia and that modifying the amount and type of damage and repair might provide useful insights into the neoplastic process.

Investigators have attempted to explain the mechanism of action of promoting agents and cocarcinogens by their ability to inhibit various aspects of the excision repair process. Thus Gaudin et al. (1971, 1972a, 1972b, 1974) found that a variety of cocarcinogens inhibited repair synthesis induced by UV radiation in lymphocytes. Teebor et al. (1973) found that phorbol myristate acetate inhibited the removal of thymine dimers in HeLa cells. More recent investigations have cast doubt on the interpretation of these findings. Results from four different laboratories (Meneghini, 1974; Cleaver and Painter, 1975; Langenbach and Kuszynski, 1975; Poirier et al., 1975) confirmed the inhibition of repair synthesis by a variety of promotors and cocarcinogens; however, at equimolar concentrations these agents were found to be as active or more active in suppressing replicative synthesis. Poirier et al. (1975) also found that these agents inhibited RNA and protein synthesis and produced cell toxicity at the same concentrations that inhibited DNA repair and DNA replicative synthesis. In addition, analogues of promotors that failed to inhibit repair had no effect on these other cellular functions. These data, combined with the wealth of other known biochemical effects of promotors, have suggested that promotors are not specific in their inhibition of repair synthesis.

Cleaver and Painter (1975) looked at many compounds that have been proposed as specific inhibitors of excision repair and found no evidence that any of them specifically inhibited excision-repair synthesis. One interesting exception to the lack of specificity of inhibitors of repair is the effect of methylated xanthines (caffeine and theophylline) on postreplication repair. It is now clear that caffeine and theophylline inhibit postreplication repair in rodent cells (Cleaver and Thomas, 1969; Fujiwara, 1972, 1975; Trosko and Chu, 1973; Lehmann and Kirk-Bell, 1974). This effect appears to be relatively specific for postreplication repair at the concentrations of the agents studied, since there was only a small effect on replicative synthesis; in addition, excision of thymine dimers appears to be relatively unaffected by caffeine (Trosko and Chu, 1973; Lehmann and Kirk-Bell, 1974). Postreplication repair in human cell lines is apparently unaffected by xanthine alkaloids; however, a recent report (Lehmann et al., 1975) indicates that some xeroderma variants (patients with XP who have normal excision repair) have a postreplication repair system that is dramatically inhibited by caffeine. This finding provides a useful tool for the study of the molecular biology involved in postreplication repair and may be of importance in helping to assess the risk of human populations exposed to foreign compounds. One wonders whether caffeine and theophylline, while probably not posing a risk to the population at large, might have effects on some individuals within the population. Furthermore, it is worth keeping in mind that if potent inhibitors of repair processes are present in the environment, their effects could be similar to those of environmental mutagens and carcinogens.

REPAIR AS PART OF THE TOXICOLOGIC PROFILE AND ITS RELATION TO RISK ASSESSMENT

So far I have dealt with repair in mammalian cells as an aspect of cell and molecular biology; perhaps of equal importance, however, is the question of the usefulness of repair as a method of identifying hazardous or potentially hazardous agents in the environment and our therapeutic armamentarium.

It is clear that the key to the development of effective tests for environmental mutagens and carcinogens is the development of effective activation systems. This development must be directed toward identifying new types of metabolic activation. Simple improvement of existing systems, while important, is unlikely to expand the breadth of screening efforts. Along these lines, work on the sequestration and transport of activated species would be of interest. Unlike toxicity, which in some cases may be primarily cytoplasmic, genetic damage implies entry into the nucleus by activated agents. Analysis of nuclear entry by cytoplasmically activated compounds has been neglected.

What remains in doubt, however, is whether repair tests (i.e., those based on unscheduled DNA synthesis) are likely to be any more sensitive than classic genetic screening methods (Malling and de Serres, 1969; Corbett et al., 1970; de Serres and Malling, 1971; Ames et al., 1973).

Table 2 compares the sensitivity of two *in vitro mammalian* specific locus tests with that of repair synthesis for the detection of several *direct-acting* agents. The conclusions drawn from these data must be tempered by the realization that they were gathered by a number of laboratories, using a variety of cell types and techniques. To date, no one laboratory has attempted a systematic comparison of repair tests and specific locus tests. These data suggest, however, that repair synthesis and specific locus tests in *mammalian* cells may be about equally sensitive. Thus, for instance, with ethyl methane-sulfonate (Table 2) a repair synthesis assay was able to detect activity easily at 1.0 mM and marginally at 0.1 mM, while the $TK^{+/-} \rightarrow TK^{-/-}$ (thymidine kinase) assay in mouse lymphoma cells showed activity at 0.5–1.0 mM and marginal activity at 0.25 mM. Surprisingly, activity was not seen in one set of experiments at 20 mM in the $HGPRT^{+} \rightarrow HGPRT^{-}$ system in Chinese hamster cells. Maher has begun mutagenesis studies on repair-deficient human cells (XP), and these apparently have higher induced mutation frequencies than normal fibroblasts (Maher et al., 1976). Hence this approach may lead to a successful way to increase the sensitivity of assay systems using human cells.

In one respect, repair synthesis, at least as it is analyzed by autoradiography, has a distinct advantage: it requires much less skill and specialized training to do autoradiography than to do somatic cell genetics. In addition, much less fastidious cell culture methods are needed for these repair studies. The repair synthesis assay is probably faster than the HGPRT assay in human cells and as fast as or faster than the TK system or HGPRT system in rodent cells.

In terms of rapidity of assay, however, none of them compares with the *Salmonella* system perfected by Ames et al. (1973). While one may argue the merits of demonstration of genetic activity in human cells as a prerequisite for administrative action, it seems unlikely that a human culture system will replace a prokaryotic one as a first screen.

An advantage mammalian systems have is the potential for using the intracellular activation system for metabolizing the compound of interest. The possibility of using human liver cells in culture for repair and mutagenesis screening studies has been suggested (Lieberman, 1976b), and it is not unlikely that the near future may see a variety of *in vitro* systems for examining the organ specificity of xenobiologic compounds.

The problem of aging in relation to mutagenesis and carcinogenesis is a subject of considerable interest. To date, there is little evidence from cell culture work that aging (as defined by an increase in the number of cell generations) affects repair (for a more extensive discussion, see Lieberman, 1976a); however, to date, the tests have been relatively crude quantitative ones (grain counts, DNA strand breaks, etc.), and more refined qualitative tests have yet to be developed. Studies indicate that with increasing cellular

TABLE 2 Comparison of Sensitivity of Repair Synthesis and Specific Locus Systems for Detecting Direct-Acting Mutagens and Carcinogens[a]

Agent	Repair synthesis[b]	TK$^{+/-}$ → TK$^{-/-}$	HGPRT^{+} → HGPRT^{-}
Ethyl methanesulfonate	0.1 mM, marginal[c] 1.0 mM, clear[c]	0.25 mM, marginal[d] 0.5–1 mM, clear[d]	20 mM, not detected[e]
Methyl methanesulfonate	0.01 mM, marginal[c] 0.1 mM, clear[c]	0.1–0.25, clear[d]	1.0 mM, clear[e]
N-Acetoxy-2-acetylaminofluorene	0.01 mM, marginal[c] 0.1 mM, clear[c] 0.001 mM, clear[g,h]		0.0015–0.002 mM[f] 0.0025 mM, clear[i]
7-Bromomethylbenz[a]anthracene	0.001 mM, clear[h,j]		0.0001 mM, clear[k]
Methylnitrosourea	2 mM, clear[l] 0.2 mM, clear[n]		0.05 mM, marginal[m] 0.10 mM, clear[m]
N-Methyl-N'-nitro-N-nitrosoguanidine	0.02 mM, clear[l]	0.02 mM, clear[o]	

[a]The designations marginal, clear, or not detected usually refer to the lowest dose examined, or, if the lowest dose was marginal or not detected, the next highest dose examined is listed. TK$^{+/-}$ → TK$^{-/-}$ refers to the thymidine kinase locus (see Clive, 1973); HGPRT^{+} → HGPRT^{-} refers to the hypoxanthine-guanine phosphoribosyltransferase locus.

[b]Repair synthesis was measured by a variety of means listed in the references cited.

[c]Lieberman et al., 1971.

[d]Clive, 1973.

[e]Chu et al., 1974.

[f]Maher and Wessel, 1975.

[g]Stich et al., 1972b.

[h]Lieberman and Poirier, 1974a.

[i]Huang and Lieberman, in press.

[j]Lieberman and Dipple, 1972.

[k]Duncan and Brookes, 1973.

[l]Roberts et al., 1971.

[m]Roberts and Sturrock, 1973.

[n]Harris et al., 1974.

[o]Clive, personal communication.

age, increasing percentages of variant enzymes accumulate (for two recent papers, see Fulder and Holliday, 1975; Goldstein and Moerman, 1975). These are presumably the result of accumulation of errors in the protein-synthesizing machinery, but the relation of repair to this phenomenon remains unclear. At present we have too little information in this area to begin to assess risk on the basis of age.

On the other hand, we now know from the study of human repair-deficient strains (XP) that groups within the human population may have a substantially higher risk after exposure to "genetically active agents" than does the population at large. With XP the screening problem is easy, since the effects manifest themselves clinically at an early age. Detection of other individuals who have less severe repair deficiencies but who nevertheless are at substantial risk is difficult. The variety of types of repair deficiencies that constitute the xeroderma syndrome suggests immediately that a battery of tests including unscheduled DNA synthesis, postreplication repair, host cell reactivation, and photoreactivation would have to be included. Since non-XP individuals might be expected to have less severe repair deficiencies than xeroderma patients, quantitative methods would have to be more precise. It is difficult to estimate how many individuals might be at risk. It is interesting to note, however, that in the United States the frequency of the xeroderma syndrome (homozygous for some deficiency) is 1–4 per 10^6 individuals; in Japan, however, it is 50–100 times more frequent (Takebe, 1976)! Although meager, these data, along with the unavailability of a truly rapid screening procedure, indicate that the problem of risk estimation on a worldwide or even a national level would be very difficult, if not impossible, at this time.

Several other issues should be mentioned in connection with the problem of risk assessment. As discussed previously, we must be aware that some environmental agents may act indirectly by inhibiting repair in response to damage by other compounds. An effort to develop methods to identify such inhibitors must be made. Some evaluation of the specificity of the inhibition is important, since it is necessary to be sure that simple toxicity is not being measured. Another area that deserves attention is potential virus-mutagen and virus-carcinogen interactions. Several groups have reported enhancement of viral integration and *in vivo* transformation by mutagens and strand-breaking agents (Freeman et al., 1970; Stich et al., 1972a; Casto et al., 1974). Whether these phenomena have any practical consequences remains to be seen; however, enzymatic nicking secondary to DNA damage by environmental compounds and its role in viral neoplasia might be a fertile area for investigation.

REFERENCES

Amacher, D. E., and Lieberman, M. W. 1977. Removal of acetylaminofluorene from the DNA of control and repair-deficient human fibroblasts. *Biochem. Biophys. Res. Commun.* 74:285–290.

Amacher, D. E. Elliott, J. A. and Lieberman, M. W. 1977. Differences in removal of acetylaminofluorene and pyrimidine dimers from the DNA of cultured mammalian cells. *Proc. Natl. Acad. Sci. U.S.A.* 74:1553–1557.

Ames, B. N., Lee, F. D. and Durston, W. E. 1973. An improved bacterial test system for the detection and classification of mutagens and carcinogens. *Proc. Natl. Acad. Sci. U.S.A.* 70:782–786.

Beers, R. F., Jr., Herriott, R. M. and Tilghman, R. C., eds. 1972. *Molecular and cellular repair processes.* Baltimore: Johns Hopkins.

Berliner, J., Himes, S. W., Aoki, C. T. and Norman, A. 1975. The sites of unscheduled DNA synthesis within irradiated human lymphocytes. *Radiat. Res.* 63:544–552.

Boutwell, R. K., Colburn, N. H. and Muckerman, C. C. 1969. *In vivo* reactions of β-propiolactone. *Ann. N.Y. Acad. Sci.* 163:751–764.

Bowden, G. T., Trosko, J. E., Shapas, B. G. and Boutwell, R. K. 1975. Excision of pyrimidine dimers from epidermal DNA and nonsemiconservative epidermal DNA synthesis following ultraviolet irradiation of mouse skin. *Cancer Res.* 35:3599–3607.

Burk, P. G., Lutzner, M. A., Clarke, D. D. and Robbins, J. H. 1971. Ultraviolet-stimulated thymidine incorporation in xeroderma pigmentosum lymphocytes. *J. Lab. Clin. Med.* 77:759–767.

Capps, M. J., O'Connor, P. J. and Craig, A. W. 1973. The influence of liver regeneration on the stability of 7-methylguanine in rat liver DNA after treatment with N,N dimethylnitrosamine. *Biochim. Biophys. Acta* 331:33–40

Casto, B. C., Pieczynski, W. J. and DiPaolo, J. A. 1974. Enhancement of adenovirus transformation of hamster embryo cells with diverse chemical carcinogens. *Cancer Res.* 34:72–78.

Chu, E. Y. H., Brimer, P. A., Schenley, C. K., Ho, T. and Malling, H. V. 1974. Reversion studies of chemically induced mutants in Chinese hamster cells. In *Molecular and environmental aspects of mutagenesis*, eds. L. Prakash, F. Sherman, M. W. Miller, C. W. Lawrence, and H. W. Taber, pp. 178–195. Springfield, Ill.: Thomas.

Clark, R. J. and Felsenfeld, G. 1974. Chemical probes of chromatin structure. *Biochemistry* 13:3622–3628.

Clayton, D. A., Doda, J. N. and Friedberg, E. C. 1974. The absence of a pyrimidine dimer repair mechanism in mammalian mitochondria. *Proc. Natl. Acad. Sci. U.S.A.* 71:2777–2781.

Cleaver, J. E. 1973. DNA repair with purines and pyrimidines in radiation- and carcinogen-damaged normal and xeroderma pigmentosum human cells. *Cancer Res.* 33:362–369.

Cleaver, J. E. 1974. Repair processes for photochemical damage in mammalian cells. *Adv. Radiat. Biol.* 4:1–75.

Cleaver, J. E. and Painter, R. B. 1975. Absence of specificity in inhibition of DNA repair replication by DNA-binding agents, cocarcinogens, and steroids in human cells. *Cancer Res.* 35:1773–1778.

Cleaver, J. E. and Thomas, G. H. 1969. Single strand interruptions in DNA and the effects of caffeine in Chinese hamster cells irradiated with ultraviolet light. *Biochem. Biophys. Res. Commun.* 36:203–208.

Clive, D. 1973. Recent developments with the L5178Y heterozygote mutagen assay system. *Environ. Health Perspect. Exp. Issue* 6:119–126.

Connor, W. G. and Norman, A. 1971. Unscheduled DNA synthesis in human lymphocytes. *Mutat. Res.* 13:393–402.

Corbett, T. H., Heidelberger, C. and Dove, W. F. 1970. Determination of the mutagenic activity to bacteriophage T4 of carcinogenic and noncarcinogenic compounds. *Mol. Pharmacol.* 6:667–679.

Cox, R. and Irving, C. C. 1975. Damage and repair of DNA in various tissues of the rat induced by 4-nitroquinoline-1-oxide. *Proc. Am. Assoc. Cancer Res.* 16:150.

Cox, R., Damjanov, I., Abanobi, S. E. and Sarma, D. S. R. 1973a. A method for measuring damage and repair in the liver *in vivo. Cancer Res.* 33:2114–2121.

Cox, R., Damjanov. I. and Irving, C. C. 1973b. Damage and repair of hepatic DNA by ethylating carcinogens. *Proc. Am. Assoc. Cancer Res.* 14:28.

Damjanov, I., Cox, R., Sarma, D. S. R. and Farber, E. 1973. Patterns of damage and repair of liver deoxyribonucleic acid induced by carcinogenic methylating agents *in vivo. Cancer Res.* 33:2122–2128.

de Serres, F. J. and Malling, H. V. 1971. Measurements of recessive lethal damage over the entire genome and at two specific loci in the *ad*-3 region of *Neurospora crassa* with a two component heterokaryon. In *Chemical mutagens: Principles and methods for their detection*, ed. A. Hollaender, pp. 311–342. New York: Plenum.

Duncan, M. E. and Brookes, P. 1973. The induction of azaguanine-resistant mutants in cultured Chinese hamster cells by the reactive derivatives of carcinogenic hydrocarbons. *Mutat. Res.* 21:107–118.

Epstein, J. H., Fukuyama, K., Reed, W. B. and Epstein, W. L. 1970. Defect in DNA synthesis in skin of patients with xeroderma pigmentosum demonstrated *in vivo. Science* 168:1477–1478.

Epstein, W. B., Fukuyama, K. and Epstein, J. H. 1971. Ultraviolet light, DNA repair and skin carcinogenesis in man. *Fed. Proc.* 30:1766–1771.

Evans, R. G. and Norman, A. 1968. Radiation stimulated incorporation of thymidine into the DNA of human lymphocytes. *Nature (Lond.)* 217:455–456.

Freeman, A. E., Price, P. J., Igel, H. J., Young, J. C., Maryak, J. M. and Huebner, R. J. 1970. Morphological transformation of rat embryo cells induced by diethylnitrosamine and murine leukemia viruses. *J. Natl. Cancer Inst.* 44:65–78.

Frey-Wettstein, M., Longmire, R. and Craddock, C. G. 1969. Deoxyribonucleic acid (DNA) repair replication of ultraviolet (UV) irradiated normal and leukemic leukocytes. *J. Lab. Clin. Med.* 74:109–118.

Fujiwara, Y. 1972. Characteristics of DNA synthesis following ultraviolet light irradiation in mouse L cells. *Exp. Cell Res.* 75:483–489.

Fujiwara, Y. 1975. Post replication repair of alkylation damage to DNA of mammalian cells in culture. *Cancer Res.* 35:2780–2789.

Fulder, S. J. and Holliday, R. 1975. A rapid rise in cell variants during senescence of populations of human fibroblasts. *Cell* 6:67–73.

Gaudin, D., Gregg, R. S. and Yielding, K. L. 1971. DNA repair inhibition: A possible mechanism of action of co-carcinogens. *Biochem. Biophys. Res. Commun.* 45:630–636.

Gaudin, D., Gregg, R. S. and Yielding, K. L. 1972a. Inhibition of DNA repair by cocarcinogens. *Biochem. Biophys. Res. Commun.* 48:945–949.

Gaudin, D., Gregg, R. S. and Yielding, K. L. 1972b. Inhibition of DNA repair replication by DNA binding drugs which sensitize cells to alkylating agents and X-rays. *Proc. Soc. Exp. Biol. Med.* 141:543–547.

Gaudin, D., Guthrie, L. and Yielding, K. L. 1974. DNA repair inhibition: A new mechanism of action of steroids with possible implications for tumor therapy. *Proc. Soc. Exp. Biol. Med.* 146:401–405.

Glover, D. M., White, R. L., Finnegan, D. J. and Hogness, D. S. 1975. Characterization of six cloned DNAs from *Drosophila melanogaster* including one that contains the genes for rRNA. *Cell* 5:149–157.

Goldstein, S. and Moerman, E. J. 1975. Heat labile enzymes for Werner's syndrome fibroblasts. *Nature (Lond.)* 255:159.

Goth, R. and Rajewsky, M. F. 1974. Persistence of O^6-ethylguanine in rat-brain DNA: Correlation with nervous system-specific carcinogenesis by ethylnitrosourea. *Proc. Natl. Acad. Sci. U.S.A.* 71:639–643.

Graham, D. E., Neufeld, B. R., Davidson, E. H. and Britten, R. J. 1974. Interspersion of repetitive and non-repetitive DNA sequences in the sea urchin genome. *Cell* 1:127–137.

Grunicke, H., Bock, K. W., Becher, H., Gäng, V., Schnierda, J. and Puschendorf, B. 1973. Effect of alkylating antitumor agents on the binding of DNA to protein. *Cancer Res.* 33:1048–1053.

Han, A., Korbelik, M. and Ban, J. 1975. DNA to protein cross-linking in synchronized HeLa cells exposed to ultraviolet light. *Int. J. Radiat. Biol.* 27:63–74.

Hanawalt, P. C. and Setlow, R. B., eds. 1975. *Molecular mechanisms for repair of DNA.* New York: Plenum.

Harris, C. C., Connor, R. J., Jackson, F. E. and Lieberman, M. W. 1974. Intranuclear distribution of DNA repair synthesis induced by chemical carcinogens or ultraviolet light in human diploid fibroblasts. *Cancer Res.* 34:3461–3468.

Hart, R. W. and Setlow, R. B. 1974. Correlation between deoxyribonucleic acid excision repair and life-span in a number of mammalian species. *Proc. Natl. Acad. Sci. U.S.A.* 71:2169–2173.

Huang, A. T., Kremer, W. B., Laszlo, J. and Setlow, R. B. 1972. DNA repair in human leukemic lymphocytes. *Nature New Biol.* 240:114–115.

Huang, S. L. and Lieberman, M. W. 1978. Induction of 6-thioguanine resistance in human cells treated with *N*-acetoxy-2-acetylaminofluorene. *Mutat. Res.*, in press.

Ikenaga, M., Ishii, Y., Tada, M., Kakunaga, T., Takebe, H. and Kondo, S. 1975. The excision-repair of 4-nitroquinoline-1-oxide damage responsible for killing, mutation and cancer. In *Molecular mechanisms for repair of DNA*, eds. P. C. Hanawalt and R. B. Setlow. New York: Plenum.

Jacobs, A. J., O'Brien, R. L., Parker, J. W. and Paolilli, P. 1972. Abnormal DNA repair of 4-nitroquinoline-1-oxide-induced damage by lymphocytes in xeroderma pigmentosum. *Mutat. Res.* 16:420–424.

Janss, D. H., Moon, R. C. and Irving, C. C. 1972. The binding of 7,12-dimethylbenz(*a*)anthracene to mammary parenchyma DNA and protein *in vivo*. *Cancer Res.* 32:254–258.

Kirtikar, D. M. and Goldthwait, D. A. 1974. The enzymatic release of O^6-methylquanine and 3-methyladenine from DNA reacted with the carcinogen N-methyl-N-nitrosourea. *Proc. Natl. Acad. Sci. U.S.A.* 71:2022–2026.

Kitagawa, T., Michalopoulos, G. and Pitot, H. C. 1975. Unscheduled DNA synthesis in cells from *N*-2-fluorenylacetamide-induced hyperplastic nodules of rat liver maintained in primary culture. *Cancer Res.* 35:3682–3692.

Kondo, S. 1973. Evidence that mutations are induced by errors in repair and replication. *Genetics (Suppl.)* 73:109–122.

Kornberg, A. 1974. *DNA synthesis*, chap. 1. San Francisco: Freeman.

Kornberg, R. D. 1974. Chromatin structure: A repeating unit of histones and DNA. *Science* 184:868–871.

Kriek, E. 1972. Persistent binding of a new reaction product of the carcinogen *N*-hydroxy-*N*-2-acetylaminofluorene with guanine in rat liver DNA *in vivo. Cancer Res.* 32:2042–2048.

Langenbach, R. and Kuszynski, C. 1975. Nonspecific inhibition of DNA repair by promoting and nonpromoting phorbol esters. *J. Natl. Cancer Inst.* 55:801–802.

Lawley, P. D. and Orr, D. J. 1970. Specific excision of methylation products from DNA of *E. coli* treated with MNNG. *Chem. Biol. Interact.* 2:154–157.

Lawley, P. D. and Warren, W. 1975. Specific excision of ethylated purines from the DNA of *Escherichia coli* treated with *N*-ethyl-*N*-nitrosourea. *Chem. Biol. Interact.* 11:55–57.

Lehmann, A. R. 1972. Post replication repair of DNA in ultraviolet-irradiated mammalian cells. *Eur. J. Biochem.* 31:438–445.

Lehmann, A. R. and Kirk-Bell, S. 1974. Effects of caffeine and theophylline on DNA synthesis in unirradiated and UV-irradiated mammalian cells. *Mutat. Res.* 26:73–82.

Lehmann, A. R., Kirk-Bell, S., Arlett, C. F., Patterson, M. C., Lohman, P. H. M., De Weerd-Kastelein, E. A. and Bootsma, D. 1975. Xeroderma pigmentosum cells with normal levels of excision repair have a defect in DNA synthesis after UV-irradiation. *Proc. Natl. Acad. Sci. U.S.A.* 72:219–223.

Lett, J. T., Sun, C. and Wheeler, K. T. 1972. Restoration of the DNA structure in X-irradiated eukaryotic cells: *In vitro* and *in vivo*. In *Molecular and cellular repair processes*, eds. R. F. Beers, R. M. Herriott, and R. C. Tilghman, pp. 147–158. Baltimore: Johns Hopkins.

Lewin, B. *Gene expression—2: Eukaryotic chromosomes*. London: Wiley.

Lieberman, M. W. 1976a. Approaches to the analysis of fidelity of DNA repair in mammalian cells. *Int. Rev. Cytol.* 46:1–23.

Lieberman, M. W. 1976b. Quantitative aspects of using DNA repair to detect mutagens and carcinogens. *Ann. N.Y. Acad. Sci.* 269:37–42.

Lieberman, M. W. and Dipple, A. 1972. Removal of bound carcinogen during DNA repair in nondividing human lymphocytes. *Cancer Res.* 32:1855–1860.

Lieberman, M. W. and Forbes, P. D. 1973. Demonstration of DNA repair in normal and neoplastic tissues after treatment with proximate chemical carcinogens and ultraviolet radiation. *Nature New Biol.* 241:199–201.

Lieberman, M. W. and Poirier, M. C. 1973. Deoxyribonucleoside incorporation during DNA repair of carcinogen-induced damage in human diploid fibroblasts. *Cancer Res.* 33:2097–2103.

Lieberman, M. W. and Poirier, M. C. 1974a. Distribution of deoxyribonucleic acid repair synthesis among repetitive and unique sequences in the human diploid genome. *Biochemistry* 13:3018–3023.

Lieberman, M. W. and Poirier, M. C. 1974b. Intragenomal distribution of DNA repair synthesis: Repair in satellite and mainband DNA in cultured mouse cells. *Proc. Natl. Acad. Sci. U.S.A.* 71:2461–2465.

Lieberman, M. W. and Poirier, M. C. 1974c. Base pairing and template specificity during deoxyribonucleic acid repair synthesis in human and mouse cells. *Biochemistry* 13:5384–5388.

Lieberman, M. W., Baney, R. N., Lee, R. E., Sell, S. and Farber, E. 1971.

Studies on DNA repair in human lymphocytes treated with proximate carcinogens and alkylating agents. *Cancer Res.* 31:1297–1306.

Lieberman, M. W., Amacher, D. A., Elliott, J. A. and Huang, S. L. 1976. Removal of bound acetylaminofluorene from the DNA of mammalian cells in culture. In *Fundamentals in cancer prevention*, eds. P. N. Magee, S. Takayama, T. Sugimura and T. Matsushima, pp. 335–345. Tokyo: University of Tokyo Press.

Maher, V. M., Curren, R. O., Ouellette, L. M. and McCormick, J. J. 1976. Effect of DNA repair on the frequency of mutations induced in normal human skin fibroblasts and in strains of xeroderma pigmentosum by ultraviolet irradiation and by chemical carcinogens. In *Fundamentals in cancer prevention*, eds. P. N. Magee, S. Takayama, T. Sugimura and T. Matsushima, pp. 363–379. Tokyo: University of Tokyo Press.

Maher V. M. and Wessel, J. E. 1975. Mutations to azaguanine resistance induced in cultured diploid fibroblasts by the carcinogen, N-acetoxy-2-acetylaminofluorene. *Mutat. Res.* 28:277–284.

Maher, V. M., Birch, N., Mittlestat, M., Otto, J., Ouellett, L., Schnur, T. and McCormick, J. J. 1975. Effect of excision and post replication DNA repair on the cytotoxicity and mutagenicity of UV in human skin fibroblasts. *Proc. Am. Assoc. Cancer Res.* 16:158 (abstract).

Malling, H. V. and de Serres, F. J. 1969. Mutagenicity of alkylating carcinogens. *Ann. N.Y. Acad. Sci.* 163:788–800.

McGrath, R. A. and Williams, R. W. 1966. Reconstruction *in vivo* of irradiated *Escherichia coli* deoxyribonucleic acid: The rejoining of broken pieces. *Nature* (*Lond.*) 212:534–535.

Meltz, M. L. and Painter, R. B. 1973. Distribution of repair replication in the HeLa cell genome. *Int. J. Radiat. Biol.* 23:637–640.

Meneghini, R. 1974. Repair replication of opossum lymphocyte DNA: Effect of compounds that bind to DNA. *Chem. Biol. Interact.* 8:113–126.

Metzger, G. and Daune, M. P. 1975. *In vitro* binding of N-acetoxy-N-2-acetylaminofluorene to DNA in chromatin. *Cancer Res.* 35:2738–2742.

Noll, M., Thomas, J. O. and Kornberg, R. D. 1975. Preparation of native chromatin and damage caused by shearing. *Science* 187:1203–1206.

Norman, A., Ottoman, R. E., Chan, P. and Klisak, I. 1972. Unscheduled DNA synthesis in some spontaneous human tumors. *Mutat. Res.* 15:358–360.

O'Connor, P. J., Capps, M. J. and Craig, A. W. 1973. Comparative studies of the hepatocarcinogen N,N-dimethylnitrosamine *in vivo:* Reaction sites in rat liver DNA and the significance of their relative stabilities. *Br. J. Cancer* 27:153–166.

Parrish, J. A., Fitzpatrick, T. B., Tannenbaum, L. and Pathak, M. A. 1974. Photochemotherapy of psoriasis with oral methoxsalen and longwave ultraviolet light. *N. Engl. J. Med.* 291:1207–1211.

Poirier, M. C., DeCicco, B. T. and Lieberman, M. W. 1975. Nonspecific inhibition of DNA repair synthesis by tumor promotors in human diploid fibroblasts damaged with N-acetoxy-2-acetylaminofluorene. *Cancer Res.* 35:1392–1397.

Ramanathan, R., Sarma, D. S. R., Rajalakshmi, S. and Farber, E. 1975. Non-random methylation of rat liver chromatin DNA by dimethylnitrosamine (DMN) *in vivo*. *Proc. Am. Assoc. Cancer Res.* 16:9 (abstract).

Rayman, M. P. and Dipple, A. 1973. Structure and activity in chemical carcinogenesis. Comparison of the reactions of 7-bromomethylbenz(*a*)anthracene and 7-bromomethyl-12-methylbenz(*a*)anthracene with mouse skin deoxyribonucleic acid *in vivo*. *Biochemistry* 12:1538–1542.

Regan, J. D. and Setlow, R. B. 1974. Two forms of repair in the DNA of human cells damaged by chemical carcinogens and mutagens. *Cancer Res.* 34:3318–3325.

Roberts, J. J. and Sturrock, J. E. 1973. Enhancement by caffeine of *N*-methyl-*N*-nitrosourea-induced mutations and chromosome aberrations in Chinese hamster cells. *Mutat. Res.* 20:243–255.

Roberts, J. J., Pascoe, J. M., Smith, B. A. and Crathorn, A. R. 1971. Quantitative aspects of the repair of alkylated DNA in cultured mammalian cells. *Chem. Biol. Interact.* 3:49–68.

Setlow, R. B., Regan, J. D. and Carrier, W. L. 1972. Different levels of excision repair in mammalian cell lines. *Biophys. Soc. Abstr.* 12:19a.

Slor, H. 1973. Induction of unscheduled DNA synthesis by the carcinogen 7-bromomethylbenz(*a*)anthracene and its removal from the DNA of normal and xeroderma pigmentosum lymphocytes. *Mutat. Res.* 19:231–235.

Sollner-Webb, B. and Felsenfeld, G. 1975. A comparison of the digestion of nuclei and chromatin by staphylococcal nuclease. *Biochemistry* 14:2915–2920.

Stewart, B. W., Farber, E. and Mirvish, S. S. 1973. Induction by an hepatic carcinogen, 1-nitroso-5,6-dihydrouracil, of single and double strand breaks of liver DNA with rapid repair. *Biochem. Biophys. Res. Commun.* 53:773–779.

Stein, G. S., Park, W. D., Stein, J. L. and Lieberman, M. W. 1976. Synthesis of nuclear proteins during DNA repair synthesis in human diploid fibroblasts damaged with ultraviolet radiation or a chemical carcinogen. *Proc. Natl. Acad. Sci. U.S.A.* 73:1466–1470.

Stich, H. F. and Kieser, D. 1974. Use of DNA repair synthesis in detecting organotropic actions of chemical carcinogens. *Proc. Soc. Exp. Biol. Med.* 145:1339–1342.

Stich, H. F., Hammerberg, O. and Casto, B. C. 1972a. Combined effect of chemical mutagen and virus on DNA repair, chromosome aberrations, and neoplastic transformation. *Can. J. Genet. Cytol.* 14:911–917.

Stich, H. F., San, R. H. C., Miller, J. A. and Miller, E. C. 1972b. Various levels of DNA repair synthesis in xeroderma pigmentosum cells exposed to the carcinogens N-hydroxy and N-acetoxy-2-acetylaminofluorene. *Nature New Biol.* 238:9–10.

Stockdale, F. E. 1971. DNA synthesis in differentiating skeletal muscle cells: Initiation by ultraviolet light. *Science* 171:1145–1147.

Sutherland, B. M., Runge, P. and Sutherland, J. C. 1974. DNA photoreactivating enzyme from placental mammals. Origin and characteristics. *Biochemistry* 13:4710–4714.

Szafarz, D. and Weisburger, J. H. 1969. Stability of the binding of label from *N*-hydroxy-*N*-fluorenylacetamide to intranuclear targets, particularly deoxyribonucleic acid in rat liver. *Cancer Res.* 29: 962–968.

Takebe, H. 1976. Genetic complementation tests of Japanese xeroderma pigmentosum patients and their characteristics of repair and skin cancer. In *Fundamentals in cancer prevention*, eds. P. N. Magee, S. Takayama, T. Sugimura and T. Matsushima, pp. 383–394. Tokyo: University of Tokyo Press.

Takebe, H., Nii, S., Ishii, M. I. and Utsumi, H. 1974. Comparative studies of host cell reactivation, colony forming ability and excision repair after UV irradiation of xeroderma pigmentosum, normal human and some other mammalian cells. *Mutat. Res.* 25:383–390.

Teebor, G. W., Duker, N. J., Ruacan, S. A. and Zachary, K. J. 1973. Inhibition of thymine dimer excision by the phorbol ester, phorbol myristate acetate. *Biochem. Biophys. Res. Commun.* 50:66–70.

Trosko, J. E. and Chu, E. H. Y. 1973. Inhibition of repair of UV-damaged DNA by caffeine and mutation induction in Chinese hamster cells. *Chem. Biol. Interact.* 6:317–332.

Turberville, C. and Craddock, V. M. 1971. Methylation of nuclear proteins by dimethylnitrosamine and methionine in the rat *in vivo. Biochem. J.* 124:725–739.

Venitt, S. and Tarmy, E. M. 1972. The selective excision of arylalkylated products from the DNA of *Escherichia coli* treated with the carcinogen 7-bromomethylbenz(*a*)anthracene. *Biochim. Biophys. Acta* 287:38–51.

Wilkins, R. J. and Hart, R. W. 1974. Preferential DNA repair in human cells. *Nature (Lond.)* 247:35–36.

Witkin, E. M. 1975a. Thermal enhancement of ultraviolet mutability in a dnaB or uvrA derivative of *Escherichia coli* B/r: Evidence for inducible error-prone repair. In *Molecular mechanisms for repair of DNA*, eds. P. C. Hanawalt and R. B. Setlow. New York: Plenum.

Witkin, E. M. 1975b. Terminal transferase and error-prone repair of DNA in bacteria. *N. Engl. J. Med.* 292:1407.

Witkin, E. M. and George, D. L. 1973. Ultraviolet mutagenesis in polA and uvrA polA derivatives *of Escherichia coli* B/r: Evidence for an inducible error-prone repair system. *Genetics (Suppl.)* 73:91–108.

Witschi, H., Epstein, S. M. and Farber, E. 1971. Influence of liver regeneration on the loss of fluorenylacetamide derivative bound to liver DNA. *Cancer Res.* 31:270–273.

CHAPTER 4

NUTRITION, CARCINOGENESIS, AND MUTAGENESIS

Paul M. Newberne
Department of Nutrition and Food Science
Massachusetts Institute of Technology
Cambridge, Massachusetts

Errol Zeiger
National Institute of Environmental Health Sciences
Research Triangle Park, North Carolina

NUTRITION AND CARCINOGENESIS

There are sufficient data available today to state unequivocally that nutrition and cancer are related and that opportunities for cancer prevention, based on knowledge of nutrition, are rapidly emerging. A recent symposium (Symposium on Nutrition in the Causation of Cancer, 1975) brought together international experts to examine the issues, and from the published results of this gathering a number of questions can now be formulated and strategies prepared to pursue this most natural mode of attack on the overall problem of cancer cause and prevention.

Dietary deficiencies, excesses, and imbalances and the implications of these factors for the metabolism of the host are important. However, we require a better understanding of how these factors may influence susceptibility to cancer. Further, we cannot ignore other environmental factors that are inextricably woven into the overall problem of human cancer etiology. To say that dietary carcinogens present in foods as contaminants are of little if any importance (Wynder, 1975, 1976) in human carcinogenesis is to ignore the facts presented in the current literature. Some of the best examples of an association between dietary contamination and human cancer are those presented by Alpert et al. (1971) for Uganda, Keen and Martin (1971) for Swaziland, Shank et al. (1972) for Thailand, Peers and Linsell (1973) for Kenya, and van Rensburg et al. (1974) for Mozambique. The earlier observations (Newberne, 1965) that aflatoxins contaminate peanut meal in the United States and continue to appear in corn and other cereal grains in this country make the mycotoxins an important example of environmental factors.

It is most interesting that in all the areas and population groups referred to above, except for the United States, there is a remarkable association between a high incidence of cancer, malnutrition, and dietary contamination. Thus, we cannot assign a singular role for nutrition in human cancer, but must consider it as a significant component of a larger complex of etiologies comprised of many environmental factors, the interaction of which can undoubtedly modify the susceptibility of humans and animals to carcinogens. This concept will be borne out in the epidemiologic and experimental studies reported here. The wide variation in cancer incidence in some populations or ethnic groups living in the different geographic locations referred to above and the change in risk to migrant populations as they relocate and assume the dietary habits and nutritive status of low- or high-risk groups strongly support this concept. Factors that complicate the problem are real or potential carcinogens found in foods as contaminants. In addition to the aflatoxins and other mycotoxins, there are the nitrosamines, pesticides, synthetic hormones, and intentional food additives used to improve the texture, flavor, color, or nutritive value of foods, all of which are suspect.

Nutritional effects on carcinogenesis in experimental animals support much of the data suggested by epidemiologic studies. The effects of nutrition on induced cancer in animals are sometimes conspicuous and easily recognized; more often, however, they are subtle and may be expressed only as changes in induction time or in the distribution or type of tumors. There is no reason to believe that nutritional effects on cancer in humans differ from those observed in animals; the relevance of nutritive status to human cancer is probably marginal, which makes the job of identifying the important nutritional factors difficult indeed. Some of the nutritional factors and conditions about which most is known in regard to modulation of carcinogenesis will be presented, using specific organ sites as primary reference points.

Gastric Cancer

Cancer of the stomach has a remarkable variability in incidence according to geographic location. Populations in Japan, Chile, Colombia, Austria, Iceland, and Finland exhibit a high incidence; a low incidence is recorded in the United States and Canada (Levin et al., 1974). A number of dietary factors have been implicated in its etiology, but studies of dietary practices in gastric cancer patients have yielded little in the way of differences in patients compared with control groups (Chu and Malmgren, 1965; Graham et al., 1967, 1972; Acheson and Doll, 1964; Higginson, 1966; Dungal and Sigurjonsson, 1967; Merliss, 1971; Lilienfeld, 1972; Haenszel et al., 1972; Ackerman, 1972; Phillips, 1975; Haenszel and Correa, 1975). The high incidence of this tumor in Iceland has been associated with the large intake of smoked food, but this has not been substantiated (Dungal and Sigurjonsson, 1967). Talc that contains asbestos has been assigned a role in stomach cancer in

Japan (Merliss, 1971), but the evidence accumulated to date is less than convincing.

Mortality from gastric cancer in the United States has declined markedly during the past four decades. There is a gradient of increasing frequency with decreasing socioeconomic status, with the lowest socioeconomic groups having three times the incidence of the upper social groups (Lilienfeld, 1972). Japanese migrants to Hawaii have an incidence of stomach cancer about equal to that of their native Japanese cohorts in high-risk areas, even though the immigrants eat Western-style diets; but their offspring have lower risks (Haenszel et al., 1972). Elevated risks were found for Issei and Nisei, users of pickled vegetables and dried and salted fish, and low risks were associated with eating raw vegetables.

In another epidemiological study, Graham et al. (1972) observed that gastric cancer patients ate raw vegetables less often than controls, but that fried food, meat, or alcohol consumption had no relation to the disease.

Other studies have established a clear relationship between cancer of the stomach and other segments of the gastrointestinal tract and migration from a high-risk area (for stomach cancer) in Japan to a relatively low-risk area in California (Ackerman, 1972). On the other hand, the reverse was true for colon cancer. In both cases, the cancer incidence in the migrants moved toward that of the natives in the area to which they moved (Table 1). Seventh-Day Adventists, who neither smoke nor consume alcoholic beverages, and particularly those who consume a lacto-ovo vegetarian diet, have 50–70% cancer mortality rates for most cancer sites that are unrelated to smoking and drinking (Phillips, 1975). Interestingly, this study revealed that Seventh-Day Adventists and Seventh-Day Adventist physicians had equal cancer mortalities, suggesting that the apparent reduced risk of cancer death in all Adventists may result from selective factors.

TABLE 1   Rates of Mortality from Cancer of Gastrointestinal Sites at Ages 0–74 yr for Japanese in Japan and Japanese and Caucasians in California[a]

| | Japan | | California | | | | | |
| | Japanese | | Foreign-born Japanese | | U.S.-born Japanese | | Caucasian | |
Site	Men	Women	Men	Women	Men	Women	Men	Women
Stomach (151)[b]	58.4	30.9	29.9	13.0	11.7	11.3	8.0	4.0
Colon (153)	1.9	2.1	6.1	7.0	6.3	10.4	7.9	8.3
Rectum (154)	3.3	2.8	4.0	4.0	3.1	2.0	4.2	2.8
Total	63.6	35.8	40.0	24.0	21.1	23.7	20.1	15.1

[a]From Ackerman, 1972. Adapted with permission of *Nutrition Today* magazine, 101 Ridgely Avenue, Annapolis, Maryland, 21404 © January/February 1972.
[b]Numbers in parentheses are total number of cases.

Although there is convincing epidemiologic evidence that environmental factors, probably nutritional, are important in the etiology of gastric carcinoma, experimental evidence is mostly equivocal. Tatematsu et al. (1975) have shown that sodium chloride increased the incidence of gastric carcinoma induced by N-methyl-N'-nitro-N-nitrosoguanidine (MNNG) or 4-nitroquinoline-1-oxide (4NQO), but the manner in which the salt was administered clearly influenced the results. Weekly doses of saturated NaCl were more effective in enhancing gastric cancer than continuous administration in either water or diet (Table 2). Sodium chloride was not carcinogenic under these conditions, but it enhanced the effects of the two carcinogens. Furthermore, although these authors were unable to correlate erosion and ulceration of gastric epithelium by salt with cancer incidence, they suggest that salt may have modified the mucopolysaccharides and mucosal barrier, rendering the stomach lining more permeable to the carcinogen.

In our own laboratories (Smith et al., 1975a), we have found that increased intakes of vitamin A reduced the number of papillomas of the forestomach in hamsters given carcinogenic doses of benzo[a]pyrene intratracheally. However, the increased vitamin A enhanced cancer of the respiratory tree.

Other studies in our laboratory (Rogers, 1975) have revealed that a diet marginal in lipotropes and high in fat had no effect on the incidence of gastric carcinoma induced by MNNG in rats.

Wattenberg (1972a) has shown that antioxidant food additives can reduce the incidence of gastric tumor in mice, which opens up an additional approach to the study of stomach cancer.

TABLE 2 Influence of Sodium Chloride on Gastric Carcinoma[a]

Treatment	Total malignant tumors	
	No.	%
1. 50 mg MNNG/l drinking water, 6 g NaCl/l drinking water, stock diet + 10% NaCl	11/18	61.1
2. 50 mg MNNG/l drinking water, 1 ml saturated NaCl once weekly, stock diet	12/15	80.0
3. 50 mg MNNG/l drinking water, stock diet	12/27	44.4
4. 1 mg 4NQO once weekly, stock diet + 10% NaCl	7/18	38.9
5. 1 mg 4NQO, saturated NaCl, once weekly, stock diet	9/17	52.9
6. 1 mg 4NQO, once weekly, stock diet	0/18	0.0
7. 6 g NaCl, stock diet + 10% NaCl	0/10	0.0
8. 1 ml saturated NaCl, stock diet	0/10	0.0
9. Untreated: stock diet + tap water	0/10	0.0

[a]Abridged from Tatematsu et al., 1975. MNNG induced adenocarcinomas of the glandular stomach; 4NQO induced tumors of the forestomach.

It thus appears that although there is highly suggestive evidence that nutrition is related to cancer in some human populations, specific agents are still unknown and, in the case of animal experiments, the evidence is variable and sometimes conflicting.

Colon Cancer

There is a strong negative correlation between gastric and colon cancer in humans; where one is relatively common, the other is rare. Cancer of the colon is associated with environmental factors, and a number of studies have suggested a role for nutrition in the etiology of this type of malignancy. The mortality from colon cancer is high in Scotland, Canada, and the United States and low in Japan and Chile (Levin et al., 1974).

Some epidemiologic studies have implicated a high-fat diet in the etiology of colon cancer. There is a tendency, however, to ignore the fact that in the same populations there is high protein intake, since most of the dietary fat is taken in along with animal protein (Wynder and Shigematsu, 1967). In Japan, where the incidence of colon cancer is low, fat intake accounts for about 12% of the calories; most of the fat is of the unsaturated type. This may be compared with the 40–44% calories from fat in immigrants from Japan to the United States (Haenszel and Kurihari, 1968; Haenszel et al., 1973), where the fat is mainly of the saturated type (beef). The children of these immigrants, however, have a much higher incidence of colon cancer than do those born in Japan (Table 1). The increased incidence of colon cancer is associated with a more Western-style diet and a higher standard of living, with immigrants eating more meat and therefore consuming more fat. It is interesting, however, that the incidence of colon cancer in the United States does not vary appreciably with race, ethnic group, or socioeconomic status (Doll, 1967; Bailar, 1965).

Most studies reveal higher relative risks for people ingesting meats with little or no nitrate content (i.e., beef), compared with people consuming preserved pork products, which contain nitrites. No associations have been demonstrated between colon cancer and consumption of dried and salted fish rich in nitrates and nitrites.

Mortality from colon cancer in migrants from Poland and Norway has increased to a level comparable to that in U.S. natives. Bjelke (1974) reported that in Norway the risk of colon cancer was particularly high in people consuming above-average amounts of processed meats (Table 3). Rose et al. (1974) found a negative correlation between blood cholesterol and colon cancer in humans. The question of protein and fat intake and its relation to colon cancer is thus still an open one.

Many authors have pointed out that populations in areas with a high incidence of colon cancer consume diets high in refined foods and low in fiber. Refined foods result in small stools and a long transit time in the intestinal tract, while high-fiber diets are associated with large stools and a

TABLE 3   Serum Cholesterol and Relative Risk Estimates for Colon Cancer
by Intakes of Processed Meats[a]

Processed meats (times/month)	No. of men	Cholesterol (mg/100 ml)	Retrospective		Prospective	
			No. of cases	Relative risk	No. of cases	Relative risk
3	94	291	29	1.0	5	1.0
3–5	211	286	83	1.4	14	2.3
6 or more	130	271	48	2.1	6	2.0

[a]From Bjelke, 1974.

rapid transit time (Oettle, 1967; Burkitt et al., 1972; Walker et al., 1970; Walker, 1975). Differences in the bacterial flora are also associated with two types of diets (Hill et al., 1971). Populations ingesting Western diets had higher concentrations of fecal steroids, which tended to be more degraded than those in people consuming vegetarian diets; it was postulated that certain metabolites of bile salts may be carcinogenic. There is, however, some disagreement on the relative amounts of some fecal bile salts in groups consuming vegetarian diets (Walker, 1971); other studies have indicated higher counts of anaerobic bacteria, lower counts of aerobic bacteria, higher levels of total neutral steroids, and more degraded cholesterol and bile acids in feces of individuals from areas of high risk for colon cancer. Thus, as more recent observations indicate (Wynder and Reddy, 1973), the relation of a number of dietary habits and constituents to colon cancer is a complex one, and epidemiologic studies should serve only as a starting point for experimental studies designed to identify etiologic agents or conditions. In a limited way this has been the case, and a few experimental studies have followed epidemiologic leads; examples are given below.

Cancer of the colon in laboratory animals can be induced by bracken fern, cycasin, or methylazoxymethanol (Hirono et al., 1973; Newberne, 1976a); dimethylhydrazine (DMH) (Newberne and Rogers, 1973a; Rogers and Newberne, 1973); and aflatoxin (Newberne and Rogers, 1973b, 1973c). It is now recognized that diet can modify the incidence of the tumor, but the mechanism(s) remain to be elucidated.

There are a number of ways in which diet may modify the induction of colon cancer. It may influence the intestinal microflora (Reddy et al., 1974a); it may change the sensitivity of the colon mucosa to carcinogens, or liberate an active metabolite or supply promoters or accelerators to act on the colon mucosa; or it may accelerate or retard the intestinal transit time of the ingesta. Rats fed a diet high in fat excreted more bile acids and steroid metabolites than rats fed a diet low in fat, and they were more susceptible to DMH-induced colon cancer. (Reddy et al., 1974b).

We have shown that a diet high in fat and marginal in lipotropes

TABLE 4   Tumor Induction by Dimethylhydrazine in Normal or Lipotrope-deficient Rats

			% Rats dead with carcinoma of		
Diet[a]	Total DMH (mg/kg)	Mortality[b] (%)	Colon[c]	Small intestine[c]	Ear duct[d]
1	300	100	86	45	75
2	300	100	100	55	44
1	150	80	56	25	56
2	150	68	85	15	15

[a]Diet 1 = control; diet 2 = lipotrope-deficient diet.
[b]40 wk after initial dose of DMH.
[c]Adenocarcinoma with varying degrees of differentiation and mucus production.
[d]Squamous carcinoma. Difference between rats fed diet 1 and those fed diet 2 is significant if two doses are combined, $p < 0.05$.

increased the incidence of colon carcinoma induced by DMH (Rogers and Newberne, 1973) (Table 4). We found that a chronic dietary deficiency of vitamin A only slightly increased the incidence of DMH-induced colon tumors and slightly decreased induction time, while a high level of vitamin A in the diet did not affect tumor incidence but did decrease the number of tumors per rat (Rogers et al., 1973) (Table 5).

Aflatoxin B_1, usually a carcinogen specific for the liver in laboratory animals, induced a significant number of colon tumors in rats fed diets low or marginal in vitamin A (Newberne and Rogers, 1973c) (Table 6); this observation has been confirmed by more recent studies (Newberne, 1976b). Chronic vitamin A deficiency in rats fed aflatoxin resulted in a highly significant incidence of colon cancer. Moreover, there was some indication that the target organ changed from the liver to the colon in some animals (Table 7). A high vitamin A intake had no effect on the incidence of either liver or colon

TABLE 5   Influence of Dietary Vitamin A on Dimethylhydrazine-Induced Colon Cancer[a]

	Tumor incidence (%)	
Vitamin A status of diet (retinyl palmitate)	275 mg DMH/ kg body wt	420 mg DMH/ kg body wt
Deficient, 0–1 μg/g	77	100
Control, 10 –g/g	56	60
Excess, 165 μg/g	60	60

[a]Abridged from Rogers et al., 1973.

                    P. M. Newberne and E. Zeiger

TABLE 6 Liver and Colon Tumors in Rats Fed 0.1 ppm
Aflatoxin B$_1$ and Varying Amounts of Vitamin A[a]

Treatment	No. of survivors, 2 yr	Liver tumors	Colon tumors	Avg. body weight (g)
Control				
50 μg RP/day[b]	35/50	0/50	0/50	594
50 μg RP/day				
+ AFB$_1$	34/50	24/50	0/50	627
5 μg RP/day				
+ AFB$_1$	23/50	11/50	6/50	397
10 μg RP/day				
+ AFB$_1$	4/20	17/20	1/20	364
500 μg RP/day				
+ AFB$_1$	31/50	19/50	0/50	483

[a]From Newberne and Rogers, 1973c.
[b]RP = retinyl palmitate.

cancer. This suggests a change in sensitivity of the colon to some as yet
unidentified carcinogen or a change in metabolite(s) associated with vitamin A
deficiency, one or more of which may act on colon epithelium. These events
may be mediated through a change in gut microflora; a change in drug-
metabolizing enzymes; a change in the quantity or quality of the secretion of

TABLE 7 Incidence of Liver and Colon Tumors in Rats Fed
Aflatoxin B$_1$ and Various Levels of Vitamin A[a]

Treatment	Animal Nos.	Sex	Liver	Colon	Both	Liver only	Colon only
Control							
3.0 μg/g RA[b]	1–24	M	0/24	0/24			
3.0 μg/g RA	25–51	F	0/26	0/26			
3.0 μg/g RA							
+ AFB$_1$	52–76	M	21/24	1/24	1/24	20/24	0/24
3.0 μg/g RA							
+ AFB$_1$	77–101	F	19/24	2/24	2/24	17/24	0/24
Low vitamin A							
0.3 μg/g RA	102–111	M	0/10	0/10	0/10	0/10	0/10
0.3 μg/g RA	112–123	F	0/12	0/12	0/12	0/12	0/12
0.3 μg/g RA							
+ AFB$_1$	124–190	M	59/66	19/66	17/66	41/66	2/66
0.3 μg/g RA							
+ AFB$_1$	191–232	F	32/42	12/42	5/42	27/42	7/42

[a]Reprinted from Newberne, 1976b, p. 129, by courtesy of Marcel Dekker,
Inc.
[b]RA = retinyl acetate.

colon glycopeptides, which are vitamin A-dependent (DeLuca et al., 1970); or a combination of these (Newberne and Suphakarn, 1977).

In regard to drug-metabolizing enzymes, which can alter the quality or quantity of metabolites, recent studies (Wattenberg, 1971, 1972b) have clearly shown that intestinal aryl hydrocarbon hydroxylase (AHH) can be modified by diet, and this in turn can modify chemical carcinogenesis. The activity of AHH in the intestine of the rat can be changed by exogenous inducers in foods including Brussels sprouts, turnips, cabbage, and alfalfa and in other dietary components. This suggests an important role for nutrients in the modulation of carcinogenesis through enzyme systems, with some important implications for human cancer. We have shown a dietary effect on liver enzymes and liver cancer induction, referred to later in this chapter. A role for immunocompetence of the gastrointestinal tract should not be ignored, and studies in this area are now in progress (Newberne and Suphakarn, 1977).

Liver Cancer

Some segments of the human populations of Africa, South China, Hawaii, Thailand, and Mozambique have a very high incidence of primary liver cancer, particularly the males (Doll, 1967; Cook and Burkitt, 1971; Higginson, 1969; Shank et al., 1972; Tuyns, 1968; van Rensburg et al., 1974). Liver cancer is the most common of all forms of neoplasia south of the African Sahara, representing 10–30% of all of the tumors in men; in the Bantu of Mozambique it accounts for two-thirds of cancer reported in males. This is 500 times the rate for the same age group in the United States, which is about 2.4 per 100,000.

Studies in Thailand (Shank et al., 1972) and reports from East and South Africa clearly implicate dietary contaminants that are carcinogenic and probably interact with nutritional deficits or imbalances to result in liver cancer (van Rensburg et al., 1974). The tumors are mainly of the hepatocellular types. Cirrhosis, which may enhance susceptibility to tumor development, has been associated with the high frequency in Africa and Asia. Cirrhosis may be induced by malnutrition, injury from dietary contaminants, viral infection, or a combination of these and other factors. A role for nutrition is indicated, but the events and conditions leading to cancer are probably a result of many different interactions. In the United States, hepatocarcinoma is associated with alcoholic cirrhosis, another disease resulting from complex interactions of diet, toxins, and possibly viral infection.

Dietary effects on chemical induction of hepatocarcinoma in experimental animals have been studied extensively in our laboratory. Increased dietary lipids, particularly the unsaturated types, are associated with increased tumor incidence (Miller and Miller, 1953). We have found that if the diet is both high in fat and deficient in the lipotropes choline, methionine, and folic acid, the induction of liver tumors by carcinogens of several chemical classes is markedly enhanced (Table 8). Aflatoxin B_1 (AFB$_1$), nitrosamines, and

TABLE 8   Effect of Marginal-Lipotrope, High-Fat Diet on Chemical
Carcinogenesis in Rats

		Tumor induction	
Carcinogen	Enhanced in	Depressed in	Not affected in
Males			
AFB₁	Liver		
DEN	Liver, Esophagus		
DBN[a]	Liver		Esophagus, lung, bladder
DMN			Liver, kidney
AAF	Liver		Zymbal's gland
DMH	Colon	Zymbal's gland	Small intestine
MNNG			Forestomach
FANFT			Bladder
Females			
AAF (Sprague-Dawley)		Mammary gland	Zymbal's gland
AAF (Fischer)	Liver		
DMBA		Mammary gland	

[a]DBN, *N*-dibutylnitrosamine.

N-2-fluorenylacetamide (AAF) all induced liver tumors earlier or in higher incidence or both in deficient rats compared with rats fed adequate, balanced lipotropes (Rogers et al., 1974; Rogers, 1975). As discussed above, the same dietary deficiency enhanced tumor induction in colon and esophagus (Rogers et al., 1974; Rogers and Newberne, 1973).

    The most likely mechanism by which the deficiency influences carcinogenesis is through alteration of carcinogen metabolism by the tissues. Deficient rats had decreased basal levels of hepatic microsomal oxidases (Table 9), which were induced by phenobarbital and in some cases by AAF but not by AFB₁ (Rogers and Newberne, 1971; Rogers et al., 1975). Deficient rats cleared diethylnitrosamine (DEN) from their blood slightly but significantly

TABLE 9   Liver Enzymes, *N*-2-Fluorenylacetamide, and
Diet in Female Rats

Diet	PNA[a] (μg *p*-nitrophenol/ g liver)	BPOH[b] (quinine Units/ g liver)
Control	142 ± 16	8 ± 4
Control + AAF	187 ± 14	13 ± 6
Marginal lipotrope	105 ± 14	7 ± 3
Marginal lipotrope + AAF	147 ± 20	5 ± 3

[a]PNA, *p*-nitroanisole.
[b]BPOH, benzpyrine hydroxylase.

TABLE 10   Blood Content of Diethylnitrosamine at
Intervals After Intraperitoneal Injection[a,b]

Time after DEN injection (min)	DEN in blood (μg/ml ± S.E.)	
	Control	Deficient
4	36.1 ± 2.0	31.2 ± 3.1
20	19.8 ± 2.6	19.0 ± 1.6
40	13.9 ± 3.0	15.0 ± 4.4
60	11.2 ± 3.0	12.1 ± 1.4
120	3.1 ± 1.5	5.5 ± 0.9
210	ND[c]	0.6 ± 0.2

[a]From Rogers et al., 1975.

[b]Rats were given 25 μg/kg DEN; four or five rats per diet were studied at each time period.

[c]None detectable; 0.05 μg/ml would have been easily detected under the experimental conditions.

less rapidly than normal rats (Table 10) and this correlated with tumor incidence (Table 11).

Preliminary studies of AAF metabolism indicate that urinary excretion of N-hydroxy-AAF, a compound on the pathway of activation of AAF, may be increased in deficient rats following prolonged feeding (L. Poirier, personal communication). The S-adenosylmethionine content in the liver of deficient rats, a direct biochemical measure of lipotrope deficiency, was decreased. It diminished in both deficient and adequately fed rats when AAF was fed, which may indicate its participation in some aspect of AAF metabolism. The

TABLE 11   Tumor Incidence in Rats
Fed Diethylnitrosamine[a]

Diet	No. of rats	% Rats with tumor in		
		Liver	Esophagus	Any organ [b]
1	25	24	12	28
2	25	60[c]	8	64

[a]From Rogers et al., 1975.

[b]One rat fed diet 2 bore a transitional cell carcinoma of the urinary bladder but no other tumor; one rat fed diet 1 bore an esophageal tumor but no hepatic tumor; two rats in each diet group bore esophageal and hepatic tumors.

[c]Difference from diet 1 significant, $p <$ 0.05.

hepatic content of reduced glutathione, which reacts with many exogenous toxic chemicals to detoxify them, was normal in deficient rats and was not affected by AAF.

In addition to its effect on hepatic enzymes, the lipotrope-deficient diet induces and maintains increased DNA synthesis and mitosis in hepatocytes; presumably this is the result of increased cell turnover, although significant necrosis is not evident histologically. Studies in collaboration with Leffert at the Salk Institute, La Jolla, have demonstrated that there is a significant drop in serum very low density lipoproteins (VLDL) in the marginally deficient animals, although it is not as marked as in those fed low-lipotrope diets (Table 12). Serum VLDL inhibit the initiation of hepatocyte DNA synthesis both *in vitro* and *in vivo* and may, in conjunction with several hormones, control cell division in the liver (Leffert, 1978). Therefore the dietary effect on VLDL may interfere with normal regulatory growth controls and render the hepatocytes more susceptible to chemical carcinogens.

These different approaches to the problem of the mechanism by which lipotrope deficiency alters hepatocarcinogenesis all indicate that carcinogen metabolism is altered in the deficient rats and also may be altered by carcinogen treatment, in some cases in a different manner in deficient rats compared with normal control rats. The complexity of the metabolic pathways and our inability in many cases to identify the proximate carcinogen make it difficult to correlate metabolic effects with carcinogenesis. Perhaps a nutritional deficit affects the hepatocyte in a manner similar to that reported by Becker (1975), whereby a subcarcinogenic dose of a hepatocarcinogen predisposed the liver to a subcarcinogenic dose of another hepatocarcinogen. The dietary model is proving useful in separating the aspects of carcinogen metabolism that correlate with carcinogenesis from those that do not.

Other nutrients that influence tumor induction in the liver include protein, riboflavin, and vitamin B_{12}. Protein deficiency, sufficient to decrease hepatic microsomal oxidases, blocked induction of hepatic tumors by dimethylnitrosamine (DMN) and enhanced induction of renal tumors, presumably because DMN was cleared from the blood less rapidly in deficient rats

TABLE 12   Effect of Lipotrope Deficiency on
Hepatocyte DNA Synthesis and Serum Very
Low Density Lipoproteins in Weanling Rats[a]

Diet	DNA synthesis[b]	Serum VLDL[b]
Control	0.5–4	75
Marginal lipotrope	1–9	50
Low lipotrope	5–20	25

[a]From Leffert, 1978.
[b]Expressed in arbitrary units as an index of DNA synthesis and concentration of VLDL.

(McLean and Magee, 1970). Diets either marginally deficient or excessive in protein have variable effects on induction of liver and other tumors, most notably bladder tumors, which may be increased by increased urinary levels of tryptophan metabolites (Clayson, 1975).

Riboflavin specifically decreases hepatic tumor induction by the amino-azobenzenes since it is a cofactor for the enzymes that metabolize those compounds.

Vitamin B_{12} in high levels has been reported to be cocarcinogenic for the induction of liver tumors by dimethylaminoazobenzene (DAB) and DEN (Poirier, 1975). No mechanism for the effect has been proposed; it may be related to an abnormality in one-carbon metabolism, as in lipotrope deficiency.

Both the feeding of stock diets and the feeding of antioxidants tend to decrease chemical induction of liver tumors (Ulland et al., 1973). As discussed above, this may be the result of induction of microsomal oxidases by vegetable compounds or by the antioxidants.

It should be remembered that daily exposure of humans and animals to environmental chemicals, some of which are real or potential carcinogens, is not a simple matter and almost never a single event. This, combined with a deranged diet, may so cloud the issue that sorting out the various contributing factors may be difficult if not impossible. In regard to experimental hepato-carcinogenesis studies, a series of earlier investigations in which nutrition was the central focus serves to illustrate the need to consider the total environment or at least the factors that can be approached.

Copeland and Salmon (1946) reported development of liver tumors in rats depleted of choline. Following this observation, a series of papers (Engel et al., 1974; Salmon et al., 1955) from the highly productive laboratory of Salmon appeared which clearly implicated a simple nutritional deficiency as presumably carcinogenic. This was accomplished in a special strain of rats with a high choline requirement. During the prolonged deficiency, the livers of the rats progressed from fatty change to fibrosis and cirrhosis, and finally a significant number of them developed frank liver cell carcinoma with metastasis to the lungs. This pattern was not unlike that associated with alcoholic cirrhosis, where liver cancer accompanies cirrhosis in many patients. This exciting area of investigation seemed to establish choline deficiency as a significant factor in experimental hepatocarcinogenesis.

During this period, in the same laboratory, in a series of experiments designed to study the nutritional quality of peanut meal as a source of protein, I observed a significant number of liver cell tumors in rats unassociated with either choline deficiency or cirrhosis (Salmon and Newberne, 1963). Although a carcinogenic agent contaminating the peanut meal was suspected at the time, it was about 2 yr later before the active agent (AFB_1) was extracted from samples of peanut meal used in earlier choline-deficiency experiments and shown to be the carcinogen (Newberne, 1965).

These observations were followed by many attempts to reproduce choline-deficiency liver cancer in rats, but without success. Although a number of insults were applied to the liver, dietary and otherwise, liver cancer could be induced only if a known carcinogen was given in concert with the other insults (Newberne et al., 1966). Fully convincing evidence that cirrhosis alone, induced by choline deficiency, did not result in liver cancer in rats was provided by experiments in which purified amino acids served as a substitute protein source (Newberne et al., 1969).

Although a severe choline deficiency, fatty liver, fibrosis, and cirrhosis were induced over prolonged periods of time, equivalent to the results reported by Copeland and Salmon with peanut meal diets, no tumors developed.

These studies, carried out over many years with carefully designed protocols and highly defined diets, established that choline-deficiency cirrhosis alone was an inadequate stress or stimulus to result in liver cancer. In retrospect, the diets of Copeland, Salmon, and Engel most likely were contaminated with aflatoxin, contained in the peanut meal used. Since methodology and circumstances had not permitted its discovery, contamination was suspected. This early work in Salmon's laboratory stimulated research that led to a better understanding of the worldwide problem of mycotoxicoses and contributed to their control.

This one example illustrates the highly complex nature of environmental carcinogenesis and the need to be cautious in our approach to studies of nutrition and cancer.

Breast Cancer

The incidence of breast cancer is correlated with socioeconomic status and has therefore been associated with overnourishment. It is not common in women in developing societies or in Japanese women, but the incidence increases in these population groups when they migrate to the United States (Buell, 1973). Breast cancer is increasing in young women in the United States, and this has been associated by some with increased fat consumption; however, there is insufficient evidence to incriminate fat per se in breast cancer; increased fat intake in the United States is almost always accompanied by increased protein intake. Breast cancer patients have been reported to be obese compared with control groups, but recent studies have indicated that the difference is more closely related to body mass—that is, it is influenced by both height and weight (de Waard, 1975). An entire issue of a recent journal is devoted to breast cancer (*Cancer Detection and Prevention,* 1976).

Mechanisms are undoubtedly complex; one suggestion is that there is increased synthesis of estrogens and altered storage of hormones in people consuming a high-fat diet (Wynder, 1976). Another mechanism suspected by some investigators is related to the intestinal flora; in people consuming a Western, high-fat diet there is a higher proportion of strictly anaerobic microflora in the intestine. These organisms can produce estrogens from biliary steroids, which are also increased in subjects consuming high-fat diets (Hill et al., 1971).

A number of other dietary factors have been associated with breast cancer in epidemiologic studies. These include iodine deficiency (Eskin et al., 1974), the cadmium content of the water (Berg and Burbank, 1972), and a high rate of beer consumption (Breslow and Enstrom, 1974). These suggestions are based on less than convincing evidence, however, and require more extensive epidemiologic and experimental support.

In experimental studies, diets high in corn oil enhanced mammary tumor induction in rats by 7,12-dimethylbenz[a]anthracene (DMBA). DMBA-induced mammary tumors were inhibited by the synthetic antioxidants butylated hydroxyanisole (BHA), butylated hydroxytoluene and ethoxyquin (Wattenberg, 1972a) and by the sulfur-containing compounds benzyl thiocyanate, disulfiram, and dimethyldithiocarbamate (Wattenberg, 1974). In mice, dietary restriction (Rowlatt et al., 1973), riboflavin deficiency (Morris, 1947), and phenylalanine deficiency (Hui et al., 1972). inhibited the formation of mammary gland tumors.

Experiments in our laboratory, using a diet marginal in lipotropes and high in fat, have yielded interesting results related to the induction of breast or liver cancer in two strains of female rats by AAF or DMBA. Dietary AAF induced fewer mammary tumors in Sprague-Dawley rats fed the low-lipotrope, high-fat diet than in rats fed an adequate diet (Table 13). Tumor incidence was lower in the marginally lipotrope-deficient rats and death from mammary tumors was 4–6 wk later than in the controls. In Fischer rats, which are resistant to AAF induction of mammary tumors, hepatic carcinomas devel-

TABLE 13 Mammary Tumor Induction in Female Rats Fed Control
or Marginal-Lipotrope, High-Fat Diet

Diet	Rat strain	No. of rats	Mammary tumors (%)		
			Carcinoma	Adenoma	Total
Acetylaminofluorene					
Control	Sprague-Dawley	31	65	3	68
Marginal-lipotrope, high-fat	Sprague-Dawley	32	41	9	50
Control	Fischer	25	0	12	12
Marginal-lipotrope, high-fat	Fischer	25	8	0	8
DMBA					
Control	Sprague-Dawley	25	40	8	48
Marginal-lipotrope, high-fat	Sprague-Dawley	27	15	0	15

oped in a significantly greater incidence in the deficient rats, a result in accord with the findings in male rats discussed above.

The incidence of mammary tumors induced by DMBA in Sprague-Dawley rats fed the marginal-lipotrope, high-fat diet was also reduced in a manner similar to that observed with AAF.

The alteration of mammary tumor incidence in rats fed the high-fat diet is particularly important because it is in contrast to previous results, which have shown enhancement of mammary carcinogenesis in experimental animals by high-fat diets. The marginal lipotrope status of the rats may account for the observed difference in tumor induction. It should be noted, however, that the marginal deficiency of lipotropes was not severe enough to depress growth or caloric intake, and therefore this mechanism can be ruled out. There was one previous report of inhibition of DMBA induction of mammary tumors in rats fed a diet severely deficient in protein and lipotropes for 10 days before treatment (Tanaka and Dao, 1965).

Cancer of the Urinary Bladder

A number of potentially carcinogenic substances present in the diet or in water appear to be associated with urinary bladder cancer in humans (Oyasu and Hopp, 1974). Excessive beer and coffee drinking (Cole, 1971) has been related to cancer of the bladder in men, and in another report (Schmauz and Cole, 1974) a relationship was found between coffee drinking and cancer of the renal pelvis and ureter. Experimental studies with coffee in rats did not confirm these implications, even over very long periods of continuous exposure (Zeitlin, 1972).

Recently there has been a resurgence of interest in nonnutritive sweeteners as potential carcinogens, based on animal experimentation (Hicks et al., 1973; Friedman et al., 1972). The animal studies have been equivocal at best, and available data from past studies did not establish the carcinogenicity of the nonnutritive sweeteners saccharin and cyclamate in experimental animals. However, more recent observations in Canada (Arnold et al., 1977) are now beginning to challenge this view as regards saccharin. It should be pointed out that these studies involve *in utero* exposures in addition to lifetime feeding of saccharin. Epidemiologic data being collected now in population groups such as diabetics are not likely to be of much value, since the time of exposure and the data base will probably be insufficient for valid judgment.

Bracken fern, a bovine forage crop contaminant, has been established as a carcinogen for urinary cancer in cattle, guinea pigs, and rats (Evans, 1968; Pamukcu et al., 1967; Pamukcu and Price, 1969; Evans and Mason, 1965). The active carcinogen is yet to be isolated and identified in mature bracken. Young fronds of some ferns are consumed by people as a delicacy, but recent animal studies have not shown any evidence for carcinogenicity (Newberne, 1976a).

Several nitrofuran derivatives have been found to be carcinogenic for the bladder in experimental animals. In Japan, 2-(2-furyl)-3-(5-nitro-2-furyl)acrylamide is used as a food additive. This nitrofuran derivative, which has been reported to be noncarcinogenic, has shown positive mutagenic and DNA-modifying effects in microbial assay systems (Yahagi et al., 1974). Oral administration of AAF alone is not a reliable means of inducing carcinoma of the bladder in the rat. Bladder cancer developed more effectively in rats fed a pyridoxine-deficient diet, and pretreatment with a single ip dose of cyclophosphamide reduced the time required for formation of invasive tumors (Koss and Lavin, 1971). In similar studies in hamsters, the addition of dietary indole had no effect when AAF was fed at high doses (0.06%), but when the AAF dose was reduced to 0.03% there was enhancement of bladder tumorigenesis (Oyasu et al., 1972). β-Naphthylamine is a potent bladder carcinogen. In one study (Alam et al., 1972), the presence of ascorbic acid in the bladder of rabbits decreased the reabsorption of β-naphthylamine metabolites. Vitamin C has also been shown to reduce uroepithelial carcinoma in mice, and a similar effect has been postulated for humans (Schlegel et al., 1969).

In our own laboratories at Massachusetts Institute of Technology (MIT), we have investigated effects of a diet marginal in lipotropes (choline-methionine) but high in fat on carcinogen-induced bladder cancer in rats (Rogers, 1975). Neither the incidence of tumors induced by N-[4-(5-nitro-2-furyl)-2-thiazolyl]formamide (FANFT) nor that induced by N-nitrosodibutylamine was influenced by the diet low in lipotropes and high in fat. The results with FANFT shown in Table 14 illustrate the lack of effect.

Carcinogenicity of chemicals for the urinary tract apparently is not enhanced by low lipotropes and high fat, despite the metabolic effects of severe lipotrope deficiency on the kidney. The marginal deficiency in rats fed diets low in lipotropes and high in fat induced no histological renal changes. The greater toxicity of FANFT to rats fed the control diet that was observed during these studies may have been the result of their slightly greater intake of the compound, but this was not reflected in tumor incidence.

TABLE 14   FANFT,[a] Diet, and Urinary
Bladder Tumors

Diet	No. of rats	% Rats with		Tumors/ tumor-bearing rats
		Polyp, papilloma	Carcinoma	
Control	26	38	15	2.4
Deficient, high-fat	31	26	35	2.3

[a]N-[4-(5-nitro-2-furyl)-2-thiazolyl]formamide.

Lung Cancer

A recent epidemiologic appraisal of respiratory carcinogenesis has detailed the enormous number of chemicals that have been causally related to lung cancer in humans (Fraumeni, 1975).

With regard to nutritional influences on lung cancer in humans, a recent dietary survey of men with lung cancer revealed a negative association with an index of vitamin A intake (Bjelke, 1975). This preliminary finding is consistent with some but not all of the results of animal experimentation (Saffiotti, 1973; Smith et al., 1975a, 1975b). Further study of nutritional factors may help to explain the elevated risk of lung cancer in the lower socioeconomic class and in people who migrate from rural to urban areas and from the South to the North (Mancuso, 1974).

Lung adenomas were induced in rats (Newberne and Shank, 1973) and in mice by concurrent administration of sodium nitrite in the drinking water and dietary secondary amines or ureas (morpholine, methylaniline, piperazine, methylurea, and ethylurea) (Mirvish et al., 1972). DEN alone did not induce lung tumors in rats, but tumors were induced when cyclopropenoid fatty acids were added to low- or high-DEN diets (Nixon et al., 1974). In one study lung tumors were induced in mice by feeding bracken fern (Pamukcu et al., 1972), and in another by feeding boiled egg white or raw egg yolk added to the standard diet (Szepsenwol, 1963). Lung cancer induction in mice by benzo-[a]pyrene (BP), DMBA, 7-OH-DMBA, urethan, or uracil mustard was inhibited by addition to the diet of the antioxidant BHA (Wattenberg, 1973). Vitamin A deficiency causes squamous metaplasia of the hamster tracheal epithelium, which is grossly similar to, but ultrastructurally different from, lesions caused by intratracheal instillations of BP-ferric oxide (Harris et al., 1972). Vitamin A administered intragastrically inhibited methylcholanthrene-induced respiratory tract tumors in rats (Cone and Nettesheim, 1973) and BP-induced squamous metaplasia and bronchogenic carcinomas in hamsters (Saffiotti et al., 1967). In contrast, three additional extensive studies showed that vitamin A did not inhibit but instead enhanced the development of BP-induced respiratory tract carcinogenesis in hamsters; these investigations cast considerable doubt on the beneficial effects of high levels of natural vitamin A on lung cancer (Smith et al., 1975a, 1975b).

Hydrocarbon carcinogenesis in the lung can be affected by dietary modification of pulmonary AHH activity. The AHH activity in the lungs of mice and rats appears to result from exogenous inducers found in foods, including some cruciferous plants (Wattenberg, 1971). Comparable findings were obtained for the aminoazo dye N-demethylase system (Billings and Wattenberg, 1972). Flavones or related compounds (natural dietary constituents) have induced in rats a marked increase in AHH activity in the lung and small intestine and a slight increase in the liver. β-Naphthoflavone inhibited pulmonary adenoma formation resulting from oral administration of DMBA or BP (Wattenberg, 1972a).

The work conducted in our laboratory over the past several years (Smith et al., 1975a, 1975b) has been aimed at exploring the hypothesis that vitamin A, in much higher doses than normal, could prevent or inhibit development of lung cancer after exposure to a carcinogen. Unfortunately, we were unable to show that natural vitamin A had any effect on preventing BP-induced lung cancer in hamsters (Table 15); on the contrary, it appeared to enhance tumor induction. The reasons for this are obscure; however, the high tumor incidence in the animals, even at very low doses of BP, may have masked any beneficial effect vitamin A may have exerted. Perhaps analogues of vitamin A, now under intensive study (Sporn et al., 1976), will prove more effective.

Discussion

It seems logical that diet and the nutritive status of an individual can have a profound influence on resistance to cancer. This is emphasized by the truism that we are the product of what we eat. While an interest in nutrition in human populations has been steadily growing in recent years, epidemiology has been slowly developing geographic patterns of various types of cancer, which implicate a role for nutrition in their etiology.

When one views the evidence presented in cancer morbidity and mortality tables (Table 16) for the year 1975, it is difficult to remain unimpressed when it is recognized that the organ sites for which there is the strongest evidence, in people and experimental animals, for a dietary effect on tumor induction and development account for nearly one-third of the cancer incidence and deaths in the United States. Identification of related dietary factors and elucidation of their mechanisms of action offer the potential for prevention of tumors in the affected sites or perhaps for alleviation of the condition when it occurs.

Epidemiologic evidence from studies of Japanese immigrants and Scandinavian populations lends strong support to the hypothesis that cancer of the

TABLE 15   Respiratory Tract Tumor Incidence[a]

Group	RA treatment (μg/wk)	No. of hamsters	No. with tumors	%	No. of tumors
1	100	83	48	58	72
2	1600	74	52	70	70
3	2400	73	59	81[b]	84
	Total	230	159	69	226

[a]From Smith et al., 1975a.

[b]Difference from hamsters given 100 μg RA/wk is significant, $p < 0.01$.

TABLE 16 Morbidity and Mortality in the
United States from Cancers Possibly
Related to Diet

	Estimated statistics for 1975	
Organ site	New cases	Deaths
Esophagus	7,400	6,500
Stomach	22,900	14,400
Colon	69,000	38,600
Breast	88,700	32,900
Liver (and bile ducts)	11,500	9,800
Total	199,500	102,200
All cancer	665,000	365,000

gastrointestinal tract has an important nutritional component. In particular, the Japanese are an interesting and rewarding population to study in comparison with that in the United States because of the striking difference in diet and in the incidence of gastric and colon cancer. With knowledge gained from the significant progress made in recent years in epidemiology in this area, it should now be possible to move forward with investigations to identify chemical, biological, endocrinological, and nutritional influences on these types of cancer. Tables 1 and 3 clearly indicate environmental factors, probably nutritive or dietary, and Tables 2, 4, 5, 6, and 7 support the human observations with animal studies. Additional evidence presented in this chapter supports our contention that nutrition and food are central to the variation in the incidence of tumors at various sites in some population groups.

Our experimental results for the nutrients most extensively studied, lipotropes and vitamin A, are interesting in that they do not coincide. Vitamin A influenced tumor induction by AFB_1 in the colon, but not in the liver; lipotropes influenced AFB_1 induction of tumors only in liver. Vitamin A did not significantly affect induction of colon tumors by DMH, whereas lipotrope deficiency had a significant effect. Vitamin A was reported by others to block induction of bladder tumors by FANFT; lipotrope deficiency had no effect. Thus, there is clearly a complicated but perhaps specific effect of some nutrients, such as the lipotropes, on some target tissues and not on others. Of equal significance is the influence of nutritive status on drug-metabolizing enzyme activity (Table 9), which in turn is reflected in a difference in clearing the system of a known carcinogen (Table 10) and in subsequent tumor incidence (Table 11). Tumors at other organ sites have been associated with nutritional factors to a greater or lesser degree than those referred to above.

When one reflects on the magnitude of the cancer problem around the world and the well-known increasing difficulty of feeding world populations, it is clear that the compelling need to provide adequate, nutritious food for the people of the United States and of the world accentuates the importance of scientific research on food supply and consumption, and this is tied in some ways to problems of cancer in some populations. The power of effectively disseminated research results to increase the productivity and efficiency of food systems is beyond question. However, with this power comes the responsibility to use it to the best possible advantage. With these thoughts in mind, we are moved to agree with delegates to the 1974 World Food Conference in their statement that "all governments should accept the removal of the scourge of hunger and malnutrition, which at present afflicts many millions of human beings, as the objective of the international community as a whole, and accept the goal that within a decade no child will go to bed hungry, that no family will fear for its next day's bread, and that no human being's future capacities will be stunted by malnutrition" (Research to Meet U.S. and World Food Needs, 1975). That this goal is possible is implied by statistics showing that in the United States since 1950 crop production per acre has risen by 45% and farm production per hour of labor has more than doubled. The number of people supplied by each farm worker has risen from 15 to 52, and the acreage harvested per consumer has been reduced by nearly one-half.

A considerable proportion of these gains can be ascribed to effective use of agricultural chemicals, primarily fertilizer and pesticides. In the case of the latter, it should be pointed out that although pesticides account for only about 3% of farm operating expenses, they are essential to commercial agriculture. For the five-state Lake Michigan area, for example, it has been estimated that without pesticides, crop and livestock production would just about cease and vegetable production would drop by about 75%. Thus there is cause for concern when well-intentioned environmentalists press regulatory agencies into banning some pesticides essential to a sustained or increased rate of production of food and fiber without weighing the risks against the benefits. This is not to infer that manufacturers should not be held responsible for assuring reasonable safety, but these factors should be based on factual data instead of opinions. Fear about cancer has a low priority when one is starving or dying of malaria or some other disease that can be controlled by pesticides.

This and other factors enter into our overall assessment of the importance of diet and nutrition in the prevention or alleviation of cancer. Indeed, it is essential for progress in cancer cause and prevention to identify nutritional factors that modify the susceptibility of an individual to environmental or endogenous carcinogens. Nutrition offers the most acceptable and direct means of attacking the cancer problem in human populations, and the current surge of interest in this area of cancer studies reflects the growing recognition of the importance of nutrition in cancer prevention.

NUTRITION AND MUTAGENESIS

Inasmuch as it is believed that a genetic event is necessary for the initiation of carcinogenesis, the study of the role of nutrition in carcinogenesis is allied with the study of the same effects on mutagenesis. However, compared to the large number of studies of carcinogenesis, the study of nutritional influences in mutagenesis has been virtually ignored.

It has been noted that the metabolism of a number of carcinogens is affected by dietary changes or dietary constituents. Since the majority of organic chemical carcinogens are mutagens (McCann et al., 1975) and the ultimate carcinogens and mutagens appear to be identical, one would expect that a change in the metabolism of a carcinogen would be reflected as a change in its mutagenicity. This has been demonstrated in bacteria and in *Drosophila;* no studies on the effects of nutritional imbalance on radiation- or chemical-induced mutation in mammals has been reported.

In a host-mediated assay, an indicator microorganism is injected into the peritoneal cavity of a mouse and the test chemical administered either orally or parenterally. After a period of time, the indicator organism is removed from the peritoneal cavity and mutational events are scored. Although this system does not measure a mutagenic effect on the mouse, it indicates the presence of mutagenic substances produced by the mouse's metabolism. These mutagenic substances are detected by an appropriate indicator organism. Using a *Salmonella typhimurium* mutant, G46, which responds to compounds inducing base-pair substitution mutations (Ames et al., 1973), Zeiger (1975) showed that the mutagenicities of dimethylnitrosamine (DMNA), N-nitrosomorpholine (NM), and N-nitrosomethylurea (NMU) were affected by dietary changes in the host animal.

The mutagenicities of both DMNA and NM were significantly lowered in mice maintained on a complete semisynthetic diet, compared with mice maintained on a chow diet. A protein-free diet, which depresses DMNA metabolism (Swann and McLean, 1971; Venkatesan et al., 1970) decreased DMNA and NM mutagenicity. NMU, which does not require metabolic activation for its carcinogenic and mutagenic activities, showed an enhanced mutagenicity under these conditions. A 24-hr pure casein diet, which enhances DMNA demethylase activity (Venkatesan et al., 1970), increased DMNA and NM mutagenicities and dramatically decreased NMU mutagenicity.

Czygan et al. (1974) demonstrated the same effects *in vitro* by incubating rat liver microsomes with *S. typhimurium* TA1535, which measures the same types of base-pair substitutions as G46 (Ames et al., 1973). In this procedure, liver microsomes from rats fed the various test diets are incubated with the test mutagen and indicator microorganisms in the presence of an NADPH-generating system. They found that liver microsomes from rats fed decreasing levels of protein in their diet (from 30 to 0%) showed corresponding decreases in DMNA mutagenicity. At the same time, the mutagenicity of MNNG, which, like NMU, does not require metabolism for its biological activity, increased with decreasing protein levels. Dietary choline deficiency, like protein deficiency, depresses microsomal enzyme activity. The metabolism of DMNA to a mutagen was even further depressed by microsomes from mice on a choline-deficient, 10% protein diet. This same diet enhanced MNNG mutagenicity above that obtained with the 10% protein diet alone.

The *in vivo* and *in vitro* mutagenicities of DMNA and NMU follow the expected course for substances whose mutagenicity is dependent on cyto-chrome P-450 mediated microsomal activation. The *in vivo* host-mediated assay can only measure the total mutagen arriving at the indicator cells in the peritoneal cavity within a relatively short time period (up to 3–4 hr). Since the liver is the primary organ for the metabolism of nitrosamines, the changes in mutagenicity probably reflect changes in liver metabolism.

Unlike DMNA and NM, the nitrosamides NMU and MNNG are potent mutagens for *Salmonella* in the absence of metabolic activation (Brusick and Zeiger, 1972) by virtue of their spontaneous hydrolysis. The response of these mutagens in the host-mediated assay and in the *in vitro* microsomal system show that they are capable of being inactivated by the liver. No studies have been reported on the breakdown of these substances by microsomes from animals fed different diets, but the results described in these studies imply that the mixed function oxidase system of the liver is responsible for the metabolism and detoxification of these nitrosamides.

In other studies, the *in vitro* metabolic activation of AAF to a mutagen for *S. typhimurium* TA1538 by rat liver fractions was increased with increasing amounts of tallow or corn oil (from 5 to 20%) added to a fat-free diet (Castro et al., 1976). Corn oil feeding produced a higher mutagenic response than tallow feeding. AAF can be metabolized to a mutagen by both the supernatant and microsomal fractions of rat liver (Stout et al., 1976); therefore the basis for the mutagenic responses to the two fats is not clear. It still has to be determined whether the effects seen were in response to increased levels of microsomal enzymes, soluble enzymes, or both. In a companion study, rats fed a grain diet and injected with AAF or 2-OH-AAF had a decreased formation of AAF adducts with RNA and an increased formation of DNA adducts compared with rats fed a commercial chow diet.

Studies are in progress at MIT, using the *in vitro* mutagenesis assay and the *Salmonella* strains and liver preparations from lipotrope-deficients rats, to determine whether the observed dietary effects on chemical carcinogenesis result from alteration of hepatic activation of carcinogens. In agreement with the data on microsomal oxidases, liver preparations from deficient rats converted only about one-third to one-half as much AFB_1 to a bacterial mutagen as preparations from adequately fed rats. Conversion of AAF was also decreased. Treatment of rats with a carcinogen altered the ability of the liver preparations to convert the carcinogen to a mutagen. These preliminary studies have further indicated that after AAF treatment, liver preparations from lipotrope-deficient rats are as effective as preparations from normal rats for conversion of AAF to mutagen. Treatment with AFB_1 either decreased the capacity of liver preparations from adequately fed rats to convert AFB_1 to a mutagen and did not affect the conversion by preparations from deficient rats, or enhanced the conversion by both groups depending on time and dose. Additional studies are required for confirmation of these results. They agree with the results of studies of microsomal oxidases and demonstrate a diet-induced difference in hepatic carcinogen activation, insofar as it is indicated by mutagen production, but they do not fully explain the enhancement of carcinogenesis in deficient rats.

Using *Drosophila melanogaster*, deMarco et al. (1975) showed that "undernourished" larvae were more sensitive to X-ray-induced chromosomal aberrations than larvae raised on an adequate diet. Geer and Reno (1976) treated choline-deficient male *Drosophila* with the mutagenic alkylating agent Trenimon. A significant increase in X-linked recessive lethals was found in deficient flies. The spontaneous X-linked recessive lethal frequency was not affected by the diet.

These studies have been concerned with the ability of various diets or dietary constituents to affect the metabolism, and therefore the mutagenicity, of chemicals. Another, and possibly more important, area of concern is the effect of nutritional state on spontaneously occurring mutation. This is an area of research that has been generally neglected—that is, the effect of nutritional imbalances on the somatic and germinal genetic material. Mutations may occur as a direct result of the nutritional imbalance through disruption of nucleic acid synthesis and cell division, or normal DNA repair processes may be interrupted, thus allowing the cell to express spontaneously occurring genetic damage that might normally be repaired. Another factor that cannot be ruled out is that the metabolic capabilities of the animal are affected sufficiently that environmental substances that would not be effective in normal individuals are activated to genetically active products or not inactivated.

In the one reported clinical study, Armendares et al. (1971) examined 10 children, aged 1–60 months, suffering from advanced protein-calorie malnutrition. They were found to have a significantly higher level of chromosome abnormalities in their circulating peripheral lymphocytes than did a matched control group. These abnormalities were primarily chromatid in nature (gaps and breaks), but also included a significant increase in dicentrics. Significantly, after 1 yr on an adequate diet, seven of the children were reexamined and still had an increased level of chromosome abnormalities—again primarily breaks and gaps, transient phenomena indicative primarily of a general toxic effect; the only significant effects from a genetic viewpoint are chromosome exchange figures. In these patients, the damaged lymphocytes may have been descendants of those originally seen, or they may have been induced by a residual metabolic imbalance.

It must be kept in mind, however, that malnourished individuals may also have a parasite, bacteria, or virus burden that may contribute to the frequency of chromosome aberrations.

A number of studies in laboratory animals have shown that DNA synthesis and mitosis are depressed in the livers of rodents on starvation or protein-deficient diets (Leduc, 1949; Montecuccoli et al., 1972; Jasper and Brasel, 1974). After the deficient animals are transferred to an adequate diet, there is a period of "catch up" during which DNA synthesis and cell division proceed at a faster than normal rate, although DNA synthesis in regenerating rat liver was not affected by the protein-free diet (Montecuccoli et al., 1972). Polyploidy and an increased mitotic index were seen in the pancreas of rats maintained on a high (2%) methionine diet for 6 months (Bourdel et al., 1971); however, the liver, which is normally polyploid, did not show an increased frequency of either polyploidy or mitoses.

Neither induction of polyploidy nor an increase in the mitotic index can be considered a mutagenic effect per se. However, enhancement of the frequency of cell division, as reflected in the increased mitotic index, has implications for increasing the spontaneous mutation rate or susceptibility to chemical mutagens in those tissues.

As can be seen, information on the relationship between nutritional state and spontaneous and induced mutation in mammals—and lower forms— is essentially nil. Yet there is increasing concern over the long-term effects of inadequate nutrition on parental and fetal health.

The large numbers of nutritional studies of laboratory animals have used biochemical or cytological effects as end points. There is also a need to perform somatic and germinal cytogenetic investigations of animals used in these studies. This would provide data on the types of effects produced (if any) and their organ distribution.

Much work must be done in the laboratory to determine whether inadequate nutrition can induce gene and chromosome mutations. At the same time, cytogenetic evaluations should be performed on malnourished populations to see whether the different types of nutritional deficiencies seen in various geographic and economic areas are associated with elevated frequencies of chromosome damage or genetic disease.

REFERENCES

Acheson, E. D. and Doll, R. 1964. Dietary factors in carcinoma of the stomach: A study of 100 cases and 200 controls. *Gut* 5:126–131.

Ackerman, L. V. 1972. Some thoughts on food and cancer. *Nutr. Today,* Jan./Feb.:2–9.

Alam, B. S., Jaramillo, F. E., Schlegel, J. U. and DeRouen, T. A. 1972. The effect of ascorbic acid upon bladder uptake of beta-naphthylamine metabolites. *Proc. Soc. Exp. Biol. Med.* 141:1008–1013.

Alpert, M. E., Hutt, M. S. R., Wogan, G. N. and Davidson, C. S. 1971. The association between aflatoxin content of food and hepatoma frequency in Uganda. *Cancer* 28:253–260.

Ames, B. N., Lee, F. D. and Durston, W. E. 1973. An improved bacterial test system for the detection and classification of mutagens and carcinogens. *Proc. Natl. Acad. Sci. U.S.A.* 70:782–786.

Armendares, S., Salamanca, F. and Frenk, S. 1971. Chromosome abnormalities in severe protein calorie nutrition. *Nature (Lond.)* 232:271–273.

Arnold, D. L., Charbonveau, S. M., Moodie, C. A. and Munro, I. C. 1977. Long term toxicity with OTS and saccharin. *Soc. Toxicol. 16th Annu. Meet.,* abstr. 78.

Bailar, J. C. 1965. Distribution of carcinoma of esophagus, stomach and large bowel. In *Carcinoma of the alimentary tract,* ed. W. J. Burdette, pp. 3–14. Salt Lake City: Univ. of Utah Press.

Becker, F. F. 1975. Alteration of hepatocytes of subcarcinogenic exposure to N-2-fluorenylacetamide. *Cancer Res.* 35:1734–1736.

Berg, J. W. and Burbank, F. 1972. Correlations between carcinogenic trace metals in water supplies and cancer mortality. *Ann. N.Y. Acad. Sci.* 199:249–264.

Billings, R. and Wattenberg, L. W. 1972. The effects of dietary alterations on 3-methyl-4-methylaminoazobenzene N-demethylase activity. *Proc. Soc. Exp. Biol. Med.* 139:865–867.

Bjelke, E. 1974. Colon cancer and blood cholesterol. *Lancet* June 1:1116–1117.

Bjelke, E. 1975. Dietary vitamin A and human lung cancer. *Int. J. Cancer* 15:561–565.

Bourdel, G., Girard-Globa, A. and Forestier, M. 1971. Induction of polyploidy in the rat exocrine pancreas by excess dietary methionine. *Lab. Invest.* 25:311–336.

Breslow, N. E. and Enstrom, J. E. 1974. Geographic correlation between cancer mortality rates and alcohol-tobacco consumption in the United States. *J. Natl. Cancer Inst.* 53:631–639.

Brusick, D. J. and Zeiger, E. 1972. A comparison of chemically induced reversion patterns of *Salmonella typhimurium* and *Saccharomyces cerevisiae* mutants using *in vitro* plate tests. *Mutat. Res.* 14:271–275.

Buell, P. 1973. Changing incidence of breast cancer in Japanese and American women. *J. Natl. Cancer Inst.* 51:1479–1483.

Burkitt, D. P., Walker, A. R. and Painter, N. S. 1972. Effect of dietary fiber of stools and transit times and its role in causation of disease. *Lancet* 2:1408–1412.

Cancer Detection and Prevention. 1976. 1(2):240–485.

Castro, C. E., Felkner, I. C., Yang, S. P. and Sproat, H. F. 1976. Effects of tallow and corn oil on the mutagenicity and carcinogenicity of 2-acetyl-aminofluorene (2-AAF) in rats. *Fed. Proc.* 35:519 (abstr.).

Chu, E. W. and Malmgren, R. A. 1965. An inhibitory effect of vitamin A on the induction of tumors of forestomach and cervix in the Syrian hamster by carcinogenic polycyclic hydrocarbons. *Cancer Res.* 25:884–895.

Clayson, D. B. 1975. Nutrition and experimental carcinogenesis. *Cancer Res.* 35:3292–3300.

Cole, P. 1971. Coffee-drinking and cancer of the lower urinary tract. *Lancet* 1:1335–1337.

Cone, M. V. and Nettesheim, P. 1973. Effects of vitamin A on 3-methylchol-anthracene-induced squamous metaplasia and early tumors in the respiratory tract of rats. *J. Natl. Cancer Inst.* 50:1599–1606.

Cook, P. and Burkitt, D. 1971. Cancer in Africa. *Br. Med. Bull.* 27:14–20.

Copeland, D. H. and Salmon, W. D. 1946. The occurrence of neoplasms in the liver, lungs and other tissues of rats as a result of prolonged choline deficiency. *Am. J. Pathol.* 22:1059–1079.

Czygan, P., Greim, H., Garro, A., Schaffner, F. and Popper, H. 1974. The effect of dietary protein deficiency on the ability of isolated hepatic microsomes to alter the mutagenicity of a primary and a secondary carcinogen. *Cancer Res.* 34:119–123.

DeLuca, L., Schumacher, M., Wolf, G. and Newberne, P. M. 1970. Biosynthesis of a fucose-containing glycopeptide from rat small intestine in normal and vitamin A-deficient conditions. *J. Biol. Chem.* 245:4551–4558.

deMarco, A., Belloni, M. P., Cozzi, R. and Olivieri, G. 1975. Environmental mutagens and environmental factors that can modify their action. *Mutat. Res.* 29:253 (abstr.).

de Waard, F. 1975. Breast cancer incidence and nutritional status with particular reference to body weight and height. *Cancer Res.* 35:3351–3356.

Doll, R. 1967. Worldwide distribution of gastrointestinal cancer. *Natl. Cancer Inst. Monogr.* 25:173–190.

Dungal, N. and Sigurjonsson, J. 1967. Gastric cancer and diet. A pilot study on dietary habits in two districts differing markedly in respect of mortality from gastric cancer. *Br. J. Cancer* 21:270–276.

Engel, R. W., Copeland, D. H. and Salmon, W. D. 1947. Carcinogenic effects associated with diets deficient in choline and related nutrients. *Ann. N.Y. Acad. Sci.* 49(1):49–67.

Eskin, B. A., Parker, J. A., Bassett, J. G. and George, D. L. 1974. Human breast uptake of radioactive iodine. *Obstet. Gynecol.* 44:398–402.

Evans, I. A. 1968. The radiomimetic nature of bracken toxin. *Cancer Res.* 28:2252–2261.

Evans, I. A. and Mason, J. 1965. Carcinogenic activity of bracken. *Nature (Lond.)* 208:913–914.

Fraumeni, J. F., Jr. 1975. Respiratory carcinogenesis: An epidemiologic appraisal. *J. Natl. Cancer Inst.* 55:1039–1046.

Friedman, L., Richardson, H. L., Richardson, M. E., Lethco, E. J., Wallace, W. C. and Sauro, F. M. 1972. Toxic response of rats to cyclamates in chow and semisynthetic diets. *J. Natl. Cancer Inst.* 49:751–764.

Geer, B. W. and Reno, D. L. 1976. The effects of dietary deficiencies for choline and nicotinic acid on the sensitivity of *Drosophila melanogaster* to mutagenic treatment. *Mutat. Res.* 38:407–408 (abstr.).

Graham, S., Lilienfeld, A. M. and Tidings, J. E. 1967. Dietary and purgation factors in the epidemiology of gastric cancer. *Cancer* 20:2224–2234.

Graham, S., Schotz, W. and Martino, P. 1972. Alimentary factors in the epidemiology of gastric cancer. *Cancer* 30:927–938.

Haenszel, N., Berg, J. W., Segi, M., Jurihari, M. and Locke, F. B. 1973. Large bowel cancer in Hawaiian Japanese. *J. Natl. Cancer Inst.* 51:1765–1779.

Haenszel, W. and Correa, P. 1975. Epidemiology of stomach cancer. *Cancer Res.* 35:3452–3459.

Haenszel, W. M. and Kurihari, M. 1968. Studies of Japanese migrants. I. Mortality from cancer and other diseases among Japanese in the United States. *J. Natl. Cancer Inst.* 40:43–51.

Haenszel, W., Kurihari, M., Mitsuo, S. and Lee, R. K. 1972. Stomach cancer among Japanese in Hawaii. *J. Natl. Cancer Inst.* 49:969–983.

Harris, C. C., Sporn, M. B., Kaufman, D. G., Smith, J. M., Jackson, F. E. and Saffiotti, U. 1972. Histogenesis of squamous metaplasia in the hamster tracheal epithelium caused by vitamin A deficiency on benzo(a)-pyrene-ferric oxide. *J. Natl. Cancer Inst.* 48:743–761.

Hicks, R. M., Wakefield, J. J. and Chowaniec, J. 1973. Co-carcinogenic action of saccharin in the chemical induction of bladder cancer. *Nature (Lond.)* 243:347–349.

Higginson, J. 1966. Etiological factors in gastrointestinal cancer in man. *J. Natl. Cancer Inst.* 37:527–545.

Higginson, J. 1969. The geographical pathology of liver disease in man. *Gastroenterology* 57:587–598.

Hill, M. J., Drasar, B. S., Aries, V., Crowther, J. S., Hawksworth, G. and Williams, R. E. O. 1971. Bacteria and etiology of cancer of the large bowel. *Lancet* 1:95–102.

Hironi, I., Fushimi, H., Mori, T., Miwa, T. and Haga, M. 1973. Comparative study of carcinogenic activity of each part of bracken. *J. Natl. Cancer Inst.* 50:1367–1371.

Hui, Y. H., Deome, K. B. and Briggs, G. M. 1972. The developmental noduligenic and tumorigenic potentials of transplanted mammary gland and primary ducts from C_3H mice previously fed a phenylalanine-deficient diet. *Cancer Res.* 32:57–60.

Jasper, H. C. and Brasel, J. A. 1974. Rat liver DNA synthesis during the "catch-up" growth of nutritional rehabilitation. *J. Nutr.* 104:405–414.

Keen, P. and Martin, P. 1971. Is aflatoxin carcinogenic in man? The evidence in Swaziland. *Trop. Geogr. Med.* 23:44–53.

Koss, L. G. and Lavin, P. 1971. Studies of experimental bladder carcinoma in Fischer 344 female rats. I. Induction of tumors with diet low in B_6 containing N-2-fluorenylacetamide after single dose of cyclophospha-mide. *J. Natl. Cancer Inst.* 46:585–595.

Leduc, E. C. 1949. Mitotic activity in the liver of the mouse during inanition followed by refeeding with different levels of protein. *Am. J. Anat.* 84:397–429.

Leffert, H. L. 1978. Hepatocellular growth control. In *Rat liver neoplasia*, eds. P. M. Newberne and W. H. Butler. Cambridge, Mass.: MIT Press. In press.

Levin, D. L., Devesa, S. S., Godwin, J. D. and Silverman, D. T. 1974. Cancer rates and risks. *DHEW Publ. 75-691 (NIH)*.

Lilienfeld, A. 1972. Epidemiology of gastric cancer. *N. Engl. J. Med.* 286:316–317.

Mancuso, T. F. 1974. Relation of place of birth and migration in cancer mortality in the U.S.—A study of Ohio residents (1959–1967). *J. Chronic Dis.* 27:459–474.

McCann, J., Choi, E., Yamasaki, E. and Ames, B. N. 1975. Detection of carcinogens as mutagens in the *Salmonella*/microsome test: Assay of 300 chemicals. *Proc. Natl. Acad. Sci. U.S.A.* 72:5135–5139.

McLean, A. E. M. and Magee, P. N. 1970. Increased renal carcinogenesis by dimethylnitrosamine in protein-deficient rats. *Br. J. Exp. Pathol.* 51:587–590.

Merliss, R. R. 1971. Talc-treated rice and Japanese stomach cancer. *Science* 173:1141–1142.

Miller, J. A. and Miller, E. C. 1953. The carcinogenic aminoazo dyes. *Adv. Cancer Res.* 1:339–396.

Mirvish, S. S., Greenblatt, M. and Kommineni, V. R. 1972. Nitrosamide formation *in vivo:* Induction of lung adenomas in Swiss mice by concurrent feeding of nitrite and methylurea or ethylurea. *J. Natl. Cancer Inst.* 48:1311–1315.

Montecuccoli, G., Novello, F. and Stirpe, F. 1972. Effect of protein deprivation and of starvation on DNA synthesis in resting and regenerating rat liver. *J. Nutr.* 102:507–514.

Morris, H. P. 1947. Effects of the genesis and growth of tumors associated with vitamin intake. *Ann. N.Y. Acad. Sci.* 49:119–140.

Newberne, P. M. 1965. Carcinogenicity of aflatoxin-contaminated peanut meals. In *Mycotoxins in foodstuffs,* ed. G. N. Wogan, pp. 187–208. Cambridge, Mass.: MIT Press.

Newberne, P. M. 1976a. Biologic effects on plant toxins and aflatoxins in rats. *J. Natl. Cancer Inst.* 56:551–555.

Newberne, P. M. 1976b. Environmental modifiers of susceptibility to carcinogenesis. *Cancer Detect. Prev.* 1:129–173.

Newberne, P. M. and Rogers, A. E. 1973a. Adenocarcinoma of the colon: An animal model for human disease. *Am. J. Pathol.* 72:541–544.

Newberne, P. M. and Rogers, A. E. 1973b. Primary hepatocellular carcinoma: An animal model for human disease. *Am. J. Pathol.* 72:137–140.

Newberne, P. M. and Rogers, A. E. 1973c. Rat colon carcinomas associated with aflatoxin and marginal vitamin A. *J. Natl. Cancer Inst.* 50:439–448.

Newberne, P. M. and Shank, R. C. 1973. Induction of liver and lung tumors in rats by simultaneous administration of sodium nitrite and morpholine. *Food Cosmet. Toxicol.* 11:819–825.

Newberne, P. M. and Suphakarn, V. 1977. Preventive role of vitamin A in colon carcinogenesis. *Cancer* 40:2553–2556.

Newberne, P. M., Harrington, D. H. and Wogan, G. N. 1966. Effects of cirrhosis and other liver insults on induction of liver tumors by aflatoxin in rats. *Lab. Invest.* 15:962–969.

Newberne, P. M., Rogers, A. E., Bailey, C. and Young, V. R. 1969. The induction of liver cirrhosis in rats by purified amino acid diets. *Cancer Res.* 29:230–235.

Nixon, J. E., Sinnhuber, R. O., Lee, D. J., Landers, M. K. and Harr, J. R. 1974. Effect of cyclopropenoid compounds on the carcinogenic activity of diethylnitrosamine and alfatoxin B, in rats. *J. Natl. Cancer Inst.* 53:453–458.

Oettle, A. G. 1967. Primary neoplasms of the alimentary canal of white and Bantu of the Transvaal 1949–1953. A histopathological series. *Natl. Cancer Inst. Monogr.* 25:97–109.

Oyasu, R. and Hopp, M. L. 1974. The etiology of cancer of the bladder. *Surg. Gynecol. Obstet.* 138:97–108.

Oyasu, R., Kitajima, T., Hopp, M. L. and Sumie, H. 1972. Enhancement of urinary bladder tumorigenesis in hamsters by coadministration of 2-acetylaminofluorene and indole. *Cancer Res.* 32:2027–2033.

Pamukcu, A. M. and Price, J. M. 1969. Induction of intestinal and urinary bladder cancer in rats by feeding bracken fern (*Pteris aquilina*). *J. Natl. Cancer Inst.* 43:275–281.

Pamukcu, A. M., Goksoy, S. K. and Price, J. M. 1967. Urinary bladder neoplasms induced by feeding bracken fern (*Pteris aquilina*) to cows. *Cancer Res.* 27:917–924.

Pamukcu, A. M., Erturk, E., Price, J. M. and Bryan, G. T. 1972. Lymphatic leukemia and pulmonary tumors in female Swiss mice fed bracken fern. *Cancer Res.* 32:1442–1445.

Peers, F. G. and Linsell, C. A. 1973. Dietary aflatoxins and liver cancer: A population based study in Kenya. *Br. J. Cancer* 27:473–484.

Phillips, R. 1975. Cancer in Seventh Day Adventists: Implications for the role of nutrition and cancer. *Cancer Res.* 35:3513–3522.

Poirier, L. A. 1975. Hepatocarcinogenesis by diethylnitrosamine in rats fed high dietary levels of lipotropes. *J. Natl. Cancer Inst.* 54:137–140.

Reddy, B., Weisburger, J. H., Narisawa, T. and Wynder, E. L. 1974a. Colon carcinogenesis in germ-free rats with 1,2-dimethylhydrazine and N-methyl-N'-nitro-N-nitrosoguanidine. *Cancer Res.* 34:2368–2372.

Reddy, B., Weisburger, J. H. and Wynder, E. L. 1974b. Effect of dietary fat levels and dimethylhydrazine on fecal acid and neutral sterol excretion and colon carcinogenesis in rats. *J. Natl. Cancer Inst.* 52:507–511.

Research to Meet U.S. and World Food Needs. 1975. Report of a Working Conference, Agricultural Research Policy Advisory Committee, Kansas City, Missouri, July 9–11.

Rogers, A. E. 1975. Variable effects of a lipotrope-deficient, high-fat diet on chemical carcinogenesis in rats. *Cancer Res.* 35:2369–2474.

Rogers, A. E. and Newberne, P. M. 1971. Diet and aflatoxin B_1 toxicity in rats. *Toxicol. Appl. Pharmacol.* 20:113–121.

Rogers, A. E. and Newberne, P. M. 1973. Dietary enhancement of intestinal carcinogenesis by dimethylhydrazine in rats. *Nature (Lond.)* 246:491–492.

Rogers, A. E., Herndon, B. J. and Newberne, P. M. 1973. Influence of vitamin A on dimethylhydrazine-induced colon carcinoma in rats. *Cancer Res.* 33:1003–1009.

Rogers, A. E., Sanchez, O., Feinsod, F. M. and Newberne, P. M. 1974. Dietary enhancement of nitrosamine carcinogenesis. *Cancer Res.* 34:96–99.

Rogers, A. E., Wishnok, J. S. and Archer, M. C. 1975. Effect of diet on DEN clearance and carcinogenesis in rats. *Br. J. Cancer* 31:693–695.

Rose, G., Blackburn, H., Keys, A., Taylor, H., Kamel, W., Reid, P. O. and Stamler, J. 1974. Colon cancer and blood cholesterol. *Lancet* 1:181–183.

Rowlatt, L. M., Franks, M. and Sheriff, M. U. 1973. Mammary tumor and hepatoma suppression by dietary restriction in C_3H A^{vy} mice. *Br. J. Cancer* 28:83.

Saffiotti, U. 1973. Metabolic host factors in carcinogenesis. In *Host environmental interactions in the etiology of cancer in man,* eds. R. Doll and I. Vodopija, pp. 243–252. Lyon, France: International Agency for Research in Cancer.

Saffiotti, U., Montesano, R., Sellakumar, A. R. and Borg, A. S. 1967. Experimental cancer of the lung. Inhibition by vitamin A of the induction of tracheobronchial squamous metaplasia and squamous cell tumors. *Cancer* 20:857–864.

Salmon, W. D. and Newberne, P. M. 1963. Occurrence of hepatomas in rats fed diets containing peanut meal as a major source of protein. *Cancer Res.* 23:571–575.

Salmon, W. D., Copeland, D. H. and Burns, M. J. 1955. Hepatomas in choline deficiency. *J. Natl. Cancer Inst.* 15:1549–1568.

Schlegel, J. V., Pipkin, G. E., Nishimura, R. and Shultz, G. N. 1969. The role of ascorbic acid in the prevention of bladder tumor formation. *Trans. Am. Assoc. Genito-urin. Surg.* 61:85–89.

Schmauz, R. and Cole, P. 1974. Epidemiology of cancer of the renal pelvis and ureter. *J. Natl. Cancer Inst.* 52:1331–1334.

Shank, R. C., Bhamarapravati, N., Gordon, J. E. and Wogan, G. N. 1972. Dietary aflatoxins and human liver cancer. Incidence of primary liver cancer in two municipal populations of Thailand. *Food Cosmet. Toxicol.* 10:171–179.

Smith, D. M., Rogers, A. E., Herndon, B. J. and Newberne, P. M. 1975a. Vitamin A (retinyl acetate) and benzo(a)pyrene-induced respiratory tract carcinogenesis in hamsters fed a commercial diet. *Cancer Res.* 35:11–16.

Smith, D. M., Rogers, A. E. and Newberne, P. M. 1975b. Vitamin A and benzo(a)pyrene carcinogenesis in the respiratory tract of hamsters fed a semisynthetic diet. *Cancer Res.* 35:1485–1488.

Sporn, M. B., Dunlop, N. M., Newton, D. L. and Smith, J. M. 1976. Prevention of chemical carcinogenesis by vitamin A and its synthetic analogs (retinoids). *Fed. Proc.* 35:1332–1338.

Stout, D. L., Baptist, J. N., Matney, T. S. and Shaw, C. R. 1976. N-Hydroxy-2-aminofluorene: The principal mutagen produced from N-hydroxy-2-acetylamino-fluorene by a mammalian supernatant enzyme preparation. *Cancer Lett.* 1:269–274.

Swann, P. F. and McLean, A. E. M. 1971. Cellular injury and carcinogenesis. The effect of a protein-free high-carbohydrate diet on the metabolism of dimethylnitrosamine in the rat. *Biochem. J.* 124:283–288.

Symposium on Nutrition in the Causation of Cancer. 1974. *Cancer Res.* 35:3231–3550.

Szepsenwol, J. 1963. Carcinogenic effect of egg white, egg yolk and lipids in mice. *Proc. Soc. Exp. Biol. Med.* 112:1073–1076.

Tanaka, Y. and Dao, T. L. 1965. Effect of hepatic injury on induction of adrenal necrosis and mammary cancer by 7,12-dimethylbenz(a)anthracene in rats. *J. Natl. Cancer Inst.* 35:631–640.

Tatematsu, M., Takahashi, M., Fukushima, S., Hananouchi, M. and Shirai, T. 1975. Effects in rats of sodium chloride on experimental gastric cancers induced by N-methyl-N'-nitro-N-nitrosoguanidine or 4-nitroquinoline-1-oxide. *J. Natl. Cancer Inst.* 55:101–106.

Tuyns, A. J. 1968. IARC Working Conference on the Role of Aflatoxin in Human Disease, Lyon, France, October 28–30.

Ulland, B. M., Weisburger, J. H., Yamamoto, R. S. and Weisburger, E. K. 1973. Antioxidants and carcinogenesis: Butylated hydroxy-toluene, but not diphenyl-p-phenylene diamine, inhibits cancer induction by N-2-fluorenylacetamine in rats. *Food Cosmet. Toxicol.* 11:199–207.

van Rensburg, S. J., van der Watt, J. J., Purchase, I. F. H., Pereira Coutenho, L. and Markham, R. 1974. Primary liver cancer rate and aflatoxin intake in a high cancer area. *S. Afr. Med. J.* 48:2508a–2508d.

Venkatesan, N., Arcos, J. C. and Argus, M. F. 1970. Amino acid induction and carbohydrate repression of dimethylnitrosamine demethylase in rat liver. *Cancer Res.* 30:2563–2567.

Walker, A. 1971. Diet and cancer of the colon. *Lancet* 1:593–594.

Walker, A. R. P. 1975. Effect of high crude fiber intake on transit time and the absorption of nutrients in South African Negro school children. *Am. J. Clin. Nutr.* 28:1161–1169.

Walker, A., Walker, B. and Richardson, B. D. 1970. Bowel transit times in Bantu populations. *Br. Med. J.* 3:48–49.

Wattenberg, L. 1971. Studies of polycyclic hydrocarbon hydroxylases of the intestine possibly related to cancer. Effect of diet on benzo(a)pyrene hydroxylase activity. *Cancer* 28:99–110.

Wattenberg, L. W. 1972a. Inhibition of carcinogenic and toxic effects of polycyclic hydrocarbons by phenolic antioxidants and ethoxyquin. *J. Natl. Cancer Inst.* 48:1425–1430.

Wattenberg, L. W. 1972b. Dietary modification of intestinal and pulmonary aryl hydrocarbon hydroxylase activity. *Toxicol. Appl. Pharmacol.* 23:741–748.

Wattenberg, L. W. 1973. Inhibition of chemical carcinogen-induced pulmonary neoplasia by butylated hydroxyanisole. *J. Natl. Cancer Inst.* 50:1541–1544.

Wattenberg, L. W. 1974. Inhibition of carcinogenic and toxic effects of polycyclic hydrocarbons by several sulfur-containing compounds. *J. Natl. Cancer Inst.* 52:1583–1587.

Wynder, E. L. 1975. Introductory remarks, nutrition in the causation of cancer. *Cancer Res.* 35:3238–3239.

Wynder, E. L. 1976. Nutrition and cancer. Symposium on Nutrition and Cancer. *Fed. Proc.* 35:1309–1315.

Wynder, E. L. and Reddy, B. S. 1973. Studies of large bowel cancer: Human leads to experimental application. *J. Natl. Cancer Inst.* 50:1099–1106.

Wynder, E. L. and Shigematsu, T. 1967. Environmental factors of cancer of the colon and rectum. *Cancer* 20:1520–1561.

Yahagi, T., Nzgao, M., Hara, K., Matsushima, T., Sugimura, T. and Bryan, G. T. 1974. Relationships between the carcinogenic and mutagenic or DNA-modifying effects of nitrofuran derivatives, including 2-(2-furyl-3-(5-nitro-2-furyl) acrylamide, a food additive. *Cancer Res.* 34:2266–2273.

Zeiger, E. 1975. Dietary modifications affecting the mutagenicity of N-nitroso compounds in the host-mediated assay. *Cancer Res.* 35:1813–1818.

Zeitlin, B. R. 1972. Coffee and bladder cancer. *Lancet* 1:1066.

Part 3

TEST SYSTEMS

CHAPTER 5

THE *SALMONELLA*/MICROSOME MUTAGENICITY TEST: PREDICTIVE VALUE FOR ANIMAL CARCINOGENICITY

Joyce McCann and Bruce N. Ames
Department of Biochemistry
University of California
Berkeley, California

INTRODUCTION

As eloquently documented elsewhere (Hiatt et al., 1977), there is increasing evidence that environmental chemicals, both anthropogenic and natural, play an important role in the cause of human cancer. In fact, the only known causes of human cancer aside from modifying genetic factors (Knudson, 1977; Setlow, 1977) are radiation and chemicals, either from occupational sources, such as vinyl chloride (Maltoni, 1977), asbestos (Selikoff, 1976), chloroprene (Infante and Wagoner, 1977), and coal tar (Hammond et al. 1976); from natural sources, such as aflatoxin (Hsieh et al., and cigarette smoking (Hammond, 1977); and from drug exposure. In addition, many dietary factors have been linked to human cancer and these are likely to be chemicals, both natural and manufactured. If chemicals, both manufactured and natural, are indeed the primary cause of human cancer, then pinpointing the most important offenders and minimizing human exposure to them may be the most effective means of reducing the incidence of cancer.

We have been involved over the last 10 years in the development of a simple test (Ames et al., 1975a; McCann et al. 1975a; McCann and Ames 1976; reviewed in Ames and McCann, 1976) that can be used to identify chemical carcinogens and mutagens. The test detects these chemicals by means of their mutagenicity (ability to damage DNA, the genetic material) and is about 90% accurate in detecting carcinogens as mutagens. Special strains of

This chapter originally appeared in *Origins of human cancer,* eds. H. H. Hiatt, J. D. Watson and J. A. Winsten, Cold Spring Harbor Laboratory, Cold Spring Harbor, New York, 1977.

Salmonella bacteria are used for measuring DNA damage, combined with tissue homogenates from rodents (or humans) to provide mammalian metabolism of chemicals. The compound to be tested, about 1 billion bacteria of a particular tester strain (several different histidine-requiring mutants are used), and rat (or human) liver homogenate, are combined on a petri dish. After incubation at 37°C for 2 days, histidine revertants are scored.

In Figs. 1 and 2 are examples of the type of results obtained. In the "spot test" (Fig. 1) a small amount of the chemical to be tested is placed in the center of the dish, the chemical diffuses out into the agar and revertant colonies appear as a cloud around the central spot. The spot test is limited somewhat in sensitivity (Ames et al., 1975a), but it is extremely rapid. Normally, one tests individual dose levels of a chemical in the more sensitive plate test and quantitative dose-response curves can be generated, as shown in Figs. 2 and 3. These curves are almost always linear and most mutagens are detected at very low dose levels (in some cases nanogram amounts).

The simplicity, sensitivity, and accuracy of this method for screening

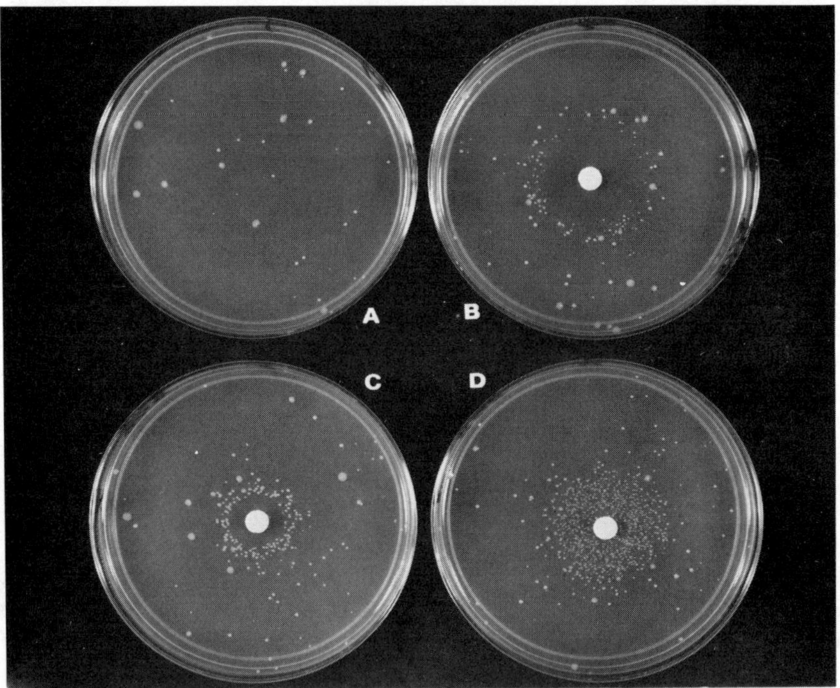

FIGURE 1 The spot test. Each petri plate contains, in a thin overlay of top agar, the tester strain TA 98 and, in the case of plates C and D, a liver microsomal activation system (S-9 mix). Mutagens were applied to 6-mm filter paper disks, which were then placed in the center of each plate: (A) spontaneous revertants; (B) furylfuramide (AF-2) (1 μg); (C) aflatoxin B_1 (1 μg); (D) 2-aminofluorene (10 μg). Mutagen-induced revertants appear as a ring of colonies around each disk. (From Ames et al., 1975a.)

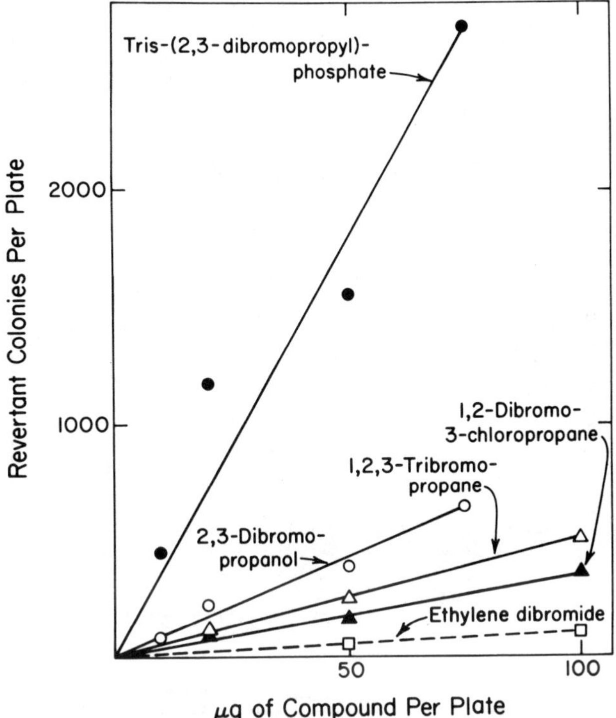

FIGURE 2 All compounds were tested on *Salmonella* strain TA100, as previously described (Ames et al., 1975a). The amount of ethylene dibromide added was 10 times that indicated on the scale. The data presented for tris, 2,3-dibromopropanol, and dibromochloropropane were obtained in the presence of rat liver homogenate (20 μl S-9 per plate, Aroclor-induced); human liver gave similar results. The potencies (revertants per nanomole) of the various chemicals are: tris (0.1; 25 with S-9), 2,3-dibromopropanol (0.15; 1.9 with S-9), 1,2,3-tribromopropane (1.4; 1.4 with S-9), 1,2-dibromo-3-chloropropane (0.5; 0.9 with S-9), ethylene dibromide (0.02; with 0.02 with S-9). (From Blum and Ames, 1977.)

large numbers of environmental sources of potential carcinogens has resulted in its current use in over 1,000 government, industrial, and academic laboratories throughout the world. The potential of this method for use as a bioassay for the development of safe, useful chemicals raises many questions about the extent to which this kind of approach should be used in a program aimed at cancer prevention. How predictive is the method? What should a regulatory agency do if a chemical is positive in the test? Should other *in vitro* tests or animal tests be initiated for a chemical that is positive in the test? Or, should the chemical be banned outright? (Italy has recently banned some hair dye ingredients, based on their positive response in our test.) These are

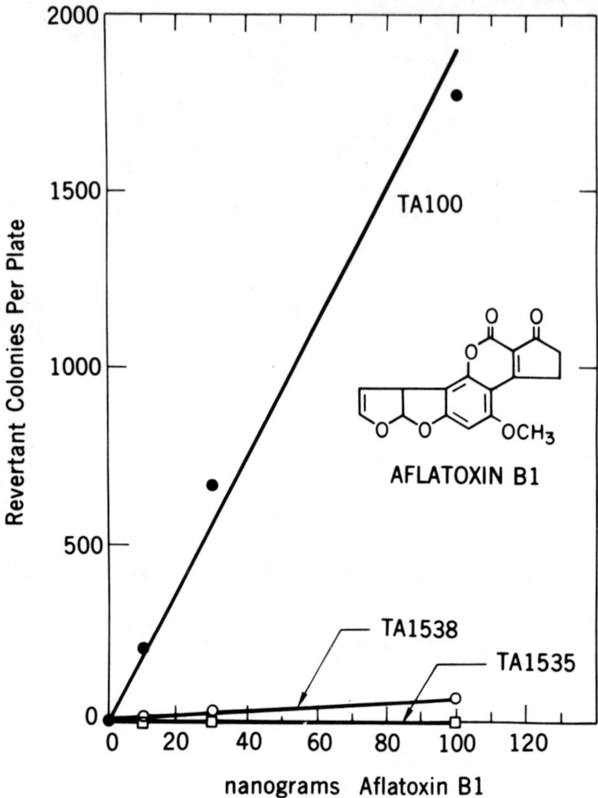

FIGURE 3 Mutagenicity of aflatoxin B_1 in the standard plate incorporation test. Spontaneous revertant colonies have been subtracted. Liver homogenate from Aroclor 1254-induced rats was added as described in Ames et al. (1975a).

difficult questions that must be addressed, and we discuss here several aspects of the experimental basis for our current assessment of the value of the test as a useful predictive tool:

1. The predictive value of the test as an indicator of carcinogenic potential, including both the strengths and weaknesses of the test at this stage in its development.

2. Current applications of the test method to problems that are not approachable using conventional animal test methods.

3. Some of the environmental chemicals that have already been pinpointed as potential carcinogens by the test and the current status of carcinogenicity tests in animals on these chemicals.

4. The evidence that the correlation between carcinogenicity and mutagenicity in the *Salmonella*/microsome test reflects more than a useful

coincidence, and fits into a compelling collection of evidence supporting a central role for somatic mutation in the initiation of human cancer.

MUTAGENIC POTENCY
VARIES OVER 1 MILLIONFOLD

One of the most striking findings to come from testing hundreds of chemicals in the *Salmonella* test is that there is a tremendously large range of mutagenic potency of carcinogens in the test—over 1 millionfold. This is illustrated in Table 1. We observed significant numbers of mutagens throughout the entire potency range. If this range has any biological reality in terms of mammals, and we think it does (see below), it has some very important implications. One is the limits it sets on what constitutes significant variability in cancer biology. For example, it may not be terribly significant if one chemical is a few times more or less carcinogenic than another, but it is important in terms of human risk if there is a 100-fold or a 1,000-fold difference. In terms of determining human risk, carcinogens with a millionfold difference in carcinogenic potency would certainly carry with them different human risks.

Mutagenic potency is dependent on the intrinsic mutagenic properties of the chemical, the efficiency of the *in vitro* microsomal activation system, and which tester strain is used (potency is calculated using results from the most active strain). Attempts are being made to see what the relation is between mutagenic potency and carcinogenic potency. Preliminary results indicate that, with a few exceptions, the *in vitro* test appears to be in rather good agreement (considering the millionfold range in mutagenic and carcinogenic potency) with the animal tests (Meselson and Russell, 1977; C. B. Sawyer, N. K. Hooper, A. Friedman and B. N. Ames, in preparation). More carcinogenic potency data are badly needed, and animal tests are not usually designed for potency calculations. Despite the complexity of the whole area of carcinogenic and mutagenic potency, we believe that it should be explored, although with great caution. For example, the mutagenic potency of a chemical in the

TABLE 1   Range of Mutagenic Potency
in the *Salmonella*/Microsome Test[a]

Chemical	Rev/nmol	Ratio
1,2-Epoxybutane	0.006	1
Benzyl chloride	0.02	3
Methyl Methanesulfonate	0.63	105
2-Naphthylamine	8.5	1,400
2-Acetylaminofluorene	108	18,000
Aflatoxin B_1	7,057	1,200,000
Furylfuramide (AF-2)	20,800	3,500,000

[a] Data from McCann et al., 1975a.

test also may be influenced by a number of additional factors and we discuss these briefly: (1) as discussed later (p. 98), we believe the activiation of a chemical by bacterial enzymes can articially elevate mutagenic potency; and (2) in the case of chemicals that are actively concentrated by cells, and which may therefore be mutagenic at very low dose levels, one wants to know, for purposes of potency comparison, whether transport systems are similar in *Salmonella* and in animals. In the bacterial test, the antibiotic carcinogen azaserine is an example of a chemical that is actively transported by the bacteria through an amino acid transport system (see McCann and Ames, 1976), such that its effective concentration in the cells is much greater than in the surrounding medium. This is most likely the explanation for the very high mutagenic potency (12,000 revertants per nanomole) of this carcinogen. Azaserine may well be transported through a similar system in animal cells. Antibiotics, in general, are polar molecules that enter cells through active transport systems and many plant toxins may fall into a similar category.

VALIDATION OF THE TEST AGAINST KNOWN ANIMAL CARCINOGENS AND NONCARCINOGENS

Ideally, one would like to validate the efficiency of a test such as this for use as a predictive tool for the detection of potential human carcinogens by testing a large number of human carcinogens. There are, however, very few data available on chemicals that cause cancer in humans, although almost all of the organic chemicals that are known or suspected human carcinogens are mutagenic in this test (Table 2). However, this is by no means sufficient to

TABLE 2 Organic Chemicals Known or Suspected
as Human Carcinogens[a]

Mutagens in the Salmonella/*Microsome Test*

Aflatoxins	Coal Tar
4-Aminobiphenyl	Cyclophosphamide
Benzidine	Melphalan
Chlornaphazine	Mustard Gas
Bis(chloromethyl) ether	2-Naphthylamine
Chloroprene	4-Nitrobiphenyl
Cigarette smoke condensates	Soot
Vinyl chloride	

Others

Auramine dye mixture (pure auramine O negative)[b]
Benzene (not tested yet)[b]
Diethylstilbestrol (nonmutagenic, but incomplete
    test because of toxicity)

[a]See McCann and Ames, 1976, for discussion.
[b]Benzene has now been tested and is not mutagenic, and auramine dye mixture was found to be mutagenic (Ames, Yamasaki, and Maron, unpublished).

validate the test because of the small number of chemicals, and also because the test must not only positively respond to carcinogens, it must also give a *negative* response with noncarcinogens. We have therefore validated the test using a large number (about 300) of organic chemicals, of many chemical classes, which have been tested in the conventional animal (usually rodent) carcinogenicity tests. This procedure is not completely ideal, since there is some degree of uncertainty surrounding the adequacy of the animal tests themselves for assessment of carcinogenic risk to humans, although with the exception of arsenic, chemicals known to cause cancer in humans also cause cancer in animals (Tomatis, 1976). This inadequacy of animal tests is especially apparent in the designation of a chemical as a noncarcinogen. Negatives are difficult to prove in the best of systems, and the statistical limitations of the animal tests make them particularly vulnerable to error in the designation of a chemical as a noncarcinogen. This problem is compounded by the great heterogeneity of animal cancer tests in the past, which differed enormously in degree of thoroughness, quality, and protocol. Out of this variety of tests, most of which are inadequate by current standards, where does one draw the boundary for defining a noncarcinogen? Some method is clearly needed that would permit a more quantitative evaluation of negative cancer data. Some kind of completeness index might be useful that would permit expression of negative data as a "less-than" figure, which would take into account limitations of the particular experimental system, such as duration of the experiment, numbers of animals used, and dose.

Thus, in a validation such as ours, one expects some noncorrelation between mutagenicity and carcinogenicity because of the inadequacies of the animal cancer tests, especially involving "noncarcinogens" that show some mutagenic activity. In the interpretation of the results it is therefore crucial to determine what proportion of any noncorrelation is likely to result from the animal tests and what proportion results from the bacterial test. Even without such a determination, and in spite of the uncertainities related to animal tests, the results show a striking correlation between carcinogenicity and mutagenicity. We found that 90% (157 of 175) of the carcinogens tested were mutagenic in the test, and 87% (94 of 108) of the noncarcinogens were nonmutagens. In almost all cases the test discriminated very well between carcinogens and noncarcinogens. This is especially striking for a number of close chemical relatives where one is a potent carcinogen and the other is an extremely weak carcinogen or a noncarcinogen (Fig. 4). The relative mutagenicity of these chemicals in the test illustrates the ability of the test to distinguish efficiently between subtle differences in chemical structures that also drastically effect carcinogenicity.

Our test system has been independently validated, with similar results, in a blind study by Imperial Chemical Industries (Purchase et al., 1976) and in a study at the National Cancer Research Institute in Tokyo (see Sugimura et al., 1977).

J. McCann and B. N. Ames

We have not reported on any metal carcinogens, physical carcinogens such as asbestos, or radiations [although X-rays, fast neutrons, and UV light do mutate *Salmonella* bacteria (Hartman et al., 1971)]. The standard test system is not suitable for metals entering the bacteria because of the large amounts of Mg salts, citrate, sulfate, and phosphate in the minimal medium. A number of carcinogenic metals have been shown to be mutagens in bacteria by a methodology somewhat different from our standard procedure (Venitt and Levy, 1974; Nishioka, 1975). At least some of the metals, such as chromate, mutate the *Salmonella* strains when salts in the medium are lowered (S. Rogers and G. Löfroth, personal communication).

	Carc	Rev/nMole	Ratio
2-Acetylaminofluorene (AAF)	+	108	
1-Hydroxy-2-AAF	0	<0.02	>5400
3-Hydroxy-2-AAF	0	<0.02	>5400
5-Hydroxy-2-AAF	0	<0.04	2700
7-Hydroxy-2-AAF	c0	<0.03	>3600
4-Acetylaminofluorene	0	0.3	360
2-Aminoanthracene	+	510	
1-Aminoanthracene	w+	22	23
β-Naphthylamine	+	8.5	
α-Naphthylamine	c0	0.42	20

FIGURE 4 Chemicals are rated as: + carcinogen; 0, noncarcinogen; w+ weak carcinogen; c0, noncarcinogen in most studies, with some reports of weak or marginal activity; or ?, inadequate data available for classification, but generally regarded as a noncarcinogen based on structural considerations. [Data from McCann et al. (1975a); for discussion see McCann and Ames (1976) and Donahue et al. (1978).]

		Carc	Rev/nmole	Ratio
4-Aminobiphenyl	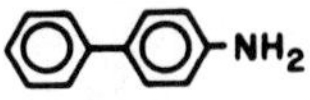	+	31	61
2-Aminobiphenyl	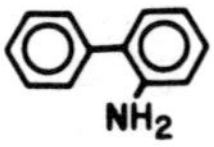	+	0.51	
Benzo(a)pyrene	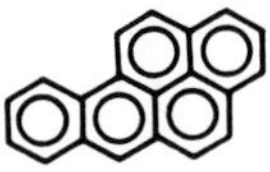	+	121	202
Benzo(e)pyrene	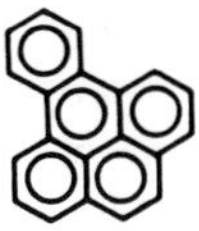	w+	0.6	
15,16-Dihydro-11-methyl cyclopenta(a)phenanthrene-17-one	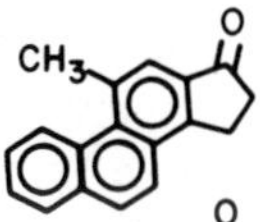	+	84	>2800
15,16-Dihydro-3-methyl-cyclopenta(a)phenanthrene-17-one	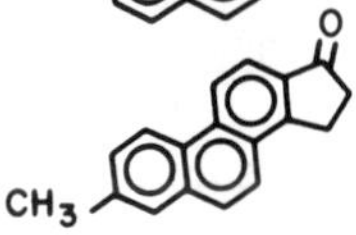	0	<0.03	
Aflatoxin B_1	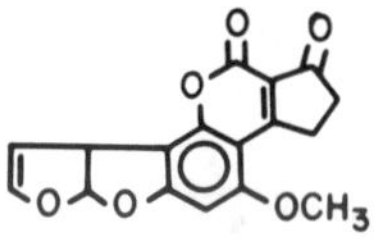	+	7057	3360
Aflatoxin B_2	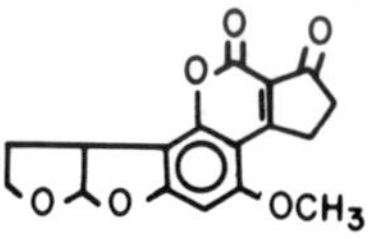	w+	2.1	

FIGURE 4 Chemicals are rated as: + carcinogen; 0, noncarcinogen; w+ weak carcinogen; c0, noncarcinogen in most studies, with some reports of weak or marginal activity; or ?, inadequate data available for classification, but generally regarded as a noncarcinogen based on structural considerations. [Data from McCann et al. (1975a); for discussion see McCann and Ames (1976) and Donahue et al. (1978).] *(Continued)*

FALSE POSITIVES AND NEGATIVES

We have previously discussed in detail the false positives and negatives in the test (McCann and Ames, 1976). In general, we believe most of these are explainable by either inadequate animal carcinogenicity tests, or inadequacies in our *in vitro* metabolic activation system. Here we would like to concentrate on a few general concepts that have arisen from our evaluation of the false positives and negatives.

Types of Problems That Can Lead to False Negatives

Role of toxicity in animal and bacterial tests. The limitations of both the animal cancer tests and the bacterial test in terms of maximum tolerated dose are defined by the toxicity of the chemical. In general, we have found that the expression of mutagenic activity occurs at concentrations well below the toxic level, and that toxicity is almost always associated with excessive DNA damage. However, the bacterial test could fail to detect chemicals that are very toxic to the bacteria for reasons not related to their mutagenic properties—for example, antibiotics. In fact, there was a small number (about 3%) of carcinogens and noncarcinogens that we could test only at very low dose levels because of their extreme toxicity (McCann and Ames, 1976). This is also true of the animal tests, and some chemicals, such as 2,3,7,8-tetra-chlorodibenzo-*p*-dioxin and many of the chlorinated pesticides, can be tested in the animal systems only at extremely low doses for this reason.

In vitro *metabolic activation system.* We believe a number of the false negatives result from technical inadequacies of the *in vitro* metabolic activation system, which, for the most part, should be relatively simple problems to solve. For example, safrole is a carcinogen that is not detected in the standard test, while we do detect 1′-acetoxysafrole, a carcinogenic metabolite. This strongly suggests that the *in vitro* metabolic activation system is simply not activating safrole efficiently. This could be related to the fact that our *in vitro* system does not contain the cofactors for acetylation. Another difficulty that can arise appears to be involved in the case of the short-chain nitrosamines, such as dimethylnitrosamine, which is a potent carcinogen but is very poorly detected in our standard plate assay. It can be detected more efficiently, although it is still of low potency, by a modification of the method that adds a preincubation step at high enzyme concentration (see Ames et al., 1975a, for references). The activation of the chemical is nonlinear (about second order) with increasing amounts of liver extract, indicating that its activation requires at least two independently acting events. The dilution effect involved in preparing the *in vitro* liver extract is most likely responsible for the relative inactivity of the activating enzymes in the *in vitro* test compared with their high efficiency *in vivo*. In addition, a new tester strain, TA92 (Ames, et al., 1975a; L. Haroun and B. N. Ames, in preparation) is more sensitive for DMN detection than TA1535. Cycasin is a carcinogen of plant origin that occurs in nature as an inactive glucoside. In mammals the active metabolite, methylazoxymethanol, is generated by action of β-glucosidases in the gut flora. Such enzymes are not present in mammalian tissue, nor are they active in *Salmonella*. Therefore, to detect this carcinogen in the test one must add β-glucosidase to the test plates (L. Haroun and B. N. Ames, unpublished; Sugimura et al., 1977). Many plant substances occur as β-glucosides (or other glycosides), and it will most likely be necessary to adapt the test for detection of these substances by adding β-glucosidase or other enzymes.

New tester strains. Tester strains have been continually improved for over 10 yr and we believe that further improvements will permit us to detect more of the remaining false negatives. For example, a few chemicals, such as the carcinogen mitomycin C (Kondo et al., 1970; McCann et al., 1975b) and malondialdehyde (Mukai and Goldstein, 1976) require an intact *uvrB* repair system to be detected as mutagens. A new strain TA94 (*hisD3052/pKM101*) is useful for their detection (B. N. Ames and L. Haroun, unpublished). A number of other improvements are under investigation.

What percentage of organic chemicals carcinogenic in animals will be mutagenic in the Salmonella *test?* The test is currently detecting about 90% of organic carcinogens as mutagens. We expect that with further improvements in both the tester strains and the metabolic activation system, as discussed above, the test will detect at least 95% of all carcinogens. McCann and Ames (1976) discuss the false negatives in the *Salmonella* test that are mutagenic in other systems. The remaining few percent will never be detected by the *Salmonella*/microsome type of bioassay. We believe that most of these will fall into the hormone and promotor category or will be a class of mutagens that are unique to animal cells. Many hormones, or hormone analogues such as diethylstilbestrol, can cause cancer in animals and are presumably active by affecting cell growth rather than by a mutagenic mechanism. Some of the promoting chemicals such as the phorbol esters appear to have hormonal-type effects and presumably will also not be active as mutagens. In addition, there should be a class of carcinogens with mutagenic activity unique to animal cells. For example, the carcinogen griseofulvin (which is negative in *Salmonella*) is known to interfere with microtubule formation (Weber et al., 1976). Microtubules are involved in mitosis in the distribution of chromosomes to daughter cells and interference with this process could result in chromosome abnormalities. Thus one can imagine a class of indirect mutagens interfering with mitosis that would not be detected in a bacterial assay.

Why is it that over 90% of chemicals that cause cancer in animals appear to be mutagens that interact with DNA rather than hormones or more indirect mutagens? A possible explanation is that a specific interaction of a chemical with a hormonal receptor places much more stringent requirements on chemical structure than does an electrophilic interaction of a chemical with DNA. A similar argument for a stringent structural requirement could be made for chemicals causing misfunction of the proteins of DNA repair systems or the mitotic apparatus. The percentage of carcinogens that act as mutagens by interacting with DNA may well be lower for natural products such as antibiotics and plant toxins. Many of these chemicals have been designed during evolution for specifc biological interactions, and one does not know what percentage of these carcinogens may act through a DNA interaction. Thus even though the test is doing extremely well, one must view with some degree of caution negatives in classes of new chemicals for which the test has not yet been validated. It is also clear that we will need rapid and accurate test systems for promoter-like carcinogens and other carcinogens that do not interact directly with DNA. Peto (Peto, 1977) emphasizes the importance of not neglecting these other types of carcinogens.

Types of Problems That Could Lead to False Positives

Bacterial activation of chemicals. If the bacterial tester strains contain enzymes capable of metabolizing chemicals tested to active mutagenic forms, this could obviously generate false positives in the test *if* the same enzymes are not functional in mammals. There are a few cases (discussed below) of carcinogens that are (or may be) activated by the bacteria, although in general bacteria have few enzymes for metabolic activation and do not have cytochrome P-450 type oxidizing systems. In every case so far the bacterial enzymes also appear to be present in mammals, either in the liver or in the gut flora (the gut bacterium *Escherichia coli* is a close relative of *Salmonella*).

As a group, nitro carcinogens represent the largest and best-documented class of chemicals activated to mutagens by bacterial enzymes (see McCann and Ames, 1976, for references). The chemicals are reduced by nitroreductases in the bacteria to their active forms. Mammalian liver is known to contain nitroreductase enzymes, as are the bacterial flora in the gut, which may play a significant role in the activation of nitro carcinogens *in vivo*. A likely effect of "in situ activation" by bacterial enzymes is to greatly increase the mutagenic potency of a chemical, since the active form is generated inside the bacteria and has a lower probability of reacting with non-DNA components, diffusing and so on, before reaching the DNA target. Therefore, we suspect that our test is extraordinarily sensitive for the detection of nitro carcinogens, many of which are known to be very weak carcinogens and difficult to detect in the animal tests, which may account for the few false positives in this class. All the carcinogenic nitro compounds we have tested have been mutagenic. Nevertheless, the predictive value of the test for this class of chemicals must be viewed with some degree of caution until we have more noncarcinogenic nitro compounds to test and more information about the nitroreductase enzymes in *Salmonella,* human gut bacteria, and human tissue. Nitroreductase-deficient mutants in our tester strains may be useful (see McCann and Ames, 1976, for a discussion of the work in this field).

Several active carcinogenic forms of 2-acetylaminofluorene (AAF) have been suggested, and on the basis of a considerable amount of physiological evidence accumulated by the Millers, the ultimate carcinogen is thought to be the highly reactive sulfate ester of the N-hydroxylated metabolite of AAF (Miller and Miller, 1977). Bacteria cannot N-hydroxylate AAF, but are known to contain enzymes capable of sulfate esterification, and it is possible that they could play a role in the activation of AAF-like carcinogens.

Repair systems and possible false positives. Our bacterial tester strains contain a mutation that deletes the capacity for excision (accurate) repair, and two of our strains also contain an increased capacity for error-prone repair (Ames et al., 1975a). The effect of removing the excision repair ability from the tester strain is to quantitatively enhance the sensitivity of the system rather than to qualitatively alter the response. In humans a similar situation appears to operate, as exposure to UV light is known to cause cancer in humans with functional excision repair enzymes. Some individuals, however, are born with defective DNA repair (see Setlow, 1977, for references), and these individuals are sensitized to cancer caused by UV light.

False positives that may result from the limitations of animal carcinogenicity tests: weak mutagens. There is a concentration of very weak mutagens among the false positives. Among all the chemicals that were positive in the test, about 25% have a mutagenic potency less than 0.6 rev/nmol, whereas among the false positives more than 60% are weak. We believe this suggests that most of the false positives may simply be weak carcinogens that have gone undetected in the animal tests. The work of Meselson and Russell (1977) and C. B. Sawyer, N. K. Hooper, A. Friedman, and B. N. Ames (unpublished) indicates that there may be a rough correlation between carcinogenic and mutagenic potency. Thus a weak mutagen may actually be a weak carcinogen, and the statistical limitations of the animal tests make it more difficult to detect weak activity.

Two of the false positives were borderline cases as to their classification as noncarcinogens. For example, in the case of styrene oxide there were several rather incomplete carcinogenicity studies (see McCann et al., 1975a, for references). In one, tumors were reported but no control data were given. In another, the authors actually concluded that the chemical was a carcinogen; however, our analysis of the data indicated that this was by no means clear, and this, together with the presence of another negative study, led us to classify the chemical as a noncarcinogen. *a-Naphthylamine* is a similar case. These chemicals may in fact be weak carcinogens and at the borderline of detectability in the standard animal tests.

Mutagenic impurities. We are finding that mutagenic impurities can play a significant role in mutagenesis testing. The millionfold range of mutagenic potency in the test (Table 1) indicates that only a tiny impurity of a potent mutagen could cause a significant mutagenic response in the test. We have found in our work a number of examples of mutagenic impurities, and we have discussed these and a number of other examples (Donahue et al., 1978). As discussed by McCann and Ames (1976), two noncarcinogens, originally thought to be false positives, were found to be nonmutagens containing mutagenic impurities.

Several industries using the test have also reported mutagenic impurities, and this has made clear the usefulness of the test method as a batch process monitor. American Cyanamid's Agricultural Division found mutagenic activity in some batches of a potentially useful chemical but not others, and it was possible to identify the step in the synthetic process that introduced the impurity. The batch process now in use removes the impurity (R. Gustafson, personal communication).

Are there any mutagens in the Salmonella ***test that are clearly noncarcinogens?*** The National Cancer Institute (NCI) recently published criteria for adequate carcinogenicity tests (Sontag et al., 1975). The test should be of adequate size and duration (lifetime preferred in rodents) in at least two animal species, at several dose levels, and positive controls should be of the same general chemical type as the chemical under test. The application of such criteria in evaluating noncarcinogenicity would mean that virtually no chemicals classified as noncarcinogens in this study could be considered noncarcinogens with a high degree of certainty. Of the 14 false positives reported and discussed by McCann and Ames (1976), most are weak mutagens where the limitations of the animal carcinogenicity tests are particularly relevant (see above). Even with the five fairly strong mutagens (folpet, ICR-191, nitrofurantoin, dibenz[a,h]anthracene-5,6-oxide, and sodium azide) the demonstration of the noncarcinogenicity is not convincing. Sodium azide was the only chemical for which the carcinogenicity test approximated the current NCI criteria, although it was tested in only one species, but even in this case the test is complicated by the fact that a high percentage (in some cases 100%) of control animals had tumors. The dibenzanthracene epoxide was tested by subcutaneous injection in newborn mice (Grover et al., 1975), and ICR-191 was tested in the lung adenoma test in strain A mice (Peck et al., 1976). Although both of these tests are useful, they cannot be considered at all definitive in relation to the NCI criteria. The high mutagenic potency of nitrofurantoin is most likely influenced by its activation by *Salmonella* nitroreductases (see above). We have previously discussed it and the pesticide folpet (McCann and Ames, 1976). We discuss captan, a pesticide related to folpet, below.

Designating a chemical a noncarcinogen is meaningless unless one couples this with a description of the thoroughness of the data used to reach this conclusion. What one really needs is a less-than figure (in a carcinogenic potency index) that describes the animal cancer tests in terms of the weakest carcinogenic potency that the test could detect. This index would incorporate information on dose, time, and number of animals used. We will discuss this concept in more detail at a later time. One needs this type of index in human risk assessment because of the millionfold range in carcinogenic potency and the statistical limitations in animal cancer tests that are done on a very few animals compared with the human population at risk.

APPLICATIONS OF THE *SALMONELLA* TEST

We believe that the test can play a central role in a long-term program of cancer prevention aimed at identifying and minimizing human exposure to environmental carcinogens and mutagens. It is a complement to traditional animal carcinogenicity tests (which take 2–3 yr and cost about $150,000) as it can be used in a variety of ways not feasible with the animal tests. (1) Chemical and drug companies can now afford to test routinely all new compounds at an early stage of development so that mutagens can be identified, and this information can be taken into consideration before there is a large vested interest in the compound. The *Salmonella* test is now being used by about 150 major chemical and drug companies. (2) If a drug is found to be mutagenic, a variety of derivatives can be synthesized to find a nonmutagenic form (Bueding and Batzinger, 1977). (3) The mutagenicity of a chemical may result from a trace of impurity, and such knowledge could save a useful chemical (see p. 99). (4) Complex mixtures or natural products with carcinogenic activity can be investigated, using the test as a bioassay for identifying the mutagenic ingredients; for example, cigarette smoke condensate is mutagenic (Kier et al., 1974) and tobacco companies are trying to identify the chemicals responsible, using *Salmonella* as a bioassay. (5) Human feces (Bruce et al., 1977) and urine (Bueding and Batzinger, 1977) (see Ames et al., 1975a, for references) can be examined to see if ingested products or drugs are giving rise to mutagens. (6) The variety of substances that humans are exposed to, both pure chemicals and mixtures, are being assayed for mutagenicity by hundreds of laboratories; for example, water supplies, soot from city air, hair dyes (Ames et al., 1975b) and cosmetics, drugs, food additives, food, mold toxins, pesticides, industrial chemicals, and fumigants. (7) The active metabolic forms of chemical carcinogens, and their metabolic routes, can be determined using the test as a bioassay (see Hiatt et al., 1977). (8) The test system is useful in clarifying basic mechanisms of mutagenesis by chemical carcinogens; for example, the demonstration that many aromatic carcinogens are reactive frameshift mutagens with particular base sequence specificity, and the clarification of the role of different repair systems in mutagenesis by various carcinogens (see McCann and Ames, 1976, for discussion). (9) The sensitivity of the *Salmonella* test may make it particularly useful for detecting chemicals that have weak carcinogenic activity and would be difficult to identify in animal tests because of statistical limitations. (10) The test is being used for setting priorities in selecting chemicals for carcinogenesis bioassay in animals.

BACTERIAL MUTAGENS THAT MIGHT BE HUMAN HAZARDS

A number of environmental chemicals that have been detected as mutagens in *in vitro* tests have subsequently been identified as animal carcinogens. We have previously discussed (McCann and Ames, 1976) the major Japanese food additive furylfuramine (AF-2) (now banned) (see also Sugimura et al., 1977) and the widely used industrial chemical and grain fumigant ethylene dibromide. Two hair dye components, 4-nitro-*o*-phenylenediamine and 2-nitro-*p*-phenylenediamine, which we found to be mutagenic (Ames et al., 1975b), have been shown to cause cell transformation and to break mammalian chromosomes (Searle et al., 1975; Benedict, 1976). Results from completed NCI carcinogenicity tests in rats and mice on a number of mutagenic hair dye ingredients have been released in 1978. Fractions of cigarette smoke condensate first shown to be mutagenic (Kier et al., 1974) have also been shown to cause cell transformation (Benedict et al., 1975).

The captan-type fungicides, including the closely related captan, folpet, and difolatan, are widely used. They are potent mutagens in the *Salmonella* test and are mutagenic and teratogenic and cause chromosome abnormalities in higher organisms, as discussed in a review by Bridges (1975). Captan was a borderline positive in a carcinogenicity study in mice and preliminary evidence from another study in mice on captan indicates it may be a potent carcinogen (H. Rosenkranz, personal communication). Ten million pounds of captan is produced every year, 100-ppm residues are still permitted in fruits and vegetables, and it has been estimated by Bridges (1975) that humans could consume as much as a few milligrams of the substance each day.

Tris(2,3-dibromopropyl)phosphate, the main flame retardant in children's polyester pajamas, is a potent mutagen in our test system, as is its metabolite, dibromopropanol, and its impurity, the carcinogen dibromochloropropane (Blum and Ames, 1977; Prival et al., 1977). Millions of children are wearing pajamas with this material added on at about 10% of the weight of the fabric. As nonpolar materials are generally absorbed through human skin at appreciable rates (see Blum and Ames, 1976, for references) we believe Tris may pose a serious hazard to children. Since its detection as a mutagen in *Salmonella*, it has been shown to be a potent mutagen in *Drosophila* (R. Valencia, personal communication) and to cause unscheduled DNA synthesis in human cells *in vitro* (H. F. Stich, personal communication). The compound is under test at NCI.[1]

Ethidium bromide is used extensively in physicochemical studies with nucleic acids as a highly fluorescent intercalating agent. It is quite mutagenic in the *Salmonella* test after metabolic activation with liver homogenate (McCann et al., 1975a). A carcinogenicity test has never been conducted on this chemical. We believe it is very likely to be carcinogenic, and should be handled with great care. We have found that propidium diiodide, which has been suggested as an alternative to ethidium bromide (Hudson et al., 1969), is virtually negative as mutagen in our test (Fig. 5). It may well be worth the effort to use propidium diiodide instead of ethidium bromide when possible, especially in gel staining, where fairly large amounts of dye are used and it is difficult to avoid human exposure. Some degree of sensitivity must be sacrificed if propidium diiodide is used, as it is somewhat less fluorescent, and at present it is considerably more expensive than ethidium bromide. Other highly fluorescent DNA intercalators are under development (B. Hudson, personal communication) and it will be of interest to determine their mutagenic properties.

A large number of laboratories are using the *Salmonella*/microsome test, and a variety of chemicals, both natural and manufactured, are showing up as mutagens. A few examples are complex mixtures (see discussion above); drugs

---

[1] *Note added in proof:* These tests have shown that Tris is a carcinogen in both rats and mice, and it has now been banned.

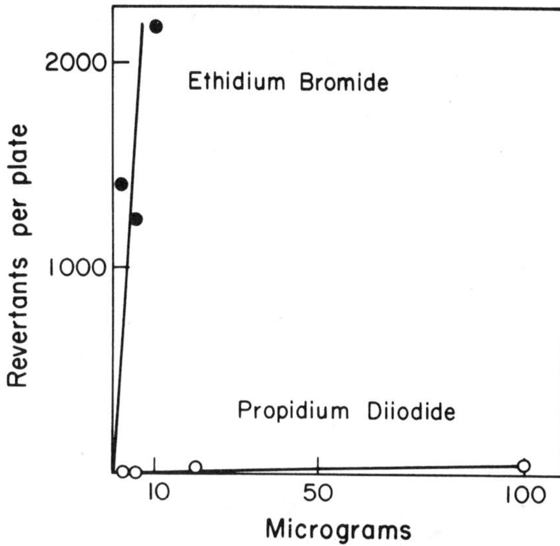

FIGURE 5 Mutagenicity of ethidium bromide and propidium diiodide on *Salmonella typhimurium* TA98. Liver homogenate (S-9 mix) from Arocolor-induced rats was used (20 μl S-9 per plate). Both chemicals are nonmutagenic in the absence of S-9 mix.

(Bueding and Batzinger, 1977), particularly the cancer chemotherapeutic agents (W. F. Benedict et al., personal communication); dietary components, and important industrial alkyl halides such as methylene chloride, vinyl bromide, and methyl bromide (V. Simmon, personal communication).

SOMATIC MUTATION AND HUMAN CANCER

It is likely that environmental factors initiate most human cancer, and it is becoming increasingly apparent that the causative agents in these environmental factors are likely to act by damaging DNA—for example, cigarette smoke (Kier et al., 1974), asbestos (Sincock, 1977), and UV light, X-rays, and known human chemical carcinogens (see above).

On the basis of our work and other evidence listed below, we find compelling the theory (see Trosko and Chu, 1975, and Miller and Miller, 1971, for historical review) that radiations and chemical carcinogens cause cancer through damage to DNA (somatic mutation). (1) It is known that cell regulation can be altered by mutation, and that a heritable change in cell regulation is a characteristic property of a cancer cell. (2) The theory is simple and consistent with facts in cancer biology (Hiatt et al., 1977). (3) It is supported by studies on the genetics of cancer (Knudson, 1977). (4) There are various human mutants with defective DNA repair systems who are extremely prone to cancer (Cleaver and Bootsma, 1975; Fujiwara and Tatsumi, 1975; Latt et al., 1975; Kuhnlein et al., 1976; Abrahams and Van der Eb, 1976; Maher et al., 1976; Lambert et al., 1976; Swift et al., 1976; Hoar and Sargent,

1976; Taylor et al., 1976. Setlow, 1977). (5) There appears to be a connection between error-prone repair function and 4-nitroquinoline-1-oxide carcinogenicity in mice (Nomura, 1976). (6) Active forms of many carcinogens are electrophiles capable of interacting with DNA (Miller and Miller, 1977). (7) Almost all carcinogens tested have been shown to be mutagens (discussed above). (8) Many potent aromatic carcinogens are unusually potent frameshift mutagens, and it is our hypothesis that the structural basis for this is that they are DNA affinity reagents containing both an aromatic ring system capable of a strong stacking interaction with DNA and an electrophilic moiety (Ames and Whitfield, 1967; Ames et al., 1972, 1973). (9) In addition to the many chemical carcinogens whose active forms have an electrophilic interaction with DNA and are mutagens, there is a diverse collection of carcinogens such as asbestos (Sincock, 1977), metal carcinogens [many of which may work by causing DNA polymerase to make errors (Nishioka, 1975; Mizutani and Temin, 1976; Sirover and Loeb, 1976)], and a variety of radiations (Hiatt et al., 1977) that have no obvious connection other than their ability to damage DNA.

It seems clear that many more chemicals will be added to the list of human carcinogens, as since the 1950s we have been exposed to a flood of chemicals that were not tested before use for carcinogenicity or mutagenicity, from flame retardants in our children's pajamas to pesticides accumulating in our body fat. In the past this problem has been largely ignored, and even very large volume chemicals, involving extensive human exposure, have been produced for decades without adequate carcinogenicity or mutagenicity tests—for example, vinyl chloride (2.5×10^9 kg/yr in the United States), ethylene dichloride (3.5×10^9 kg/yr in the United States), and a host of pesticides. A small fraction of these chemicals are now being tested in animals, but for the vast bulk of them the only experimental animals still are humans, and epidemiologic studies on humans are impractical in most cases. As the 20–30-year lag time for chemical carcinogenesis in humans is almost over, a steep increase in human cancer may be the outcome if too many of the thousands of new chemicals to which humans have been exposed turn out to be powerful mutagens and carcinogens. There is much more concern in recent years about the problem of human exposure to manufactured chemicals, and it remains to be seen how long it will take to work out an adequate system for protecting the public.

Damage to DNA by environmental mutagens (natural as well as manufactured) may be the main cause of death and disability in advanced societies. We believe that this damage, accumulating during our lifetime, initiates most human cancer and genetic defects and is quite likely a major contributor to aging (Burnet, 1974; Linn et al., 1976), and heart disease (Benditt and Benditt, 1973; Pearson et al., 1975) as well. The solution is prevention: identifying environmental mutagens and minimizing human exposures. Rapid, accurate, *in vitro* tests such as the *Salmonella*/microsome test, should play an important role in realizing this goal.

REFERENCES

Abrahams, P. J. and Van der Eb, A. J. 1976. Host-cell reactivation of ultraviolet-irradiated SV40 DNA in five complementation groups of xeroderma pigmentosum. *Mutat. Res.* 35:13.

Ames, B. N., and McCann, J. 1976. Carcinogens are mutagens: A simple test system. In *Screening tests in chemical carcinogenesis,* eds. R. Montesano, H. Bartsch, and L. Tomatis, vol. 12, pp. 493–504. Lyon, France: International Agency for Research on Cancer.

Ames, B. N. and Whitfield, H. J., Jr. 1967. Frameshift mutagenesis in *Salmonella. Cold Spring Harbor Symp. Quant. Biol.* 31:221.

Ames, B. N., Gurney, E. G., Miller, J. A. and Bartsch, H. 1972. Carcinogens as frameshift mutagens: Metabolites and derivatives of 2-acetylamino-fluorene and other aromatic amine carcinogens. *Proc. Natl. Acad. Sci. U.S.A.* 69:3128.

Ames, B. N., Durston, W. E., Yamasaki, D. and Lee, F. D. 1973. Carcinogens are mutagens: A simple test system combining liver homogenates for activation and bacteria for detection. *Proc. Natl. Acad. Sci., U.S.A.* 70:2281.

Ames, B. N., McCann, J. and Yamasaki, E. 1975a. Methods for detecting carcinogens and mutagens with the *Salmonella*/mammalian microsome mutagenicity test. *Mutat. Res.* 31:347.

Ames, B. N., Kammen, H. O. and Yamasaki, E. 1975b. Hair dyes are mutagenic: Identification of a variety of mutagenic ingredients. *Proc. Natl. Acad. Sci. U.S.A.* 72:2423.

Benditt, E. P. and Benditt, J. M. 1973. Evidence for a monoclonal origin of human atherosclerotic plaques. *Proc. Natl. Acad. Sci. U.S.A.* 70:1753.

Benedict, W. F. 1976. Morphological transformation and chromosomal aberrations produced by two hair dye components. *Nature (Lond.)* 260:368.

Benedict, W. F., Baker, M. S., Haroun, L., Choi, E. and Ames, B. N. 1977. Mutagenicity of cancer chemotherapeutic agents in the *Salmonella*/microsome test. *Cancer Res.* 37:2209.

Benedict, W. F., Rucher, N., Faust, J. and Kouri, R. E. 1975. Malignant transformation of mouse cells by cigarette smoke condensate. *Cancer Res.* 35:857.

Blum, A. and Ames, B. N. 1977. Flame retardant additives as possible cancer hazards. *Science* 195:17.

Bridges, B. A. 1975. The mutagenicity of captan and related fungicides. *Mutat. Res.* 32:3.

Bruce, W. R., Varghese, A. J. and Furrer, R. 1977. A mutagen in the feces of normal humans. In *Origins of human cancer,* eds. H. H. Hiatt, J. D. Watson and J. A. Winsten. Cold Spring Harbor, N.Y.: Cold Spring Harbor Laboratory.

Bueding, E. and Batzinger, R. 1977. Hycanthone and other antischistosomal drugs. Lack of obligatory association between chemotherapeutic effects and mutagenic activity. In *Origins of human cancer,* eds. H. H. Hiatt, J. D. Watson and J. A. Winsten. Cold Spring Harbor, N.Y.: Cold Spring Harbor Laboratory.

Burnet, M. 1974. *Intrinsic mutagenesis: A genetic approach to ageing.* Lancaster, England: Medical & Technical Publishing Co.

Cleaver, J. E. and Bootsma, D. 1975. Xeroderma pigmentosum: Biochemical and genetic characteristics. *Annu. Rev. Genet.* 9:19.

Donahue, E. V., McCann, J. and Ames, B. N. 1978. Impurities, high pressure liquid chromatography, and mutagenicity testing. *Cancer Res.* 38:431.

Fujiwara, Y. and Tatsumi, M. 1975. Repair of mitomycin C damage to DNA in mammalian cells and its impairment in Fanconi's anemia cells. *Biochem. Biophys. Res. Commun.* 66:592.

Grover, P. L., Sims, P., Mitchley, B. C. V. and Roe, F. J. C. 1975. The carcinogenicity of polycyclic hydrocarbon epoxides in newborn mice. *B. J. Cancer* 31:182.

Hammond, E. C. 1977. Smoking. In *Origins of human cancer*, eds. H. H. Hiatt, J. D. Watson and J. A. Winsten. Cold Spring Harbor, N.Y.: Cold Spring Harbor Laboratory.

Hammond, E. C., Selikoff, I. J., Lawther, P. L. and Seidman, H. 1976. Inhalation of benzpyrene and cancer in man. *Ann. N. Y. Acad. Sci.* 271:116.

Hartman, P. E., Hartman, Z., Stahl, R. C. and Ames, B. N. 1971. Classification and mapping of spontaneous and induced mutations in the histidine operon of *Salmonella*. *Adv. Genet.* 16:1.

Hiatt, H. H., Watson, J. D. and Winsten, J. A. eds. 1977. *Origins of human cancer*. Cold Spring Harbor, N.Y.: Cold Spring Harbor Laboratory.

Hoar, D. I. and Sargent, P. 1976. Chemical mutagen hypersensitivity in ataxis telangiectasia. *Nature (Lond.)* 261:590.

Hsieh, D. P. H., Wong, J. J. and Wong, Z. A. 1977. Hepatic biotransformation of aflatoxin and its carcinogenic activity. In *Origins of human cancer*, H. H. Hiatt, J. D. Watson and J. A. Winsten. Cold Spring Harbor, N.Y.: Cold Spring Harbor Laboratory.

Hudson, B., Upholt, W. B., Devinny, J. and Vinograd, J. 1969. The use of ethidium analogue in the dye-buoyant density procedure for the isolation of closed circular DNA: The variations of the superhelix density of mitochondrial DNA. *Proc. Natl. Acad. Sci. U.S.A.* 62:813.

Infante, P. F. and Wagoner, J. K. 1977. Chloroprene: Observations of carcinogenesis and mutagenesis. In *Origins of human cancer*, eds. H. H. Hiatt, J. D. Watson, and J. A. Winsten. Cold Spring Harbor, N.Y.: Cold Spring Harbor Laboratory.

Kier, L. D., Yamasaki, E. and Ames, B. N. 1974. Detection of mutagenic activity in cigarette smoke condensates. *Proc. Natl. Acad. Sci. U.S.A.* 71:4159.

Knudson, A. G. 1977. Genetic predisposition to cancer. In *Origins of human cancer*, eds. H. H. Hiatt, J. D. Watson and J. A. Winsten. Cold Spring Harbor, N.Y.: Cold Spring Harbor Laboratory.

Kondo, S., Ichikawa, H., Iwo, K. and Kato, T. 1970. Base-change mutagenesis and prophage induction in strains of *Escherichia coli* with different DNA repair capacities. *Genetics* 66:187.

Kuhnlein, U., Penhoet, E. E. and Linn, S. 1976. An altered apurinic DNA endonuclease activity in group A and group D xeroderma pigmentosum fibroblasts. *Proc. Natl. Acad. Sci. U.S.A.* 73:1169.

Lambert, B., Hansson, K., Bui, T. H., Funes-Craviota, F., Lindsten, J., Holmberg, M. and Strausmanis, R. 1976. DNA repair and frequency of X-ray and u.v.-light induced chromosome aberrations in leukocytes from patients with Down's syndrome. *Ann. Hum. Genet.* 39:293.

Latt, S. A., Stetten, G., Juergens, L. A., Buchanan, G. R. and Gerald, P. S. 1975. Induction by alkylating agents of sister chromatid exchanges and chromatid breaks in Fanconi's anemia. *Proc. Natl. Acad. Sci. U.S.A.* 72:4066.

Linn, S., Kairis, M. and Holliday, R. 1976. Decreased fidelity of DNA polymerase activity isolated from aging human fibroblasts. *Proc. Natl. Acad. Sci. U.S.A.* 73:2818.

Maher, V. M., Ouèllette, L. M., Curren, R. D. and McCormick, J. J. 1976. Frequency of ultraviolet light-induced mutations is higher in xeroderma pigmentosum variant cells than in normal human cells. *Nature (Lond.)* 261:593.

Maltoni, C. 1977. Vinyl chloride carcinogenicity: An experimental model for carcinogenesis studies. In *Origins of human cancer,* eds. H. H. Hiatt, J. D. Watson and J. A. Winsten. Cold Spring Harbor, N.Y.: Cold Spring Harbor Laboratory.

McCann, J. and Ames, B. N. 1976. Detection of carcinogens as mutagens in the *Salmonella*/microsome test: Assay of 300 chemicals: Discussion. *Proc. Natl. Acad. Sci. U.S.A.* 73:950.

McCann, J., Choi, E., Yamasaki, E. and Ames, B. N. 1975a. Detection of carcinogens as mutagens in the *Salmonella*/microsome test: Assay of 300 chemicals. *Proc. Natl. Acad. Sci. U.S.A.* 72:5135.

McCann, J., Springarn, N. E. Kobori, J. and Ames, B. N. 1975b. Detection of carcinogens as mutagens: Bacterial tester strains with R factor plasmids. *Proc. Natl. Acad. Sci. U.S.A.* 72:979.

Meselson, M. and Russell, K. 1977. Quantitative measures of carcinogenic and mutagenic potency. In *Origins of human cancer,* eds. H. H. Hiatt, J. D. Watson and J. A. Winsten. Cold Spring Harbor, N.Y.: Cold Spring Harbor Laboratory.

Miller, E. C. and Miller, J. A. 1971. The mutagenicity of chemical carcinogens: Correlations, problems, and interpretations. In *Chemical mutagens: Principles and methods for their detection,* ed. A. Hollaender, vol. 1, pp. 83–119. New York: Plenum.

Miller, J. A. and Miller, E. C. 1977. Ultimate chemical carcinogens as reactive mutagenic electrophiles. In *Origins of human cancer,* eds. H. H. Hiatt, J. D. Watson and J. A. Winsten. Cold Spring Harbor, N.Y.: Cold Spring Harbor Laboratory.

Mizutani, S. and Temin, N. M. 1976. Incorporation of noncomplementary nucleotides at high frequencies by ribodeoxyvirus DNA polymerases and *Escherichia coli* DNA polymerase I. *Biochemistry* 15:1510.

Mukai, F. H. and Goldstein, B. D. 1976. Mutagenicity of malonaldehyde, a decomposition product of peroxidized polysaturated fatty acids. *Science* 191:868.

Nishioka, H. 1975. Mutagenic activities of metal compounds in bacteria. *Mutat. Res.* 31:185.

Nomura, T. 1976. Diminution of tumorigenesis initiated by 4-nitroquinoline-1-oxide by post-treatment with caffeine in mice. *Nature (Lond.)* 260:547.

Pearson, T. A., Wang, A., Solez, K. and Heptinstall, R. H. 1975. Clonal characteristics of fibrous plaques and fatty streaks from human aortas. *Am. J. Pathol.* 81:379.

Peck, R. M., Tan, T. K. and Peck, E. B.1976. Pulmonary carcinogenesis by derivatives of polynuclear aromatic alkylating agents. *Cancer Res.* 36:2423.

Peto, R. 1977. Epidemiology, multistage models, and short-term mutagenicity tests. In *Origins of human cancer,* eds. H. H. Hiatt, J. D. Watson and J. A. Winsten. Cold Spring Harbor, N.Y.: Cold Spring Harbor Laboratory.

Prival, M. J., McCoy, E. C., Gutter, B. and Rosenkranz, H. S. 1977. Tris (2,3-dibromopropyl) phosphate: Mutagenicity of a widely used flame retardant. *Science* 195:76.

Purchase, I. F. H., Longstaff, E., Ashby, J., Styles, J. A., Anderson, D.,

Lefevre, P. A. and Westwood, F. R. 1976. Evaluation of six short term tests for detecting organic chemical carcinogens and recommendations for their use. *Nature* 264:624.

Rajwesky, M. F., Augenlicht, L. H., Biessman, H., Goth, R., Hulser, D. F., Laerum, O. D. and Ya, L. 1977. Nervous system-specific carcinogenesis by ethylnitrosourea in the rat: Molecular and cellular aspects. In *Origins of human cancer*, eds. H. H. Hiatt, J. D. Watson and J. A. Winsten. Cold Spring Harbor, N.Y.: Cold Spring Harbor Laboratory.

Searle, C. E., Harnden, D. G., Venitt, S., and Gyde, O. H. B. 1975. Carcinogenicity and mutagenicity tests of some hair colourants and constituents. *Nature (Lond.)* 255:506.

Selikoff, I. J. 1977. Cancer risk of asbestos exposure. In *Origins of human cancer*, eds. H. H. Hiatt, J. D. Watson and J. A. Winsten. Cold Spring Harbor, N.Y.: Cold Spring Harbor Laboratory.

Setlow, R. B. 1977. Xeroderma pigmentosum: Damage to DNA is involved in carcinogensis. In *Origins of human cancer*, eds. H. H. Hiatt, J. D. Watson and J. A. Winsten. Cold Spring Harbor, N.Y.: Cold Spring Harbor Laboratory.

Sincock, A. M. 1977. *In vitro* chromosomal effects of asbestos and other materials. In *Origins of human cancer*, eds. H. H. Hiatt, J. D. Watson and J. A. Winsten. Cold Spring Harbor, N.Y.: Cold Spring Harbor Laboratory.

Sirover, M. A. and Loeb, L. A. 1976. Metal-induced infidelity during DNA synthesis. *Proc. Natl. Acad. Sci. U.S.A.* 73:2331.

Sontag, J., Page, N. P. and Saffiotti, U. 1975. *Guidelines for carcinogen bioassay in small rodents*. Bethesda, Md.: Division of Cancer Cause and Prevention, National Cancer Institute.

Sugimura, T., Sato, S., Nagao, M., Yahagi, T., Matsushima, T., Seino, Y., Takeuchi, M. and Kawachi, T. 1976. Overlapping of carcinogens and mutagens. In *Fundamentals in cancer prevention*, ed. P. N. Magee et al. Tokyo: University of Tokyo Press.

Sugimura, T., Matsushima, T., Matsumoto, H., Kawachi, T., Nagao, M., Sato, S., Yahagi, T., Seino, Y., Sawamura, M. and Shirai, A. 1977. Mutagen-carcinogen and food. In *Origins of human cancer,* eds., H. H. Hiatt, J. D. Watson and J. A. Winsten. Cold Spring Harbor, N.Y.: Cold Spring Harbor Laboratory.

Swift, M., Sholman, L., Perry, M. and Chase, C. 1976. Malignant neoplasms in the families of patients with ataxia-telangiectasia. *Cancer Res.* 36:209.

Taylor, A. M. R., Metcalfe, J. A., Oxford, J. M. and Harnden, D. G. 1976. Is chromatid-type damage in ataxia telangiectasia after irradiation at G_0 a consequence of defective repair? *Nature (Lond.)* 260:441.

Tomatis, L. 1977. Value of long-term testing for the implementation of primary prevention. In *Origins of human cancer*, eds. H. H. Hiatt, J. D. Watson and J. A. Winsten. Cold Spring Harbor, N.Y.: Cold Spring Harbor Laboratory.

Trosko, J. E. and Chu, E. H. Y. 1975. The role of DNA repair and somatic mutation in carcinogenesis. *Adv. Cancer Res.* 21:391.

Venitt, S. and Levy, L. S. 1974. Mutagenicity of chromates in bacteria and its relavance to chromate carcinogenesis. *Nature (Lond.)* 250:493.

Weber, K., Wehland, J. and Herzog, W. 1976. Griseofulvin interacts with microtubules both *in vivo* and *in vitro*. *J. Mol. Biol.* 102:817.

CHAPTER 6

INDUCIBILITY BY CHEMICAL MUTAGENS OF HERITABLE TRANSLOCATIONS IN MALE AND FEMALE GERM CELLS OF MICE

W. M. Generoso, Katherine T. Cain, and Sandra W. Huff
Biology Division
Oak Ridge National Laboratory
Oak Ridge, Tennessee

D. G. Gosslee
Computer Sciences Division
Union Carbide Corporation Nuclear Division
Oak Ridge, Tennessee

INTRODUCTION

There is no longer any doubt of the need for careful and exhaustive testing and definitive evaluation of mutagenic hazards to humans because of the chromosomal aberration effects of certain chemicals. This necessity arises from the facts that (1) some chemicals are already known to be highly potent in inducing chromosomal aberrations in specific germ cells of certain laboratory mammals even at very low doses, and (2) some groups of humans have actually been exposed to chemicals (as when the use of the chemical is medically necessary) that have been shown to induce aberrations in germ cells of certain laboratory mammals (for example, Russell et al., 1974; Russell and Hunsicker, 1975). Thus the problem involves preventing human exposure to mutagenic chemicals and approximating the magnitude of genetic damage to

The research reported here was jointly sponsored by the National Center for Toxicological Research and the Energy Research and Development Administration under contract with the Union Carbide Corporation.

The authors are grateful to Mr. N. L. Cacheiro and Drs. J. G. Brewen, D. G. Hoel (National Institute of Environmental Health Sciences), and B. E. Matter (Sandoz, Ltd.) for their help in some of the studies included in this chapter, and to Drs. R. F. Kimball, E. F. Oakberg, and W. L. Russell for reviewing the manuscript.

persons who are exposed. How to solve this problem has been one of our most important concerns in environmental mutagenesis. This concern has been magnified by a number of cases in which results of tests for induction of chromosomal aberrations have not only failed to resolve the problem of mutagenicity but also created controversy over the safety of the chemicals involved. It is obvious that at present, and probably for some time to come, there will be no unanimity of opinion on the best approach to the problem of screening and evaluating chemicals for chromosomal aberration effects. However, it is reasonable to base the choice of methods and the decision about the fate of the chemicals on the benefit/risk ratio for each chemical. In any case, the most important considerations should be the reliability of data and the definitiveness of conclusions that will be drawn from the results.

If only the genetic or cytogenetic end point is used as the basis, chromosomal aberration effects can be conveniently grouped into two classes, chromosome breakage and chromosome nondisjunction. In this chapter, only studies on chromosome breakage effects of chemicals in mouse germ cells are considered, with emphasis on the information that is most pertinent to mutagenicity testing and hazard evaluation. The objective is to give an overview of the current status of research on which we base our methodology for evaluating chromosome breakage effects in mammalian germ cells. It is important to keep in mind that the problem of chemical induction of chromosome breakage in mammalian germ cells is complex, and the data presented in this chapter clearly demonstrate the futility of looking for a single best test for measurement of induced chromosome breakage in mammalian germ cells.

Nevertheless, the situation is far from hopeless. From the time chemical mutagenicity testing became a serious subject of interest to the present, there has been progress in fundamental research on mammalian *in vivo* mutagenesis directly relevant to the development of methodology. Important information comes from studies on dose-response relationships, on male and female germ-cell stage sensitivity, on comparative inducibility of various chromosome breakage effects, and on molecular dosimetry. For the most part, the information in this chapter came from our own research projects, in which one of the goals was to provide fundamental information on which to base methodology for screening and definitive evaluation of chromosomal aberration effects in mouse germ cells.

CHROMOSOME BREAKAGE IN MOUSE GERM CELLS

To date, the most striking genetic damage of known mutagenic chemicals in mammalian germ cells is chromosome breakage. Chemicals can differ greatly from one another in their effectiveness in inducing chromosome breakage and in the types of germ cells affected. The high efficacy of certain chemicals in inducing such breakage makes this class of damage a major concern when the potential hazards to humans of various chemicals are evaluated. Chromosome breakage can result in chromosome loss (which often leads to embryonic lethality and rarely to viable aneuploids) or in viable reciprocal translocations and inversions. Chromosome breakage effects in mouse germ cells may be measured by using any of the following end points: dominant-lethal mutations, sex-chromosome loss, heritable translocations, heritable inversions, and chromosome breakage scored cytologically in meiotic and gonial cells. The usefulness of these end points for chemical screening and hazard evaluation will be discussed below.

All of our heritable translocation studies in males were done by treating (101 $\times$ C3H)F_1 males with mutagen and then mating them to untreated (SEC $\times$ C57BL)F_1 females. Only male progeny from this mating were tested for translocation heterozygosity. For details of the procedure, see pp. 123–125.

Chromosome Breakage in Mammalian Male Germ Cells

Because genetic studies are generally easier to do in males than in females, the bulk of published results on mammalian chemical mutagenesis has come from studies on male mice. Consequently, the methodology for detection of induced chromosome breakage in male germ cells is considerably better developed than that for females. In trying to understand the current status of methodology in male mice and what to expect of further development, it is important to keep in mind that the most sensitive end point for measuring induced chromosome breakage can vary from one chemical to another depending on the stage in spermatogenesis affected.

Postmeiotic male germ cell. It is generally known that the alkylating chemicals effective in inducing chromosome breakage in male germ cells in mammals are most effective on postmeiotic stages—that is, spermatozoa and/or spermatids—and that the most sensitive period may vary with the chemical. In addition to radiation, a number of alkylating chemicals that are effective inducers of dominant-lethal mutations have also been found to induce heritable translocations and heritable inversions in the same postmeiotic male germ-cell stages in which the dominant lethals are induced. These findings have not only strengthened the belief that dominant-lethal mutations induced in postmeiotic male germ cells are primarily due to breaks, but have also made it possible to compare the relative usefulness of dominant lethals, translocations, and inversions as indicators of induced chromosome breakage at these germ-cell stages.

Relative sensitivities can be compared accurately by use of a range of doses that includes dose levels that do not induce a significant effect for one of the end points. Such comparative studies have been done for dominant-lethal mutations and heritable translocations. The first of these studies involved the compound ethyl methanesulfonate (EMS) (Generoso et al., 1974a). An EMS dose-effect study was performed with doses ranging from 50 to 300 mg/kg. The frequencies of dominant-lethal mutations and heritable translocations were measured in germ cells treated as early spermatozoa and late spermatids. The EMS data from Generoso et al., 1974a are shown in Tables 1 and 2. The only similar study completed so far was with the compound triethylenemelamine (TEM). Effects of TEM dose on the induction of dominant-lethal mutations and heritable translocations were studied for midspermatids. The TEM dominant-lethal data shown in Table 3 are from Matter and Generoso (1974), while the comparative heritable translocation data in Table 4 are presented here for the first time. Both the EMS and TEM comparative studies were performed on germ cells that are most sensitive to dominant-lethal induction and presumably also to induction of heritable translocations by the respective chemicals.

In the EMS and TEM studies, the lowest doses at which clear-cut increases in induced dominant-lethal mutations were detected were 150 and 0.05 mg/kg, respectively, whereas significant increases in heritable translocations were already detectable at 50 and 0.0125 mg/kg, respectively. In the 50 mg/kg EMS dose and 0.0125 mg/kg TEM dose, the translocation induction rates were 6 in 853 and 8 in 927 first-generation males tested, respectively. These rates are significantly higher ($p < 0.01$) than the cumulative spontaneous rate of 3 translocations in 2,602 males. It is expected that for these two compounds, dominant-lethal mutations were also induced at doses lower than 150 and 0.05 mg/kg (for EMS and TEM, respectively) since only a single break is required for each lethal event. In fact, although the effects were not statistically significant, there were some indications of induced dominant lethality at the 100 mg/kg EMS and 0.035 mg/kg TEM doses. Nevertheless, because of the high and variable spontaneous frequency of dead implants compared with the low spontaneous frequency of heritable translocations, it is clear that for these two compounds, heritable translocations are a much more sensitive and definitive end point of induced chromosome breakage than dominant-lethal mutations. Obviously, this difference between the two end points is particularly significant at low levels of effect, which, in practice, are the most difficult cases in mutagenicity testing.

Another consequence of chromosome breakage in postmeiotic stages of the male mouse is the production of paracentric inversions that can be passed to some of the first-generation progeny. Such progeny are thus heterozygotes for the inversion. EMS, TEM, and X-rays, which are effective in inducing heritable translocations in the postmeiotic stages in males, have also been studied for induction of heritable inversions in similar germ-cell stages (Roderick and Hawes, 1974). A comparison of the relative inducibility of the two heritable end points can be made (Table 5), even though there are some differences in the conditions under which the frequencies were obtained. First, in the inversion studies males from inbred strain DBA/2J received the mutagenic treatment, while in the translocation studies hybrid (101 $\times$ C3H)F$_1$ males were used. Second, in the inversion studies the animals scored were conceived during the first 2 wk after treatment. In the translocation studies, the X-ray data were also based on progeny conceived during the first 2 wk

TABLE 1 Effect of Ethyl Methanesulfonate Dose on the Induction of Dominant-Lethal Mutations[a]

EMS dose (mg/kg)	No. of mated females[b]	No. of fertile matings	No. of total implants (avg/fertile mating)	No. of living embryos (avg/fertile mating)	No. of dead implants (%)	Living embryos (% of control)	
						Among fertile matings	Among all mated females
0	22	22	7.7	7.1	7.1	–	–
100	25	22	7.5	7.0	7.3	99	86
150	21	21	7.2	5.9[c]	18.5	83	82
200	27	25	6.4[d]	3.5	45.3	49	46
250	29	15[c]	4.5[c]	1.1	71.2	15	8
300	21	1	2.0	0	100.0	0	0

[a]From Generoso et al., 1974a.
[b]All matings occurred 6.5–7.5 days after treatment.
[c]$p < 0.01$ for comparison with control.
[d]$p < 0.05$ for comparison with control.

TABLE 2　Effect of Ethyl Methanesulfonate Dose on the Induction
of Reciprocal Translocations[a]

EMS dose (mg/kg)	No. of male progeny tested[b]	No. of partially sterile males	No. of sterile males	Translocation frequency (%)
0	1,218	0	1[c]	0.08
50	853	2	4	0.70[d]
100	1,013	8	10	1.78
150	621	36	9	7.25
200	246	52	27	32.11

[a]From Generoso et al., 1974a.
[b]All male progeny were conceived 6.5–7.5 days after treatment.
[c]The testes weight of this animal was 0.04 g.
[d]$p = 0.022$ for comparison with control.

after irradiation, but for EMS and TEM the progeny tested were conceived during the few days when dominant-lethal, and presumably also translocation, effects are known to be maximum. Third, while the TEM dose was the same in the two studies, higher average doses of EMS and X-rays were used in the inversion study. Thus, higher frequencies of translocations could be expected at the doses of EMS and X-rays used for the inversion studies. Despite these differences in experimental conditions, on the whole there seems to be little doubt that heritable translocations are a considerably more sensitive end point than heritable inversions for detection of chromosome breakage induced in postmeiotic male germ cells.

　　Such a large difference in the observed rates is worth some comment. Both translocations and inversions are products of two breakage events; if the occurrence of a break is random within and between chromosomes, it is possible that the difference in the recovery between translocations and inversions lies in the rates at which they are formed in postmeiotic male germ cells in mammals. On the other hand, this difference may be nonexistent or much less in mammalian oocytes (see p. 118). Another possible explanation lies in the methods used for detecting the two types of aberrations. It is likely that the great majority of translocations confer partial or complete sterility in heterozygous males, and detection of such reduction in fertility is rather simple (see pp. 123–125). The method used for detecting inversion heterozygotes, on the other hand, not only involves considerable effort but is capable of detecting only large inversions. The heritable inversion method used is essentially a search for high frequencies of bridges in the first meiotic anaphase in male progeny. One of the testes is removed and histologically prepared for bridge analysis. The animal is kept alive and bred for further studies if the incidence of anaphase bridges is at least 15% (the "background"

TABLE 3 Effect of Triethylenemelamine Dose on the Induction of Dominant-Lethal Mutations[a]

Treatment	Dose (mg/kg)	No. of mated females[b]	No. of pregnant females	Total No. of implants (avg/fertile mating)	No. of living embryos (avg/fertile mating)	Dead implants (%)	Living embryos (% of control) Among fertile females	Living embryos (% of control) Among all mated females
Control[c]	—	61	59	9.2	8.7	5.5	100	100
TEM	0.035	55	55	9.3	8.3	11.1	95.4	98.8
TEM	0.05	55	54	8.9	7.4[d]	17.6	85.1	86.9
TEM	0.1	55	52	8.4[d]	5.3	36.9	60.9	59.5
TEM	0.2	54	51	6.7	2.4	64.2	27.6	27.4
TEM	0.3	54	25[d]	5.3	1.3	75.9	14.9	7.1
TEM	0.4	56	15	3.9	1.0	74.6	11.5	4.0
TEM	0.8	25	1	1.0	—	—	—	—

[a]From Matter and Generoso, 1974.
[b]All matings occurred 11.5–15.5 days after treatment.
[c]Hank's balanced salt solution (HBSS).
[d]$p < 0.05$ for comparison with control.

TABLE 4 Effect of Triethylenemelamine Dose on the Induction
of Heritable Translocations

Dose (mg/kg)	No. of male progeny tested[a]	No. of partially sterile males	No. of sterile males	Translocation frequency (%)
0.2	204	36	23	28.9
0.1	466	48	22	15.0
0.05	597	25	10	5.9
0.025	732	5	5	1.4
0.0125	927	5	3	0.86[b]
Control	2,602	0	3	0.12

[a]All male progeny were conceived 11.5–15.5 days after treatment.
[b]$p < 0.01$ for a comparison with control.

frequency is about 4%)—that is, assuming that the incidence of bridges is directly proportional to the length of inversion, the minimum length of the inverted segment is equivalent to 7.5 centimorgans. Detection of shorter inversions appears to be difficult.

Chromosome breakage in early-meiotic and differentiating spermatogonial stages. Recent studies in male mice with two mutagenic chemicals, mitomycin C and 6-mercaptopurine, have contributed significantly to our

TABLE 5 Relative Inducibility of Heritable Inversions and Heritable
Translocations in the Postmeiotic Stages of Male Mice

Treatment	Dose	No. of offspring tested	No. of progeny with aberration
		Inversions[a]	
Control	–	44	0
X-ray	700–1,000 R	1,557	15 (0.96)[b]
EMS	200–400 mg/kg	156	1 (0.64)
TEM	0.2 mg/kg	97	3 (3.09)
		Translocations	
Control	–	2,602	3 (0.12)
X-ray	700 R	151	41 (27.15)
EMS	200 mg/kg	246	79 (32.11)
TEM	0.2 mg/kg	204	59 (28.92)

[a]All data on heritable inversions were taken from Roderick and Hawes, 1974.
[b]Numbers in parentheses are percentages.

present knowledge of the overall picture of chromosome breakage effects of chemicals in male germ cells. Until results with these two compounds became available, (1) the chemicals that clearly induced chromosome breakage in male germ cells were either alkylating agents or were known to be transformed *in vivo* into alkylating forms, and (2) clear-cut chromosome breakage effects of such chemicals in males were found only when postmeiotic germ cells or late spermatocytes were treated. The antileukemic purine analogue, 6-mercapto-purine, is an exception—it is not an alkylating chemical nor is it known to be transformed into one, and the chromosome breakage effects were induced only in germ cells that were presumably in late-differentiating spermatogonial and early-meiotic spermatocyte stages. The chromosome breakage effect of this compound was first detected as clear-cut increases in induced dominant-lethal mutations (Ray and Hyneck, 1973; Generoso et al., 1977a). Subsequent cytological analysis of the germ cells in the diakinesis-metaphase I stage revealed that chromatid deletions were the likely cause of dominant lethality (Generoso et al., 1977a). The cytological study also revealed, unexpectedly, that the relative yield of chromatid interchanges was very low. We have subsequently found that 6-mercaptopurine induces virtually no heritable translocations in the same germ-cell stages (Table 6) (Generoso et al., 1977b). These findings clearly demonstrate a marked difference in the relative rates by which dominant-lethal mutations and heritable translocations are produced in postmeiotic stages on the one hand and in the early-meiotic and differen-tiating gonial stages on the other. While heritable translocations are a more sensitive end point in postmeiotic stages, the reverse seems to be true in the early-meiotic and differentiating gonial stages. However, it should be noted that the comparative inducibility of dominant lethals and heritable trans-locations in the early-meiotic and differentiating gonial stages was studied only for the compound 6-mercaptopurine. More information on these cell stages is certainly needed.

Mitomycin C is metabolized *in vivo* into alkylating intermediates, but it was the first chemical agent found to clearly induce chromosomal aberrations in differentiating spermatogonia. It was shown, by direct observation of spermatogonial metaphases, to cause a high incidence of chromatid breaks in spermatogonia that were largely in differentiating stages (Adler, 1973, 1974). At these stages this compound also induced a clearly demonstrable effect on the number of implants but not on the incidence of dead implantations (Ehling, 1971). Thus, the reduction in number of implants could conceivably result from cell killing and/or preimplantation dominant lethality. It is difficult to distinguish between these two effects, although Kratochvilova (1973) claims that there is a significant level of preimplantation dominant lethality. If mitomycin C does induce dominant lethality in these cell stages, it is interesting to point out that the lethality is expressed at a different time than with 6-mercaptopurine—that is, pre- versus postimplantation.

Chromosome breakage in spermatogonia stem cell. One of the most

TABLE 6 Chemical Induction of Heritable Translocations in Oocytes and Early-Meiotic Spermatocytes and Late-Differentiating Spermatogonia of Mice

Germ-cell stages	Posttreatment interval when male progeny were conceived (days)	Chemical treatment	Dose (mg/kg)	No. of male progeny tested	No. of partially sterile males	No. of sterile males
Dictyate oocytes	0.5–23.5[a]	IMS[b]	75	549	0	2[c]
	23.5–156.5	IMS	75	915	1	1[d]
Early-meiotic spermatocytes and late-differentiating spermatogonia	31.5–35.5	6-mercapto-purine	196	215	1	0
			150	400	0	4[e]

[a]Oocytes fertilized within 0.5 day after treatment were already in postdictyate stages at the time of treatment.
[b]Isopropyl methanesulfonate.
[c]Testes weight and cytology of these males were normal.
[d]This male died before cytological analysis was done.
[e]Cytological analysis of these males revealed that one was normal and three were XYY (Cacheiro and Generoso, 1975).

118

striking differences between radiation and chemical mutagens studied so far is that radiation is highly effective in inducing chromosome breakage in spermatogonia stem cells, while alkylating chemicals are almost ineffective. This is a paradox, because some of these chemicals, like X-rays, are potent chromosome breakers in the postmeiotic stages and affect spermatogonia stem-cell survival. This difference first became clear from the cytological studies at the diakinesis-metaphase I stage done by a number of workers, who found that radiation is effective in inducing reciprocal translocations on treated spermatogonia stem cells, but the alkylating chemicals studied so far have been virtually ineffective. It is well known, however, that very often a reciprocal translocation does not manifest itself at the diakinesis-metaphase I stage, and it is possible that certain chemicals may produce predominantly such translocations in spermatogonia stem cells. Thus there remains the possibility that chemically induced translocations not detectable cytologically can be passed through some of the progeny. To check on this possibility and to have a thorough understanding of the chemical hazard to spermatogonia stem cells, we have studied the induction of heritable reciprocal translocations at this cell stage with chemicals such as cyclophosphamide (350 and 400 mg/kg), tris(1-aziridinyl)phosphine oxide (TEPA) (20, 25, and 30 mg/kg), and TEM (3.0 and 4.0 mg/kg). These chemicals were chosen because, like radiation, they are known to be potent chromosome breakers in postmeiotic male germ cells and they affect spermatogonial survival. In this study chemically treated males were caged individually with untreated females beginning 42 days after injection.

In all experimental groups, the treated males were sterile at the time of caging with females. The sterile periods were short among cyclophosphamide-treated males (3–4 days for the two doses), while for TEM and TEPA doses the sterile periods were long (17–54 days). Combining all doses for each chemical, the incidences of partially sterile and sterile male progeny were 2 and 4 in 1,633 tested for TEM, 1 and 4 in 1,148 tested for cyclophosphamide, and 0 and 7 in 1,031 for TEPA (Table 7). The sterile males have been studied cytologically by N. L. Cacheiro, M. Swartout, and L. B. Russell in our division, and the results indicate that, unlike sterility induced in postmeiotic stages (Cacheiro et al., 1974), sterility induced in spermatogonia may have causes other than translocation heterozygosity (Cacheiro and Generoso, 1975; Cacheiro and Swartout, 1975). The three partially sterile males (two from TEM and one from cyclophosphamide) were all confirmed cytologically as translocation heterozygotes. Nevertheless, if the rates in the experimental groups are compared with the spontaneous level of 4 in 4,423 tested (pooled from controls of various experiments), none of the chemicals studied significantly induced transmissible translocations in mouse spermatogonia. On the other hand, X-rays given at optimum conditions induced unequivocal increases in heritable translocations at this cell stage (Ford et al., 1969; Reddi, 1965; Generoso et al., 1974b), although the rates were lower than would be

TABLE 7 Chemical Induction of Heritable Translocations in Mouse
Spermatogonia Stem Cells

Chemical mutagen	Dose (mg/kg)	No. of male progeny tested	No. of partially sterile males[a]	No. of sterile males
TEM	3–4	1,633	2	4
Cyclophosphamide	350–400	1,148	1	4[b]
TEPA	20–30	1,031	0	7
Control (HBSS)	(0.8 ml per mouse)	4,392	1	3[c]

[a]All partially sterile animals were confirmed cytologically as translocation heterozygotes.
[b]One was confirmed cytologically as a translocation heterozygote.
[c]These sterile males have small testes typical of sterile translocation heterozygotes produced through postmeiotic treatment of male mice with EMS, X-rays, or TEM (see Generoso et al., 1974a; Cacheiro et al., 1974).

expected on the basis of the cytological frequency determined at diakinesis-metaphase I. Thus, for both X-rays and the chemicals studied so far, there is generally good correspondence between cytologically scored and transmissible reciprocal translocations.

Induction of Heritable Translocations in Female Mice

A number of chemicals that are known to be effective dominant-lethal inducers in postmeiotic male germ cells have been found to induce dominant-lethal effects in dictyate oocytes of mice (see Generoso and Cosgrove, 1973 for review). While it is generally known that one of the consequences of chromosome breakage in postmeiotic stages in males is the formation of reciprocal translocations, no information for such chemical effects on oocytes has been available until now. We studied the inducibility by isopropyl methanesulfonate (IMS) of heritable translocations in dictyate oocytes of mice that were in various stages of follicular development. IMS was chosen because it is an effective inducer of dominant-lethal mutations both in postmeiotic stages in males and in dictyate oocytes (Ehling et al., 1972; Generoso et al., 1971a). (SEC × C57BL)F_1 female mice (10–12 wk old) were injected ip with a dose of 75 mg/kg of IMS. This dose, in addition to dominant-lethal effects on oocytes in advanced stages of follicular development, also affects survival of young oocytes (Generoso et al., 1971b). However, the degree of cytotoxicity still permits production of progeny from oocytes treated at the early stage. Treated females were caged individually with untreated males carrying the sex-linked gene *Greasy* immediately after injection. A total of 1,464 male progeny were tested for translocation heterozygosity (see Table 6). Of these, 549 were conceived within 24 days after treatment, and 915 at later periods.

It should be noted that there is a considerable dominant-lethal effect on oocytes ovulated within 24 days after treatment. Two sterile and no partially sterile males were found among progeny conceived at the early period, and one sterile and one partially sterile male were found among progeny conceived in the later period. The partially sterile male was confirmed cytologically as a translocation heterozygote. One of the sterile males died before cytological analysis was done, and the other two that were analyzed (normal testes weights) did not show cytological evidence of translocation heterozygosity. Thus, the results indicate that IMS, which is an effective inducer of dominant-lethal mutations in dictyate oocytes, does not induce a significant increase in the incidence of translocations in cells that were transmissible to male offspring.

Our results are similar to those of Russell and Wickham (1957) and Gilliavod and Leonard (1973) with X-rays in that no translocations were recovered when male progeny were scored. Searle and Beechey (1974), on the other hand, claimed that although they, too, did not detect transmissible translocations among male progeny from X-irradiated oocytes, induced translocations were recovered in female progeny (3 confirmed translocations in 294 female progeny tested). This finding must be verified, because the number of female progeny scored was rather small and because they did not find the same effect with fission neutrons.

FERTILITY OF MALE TRANSLOCATION HETEROZYGOTES

A thorough knowledge of the fertility of male translocation heterozygotes produced by various agents is essential for the development of procedures for large-scale screening of these animals (see pp. 123–125). Male translocation heterozygotes produced from treatment of male postmeiotic stages are either completely sterile or partially sterile. In Tables 2 and 4 we showed that about one-third of EMS- or TEM-induced translocations were completely sterile, while two-thirds were partially sterile. Our new data with 700 R of acute X-rays in postmeiotic stages also show a similar ratio of partially sterile to sterile translocations (30 to 18, respectively) (Generoso et al., 1974c).

Two sets of fertility data are available for the partially sterile male progeny produced from the EMS and X-ray studies. The first set was obtained by caging each male with a young female of the (SEC $\times$ C57BL)F$_1$ stock to produce at least four litters. The second set was obtained by mating each male to at least six virgin (C3H $\times$ C57BL)F$_1$ females, which were killed during pregnancy for uterine analysis (Table 8). In the case of TEM-induced partially sterile male translocation heterozygotes, only data on killed females are available (Table 8). On the basis of live births, the average fertilities of EMS- and X-ray-induced partially sterile male translocation heterozygotes were 43 and 39% that of normal males, respectively. These fertility reductions are

TABLE 8 Average Fertility of Partially Sterile Male Translocation Heterozygotes Produced from Postmeiotic Treatment of Male Mice[a]

Treatment	Class	No. of males tested	No. of implants[a] (avg)	No. of living embryos[a] (avg)	Dead implants (%)
X-ray[b]	Partially sterile	30	9.1	3.9 (43%)[c]	57
	Normal	39	9.6	9.0	6
TEM[b]	Partially sterile	119	9.2	4.2 (44%)[c]	54
	Normal	69	10.0	9.5	5
EMS[d]	Partially sterile	98	9.3	4.5 (44%)[c]	58
	Normal	39	10.7	10.2	5

[a]Six pregnancies were analyzed for each partially sterile male and three for each normal male.
[b]Data from Generoso et al., 1974c.
[c]Percentage of normal.
[d]Data from Generoso et al., 1974a.

comparable to those obtained for killed females. The average numbers of living embryos for the EMS-, TEM-, and X-ray-induced partially sterile translocation heterozygotes were 44, 43, and 44% of that of normal males, respectively. Data on killed females show that fertilization involving sperm carrying unbalanced chromosome constitutions leads to the death of embryos shortly before or shortly after implantation in most cases. This is indicated by the observation that the reduction in the number of living embryos is attributable mainly to an accompanying increase in dead implantation. However, a small proportion of embryonic loss occurred in early cleavage stages, as indicated by consistently lower numbers of implantations in the partially sterile groups.

There is overwhelming evidence that partial sterility alone can be taken as an unequivocal indicator of a reciprocal translocation (Generoso et al., 1974a). Also, there are now strong indications that at least the great majority of sterile male progeny induced from treatment of postmeiotic male germ cells are also translocation heterozygotes. The extensive cytological and histological study by Cacheiro et al. (1974) clearly showed that the great majority of sterile sons produced by fathers postmeiotically treated with EMS or X-rays were carriers of a translocation, and that a majority of the translocations were of the autosome-autosome type. Furthermore, they found that translocations that cause sterility, rather than partial sterility, in males appear to be those in which at least one of the breaks occurs close to one end of a chromosome. The great majority of sterile males with translocations had distinctly small testes (about one-third those of normals) (Generoso et al., 1974a). In most cases spermatogenesis is blocked at various stages of meiosis; for the few that had sperm in the epididymis, the number of sperm was low, most of the sperm were nonmotile, and in many cases there was a high frequency of sperm with bent tails or other abnormalities. Although the study of Cacheiro et al. on TEM-induced sterile males (Table 4) is still in progress, the situation is clearly similar to that of EMS and X-rays.

A SEQUENTIAL PROCEDURE FOR THE DETECTION OF MALE TRANSLOCATION HETEROZYGOTES

Screening for translocation heterozygosity among first-generation progeny can be done either by cytological analysis or by fertility testing; it is more readily accomplished in males than in females. Cytological screening of diakinesis-metaphase I spermatocytes of male progeny has the advantage of requiring a relatively small animal space. On the other hand, because of the mechanics involved in the cytological preparation and scoring of meiotic chromosomes, it is obviously relatively less suitable for large-scale screening than the fertility test.

Screening by fertility testing of male progeny has been accomplished by either of the following methods. The more conventional procedure is to mate each male progeny to three or more different females. Each female is killed at midpregnancy, and the living and dead implants are counted. This method is very reliable and recommended for use in small-scale studies. The procedure most suitable for large-scale screening of male translocation heterozygotes employs a sequential analysis of the litter size (Generoso, 1973; Generoso et al., 1973a). With this procedure it is esssential to know beforehand the reproductive performance of females that will be used to test the males, and it is desirable to use females of high fertility. Many stocks of female mice are suitable for use in this procedure, and the general features described below for (SEC × C57BL)F_1 females should be applicable to other stocks of comparable fertility. Each male progeny to be tested is caged with an (SEC × C57BL)F_1 female as soon as he reaches sexual maturity. The females are used for the first time when they are 10–12 wk old. Breeding pens are checked for newly born mice when they are expected (i.e., pens are examined daily during weekdays beginning 18 days after pairing and 18 days after appearance of a litter). Young are discarded immediately after they are scored. For each male, if the size of the first litter is 10 or more, the male is declared fertile and discarded immediately after scoring the litter. If the size of the first litter is less than 10, a second litter is scored. If the second litter is 10 or more, the male is declared fertile and discarded; otherwise the male is separated for further testing. Often a male has already mated before separation, and a third litter is produced. Again, if the size of the third litter is 10 or more, the male is declared fertile and discarded; otherwise the male is a suspect and is mated with three virgin females, which are killed during pregnancy. In either case, another male is placed with the female 1 wk after the litter is born, and the same procedure is followed until the last male is added no later than after the tenth litter. The lapse of 1 wk is required so that parentage of litters will not be confused.

From our study of the fertility of partially sterile translocation heterozygotes induced by EMS (Generoso et al., 1974a) or X-rays (Generoso et al., 1974c), the probabilities that a partially sterile male will sire a litter of 10 or more on (SEC $\times$ C57BL)F_1 females are estimated as 0.02 and 0.0056, respectively. In the EMS study 9 litters (which were sired by independent males) out of 462 were of sizes 10 or more. In the X-ray study, of the 177 litters (sired by 30 partially sterile males) only 1 had more than 9 offspring. Thus the probability of not detecting a translocation heterozygote with the cutoff point of 10 or more is quite small.

The reproductive data were analyzed from a sample of 428 (SEC $\times$ C57BL)F_1 females mated with 2,302 males (a very small number of these are translocation heterozygotes), where a litter size of 10 or more in the first, second, or third litter sired by a male was used as the indicator of full fertility. These females produced a minimum of 10 litters each. Females that were caged with sterile males were not included. The cumulative proportions of males that were declared fertile on the basis of one, two, and three litters were 0.65, 0.88, and 0.91 respectively. Only 9% of the males had to be mated further with three virgin females each. An average of 5.38 males were tested per female.

Thus, a large percentage of males can be declared fertile by the simple procedure of counting the number of live births in, at most, three litters, with only small risk (estimated as 0.0056–0.02) of declaring a partially sterile translocation normal. Since (SEC $\times$ C57BL)F_1 females normally produce 12 good litters, it is now possible to test several males per female instead of killing 3 or more females per male, as in the old procedure. The procedure described above is now routinely used in our laboratory for screening male translocation heterozygotes produced in chemical and radiation experiments; it can be modified depending on the reproductive nature of the stock of females used in the screening and on the efficiency desired.

At present the spontaneous frequency of heritable translocations pooled from the controls of various experiments in our laboratory is 0.0009 (4 translocations in 4,392 male progeny tested). This rate is probably higher than the actual spontaneous level because the three sterile males, although typical of sterile translocation heterozygotes, were not cytologically analyzed and may instead be carriers of other types of aberrations. By using this spontaneous rate and specified levels of significance α and power, the number of male progeny needed for testing at each given rate of induction can be calculated (Table 9). In Table 9, C is the critical (minimum) number of translocations that must be observed in a sample of N males in order to declare that the observed rate π is significantly greater than the spontaneous rate. The probability of falsely claiming significance is α. All calculations were

TABLE 9 Minimum Number (N) of Male Progeny Needed for Testing to Detect (with a Probability of at least 0.95) a Translocation Rate of π

N	C^a	α^b	π
300	2	0.031	0.020
400	2	0.052	0.015
700	3	0.026	0.010
1,800	5	0.025	0.005
2,600	6	0.033	0.004

[a]Minimum number of translocations needed to declare that the observed rate is significantly larger than the spontaneous rate of 0.000904.
[b]Actual level of significance for a nominal level of 0.05.

based on the binomial distribution and on the assumption that the spontaneous frequency of heritable translocations is known. As pointed out earlier, the spontaneous frequency was actually estimated by pooling various control groups. Because of the discrete nature of the binomial distribution, the actual level of significance changes as the sample size changes; thus it is not possible to maintain a constant level of significance, such as $\alpha = 0.05$. Values of C and N can be chosen such that $\alpha \leqslant 0.05$. However, we have arbitrarily chosen an α between 0.05 and 0.06 in cases where the alternative was to use a very small value of α, such as $\alpha < 0.01$. In all cases, sample sizes were calculated so that the level of significance was close to 0.05 and so that the probability was at least 0.95 for detecting a given translocation rate π.

For example, in the EMS comparative dominant-lethal and translocation studies (Generoso et al., 1974a) it was found that the lowest dose at which a significant increase in dominant-lethal mutations was detected was 150 mg/kg. EMS doses of 50 or 100 mg/kg, on the other hand, induced significant increases in heritable translocations at rates of 0.7 and 1.78%. From Table 9, 400 male progeny can be calculated as the minimum number that must be tested in order to detect, with a probability of 0.95, a translocation rate of $\pi = 1.5\%$, a rate that is lower than that induced by the EMS dose of 100 mg/kg. As π decreases, N increases; but the sample size of 400 males is certainly not too large to make large-scale testing difficult.

Improvement of the translocation procedure, especially in the determination of statistical limits and levels of significance, is expected as more data become available on the comparative dominant-lethal and translocation dose-effect studies with a number of mutagenic chemicals and on the spontaneous level of translocations. So far, we have studied the fertility of male translocation heterozygotes and developed a procedure for screening them on a large scale. We are presently studying the fertility of female translocation heterozygotes. It will be a great improvement if a simple procedure can be used for testing both male and female progeny for translocation heterozygosity

CONCLUSION

In the discussion above we have attempted to present an overall picture, as we see it at present, of the inducibility of heritable translocations in various germ-cell stages in mice relative to other end points of chromosome breakage effects, primarily dominant-lethal mutations, heritable inversions, and cytologically scored aberrations. The picture is not complete yet, because only a few chemicals have been tested and no information is available for some germ-cell stages. Nevertheless, it can already be said that no single end point will be adequate in the detection and evaluation of all types of chromosome breakage events induced by various mutagenic chemicals at all stages in gametogenesis. Furthermore, it appears that it will be essential to employ the heritable translocations, dominant-lethal mutations, and cytological analysis of spermatogonial metaphases and diakinesis-metaphase I spermatocytes for a comprehensive evaluation of chromosome breakage events of chemicals in the mouse.

Heritable translocations are the most reliable end point of chromosome breakage induced in postmeiotic stages in males. These stages are very important in mutagenicity testing because of their proved high sensitivity to various alkylating chemicals. For instance, the fact that TEM induced a significant increase in heritable translocations in mouse spermatids at a dose of 0.0125 mg/kg is quite significant from the practical standpoint, because it shows that a chemical can distinctly increase heritable translocations at a dose level far below the lethal dose [in this case only 1/400 of a lethal dose (Matter and Generoso, 1974)]. This finding clearly demonstrates the importance of the postmeiotic male germ cells not only in the routine screening for chromosome breakage effects but also in terms of genetic hazards to humans. It is interesting to point out that both dominant-lethal and heritable-translocation end points are markedly more sensitive than teratological end points in detecting biological damage by TEM (Matter and Generoso, 1974). Even though alkylating chemicals like TEM are considered a unique class of compounds in terms of their mutagenic potential, the human exposure to many chemical compounds, which is generally either continuous or repetitive, can often be at relatively much higher doses, and some of these chemicals may be transformed *in vivo* into mutagenic forms.

The dominant-lethal (Ray and Hyneck, 1973; Generoso et al., 1977a), cytological (Generoso et al., 1977a), and heritable-translocation data (Table 6) with 6-mercaptopurine have shown the importance of the early-meiotic male germ cells and differentiating spermatogonia in the screening of chemicals for chromosome breakage effects in mouse germ cells. Furthermore, for the first time we have a good example of a nonalkylating chemical that clearly induces chromosome breakage in the germ line of male mice. The most significant features of the 6-mercaptopurine effect are that chromosome breakage was induced only in late-differentiating spermatogonia and very early spermatocytes and that dominant-lethal mutations and cytologically scored breaks appear to be more sensitive end points than heritable translocations. This finding raises three important questions. First, what classes of chemical compounds induce chromosome breakage only at these stages? 6-Mercaptopurine is a purine analogue, and as such would be expected to affect only germ cells that are undergoing DNA synthesis. But we have no direct proof that this was the case for the chromosome breakage effects observed only in late-differentiating spermatogonia and early spermatocytes. Second, do chromosome breakage events induced at these stages always lead to lethality and not to heritable translocations—that is, predominantly deletions and very few interchanges? Third, if deletions are the predominant types, do they result in the production of viable aneuploids? To answer these three questions, we are studying these germ-cell stages and other compounds that are expected to be effective only on cells that are undergoing DNA synthesis.

All information available on the spermatogonia stem cell indicates that this germ-cell stage is virtually unaffected by the chromosome breakage effects of known mutagenic chemicals. Unless this general picture changes as more chemicals are studied, there seems to be no need for doing cytological, dominant-lethal, or heritable-translocation studies on spermatogonia stem cells in the practical screening for chromosome breakage effects of chemicals.

The use of female mice in mutagenicity testing of chemicals is now necessary in view of the extensive information available on the antischistosomal drug hycanthone (Russell et al., 1974; Russell and Hunsicker, 1975; Generoso et al., 1972) and on IMS (Generoso et al., 1973b). Hycanthone was ineffective in inducing dominant-lethal mutations in male mice (Generoso et al., 1972). However, when females were treated a few days prior to mating, presumed dominant-lethal effects were induced (Generoso et al., 1972). Subsequently, Russell and co-workers (1974, 1975) found, in the same oocyte stages but not in earlier stages, a clear-cut increase in X-chromosome loss in the offspring of mothers treated with a dose of hycanthone that produced dominant-lethal effects. Thus, like 6-mercaptopurine, hycanthone is a non-alkylating chemical that is clearly a mutagen in the mouse. Results with IMS (Generoso et al., 1973b) indicate that this compound is effective in inducing sex-chromosome loss in mouse oocytes, in addition to dominant-lethal mutations. Although the mechanisms for the induction of dominant-lethal mutations and sex-chromosome loss with hycanthone and IMS are not known, the use of these two end points in evaluating chromosome aberration effects of chemicals in female germ cells is clearly necessary. On the other hand, the evidence presented in Table 6 suggests that heritable translocations may not be a useful end point for chromosome breakage effects induced by chemicals in mouse oocytes.

REFERENCES

Adler, I. D. 1973. Cytogenetic effect of mitomycin C on mouse spermatogonia. *Mutat. Res.* 21:20–21.

Adler, I. D. 1974. Comparative cytogenetic study after treatment of mouse spermatogonia with mitomycin C. *Mutat. Res.* 23:369–379.

Cacheiro, N. L. A. and Generoso, W. M. 1975. Cytological studies of sterility in sons of mice treated at spermatogonial or early spermatocyte stages with mutagenic chemicals. *Mouse News Lett.* 53:52.

Cacheiro, N. L. A. and Swartout, M. S. 1975. Cytological studies of sterility in sons of mice treated at spermatogonial or oocyte stages with mutagenic chemicals. *Genetics* 80:s18.

Cacheiro, N. L. A., Russell, L. B. and Swartout, M. S. 1974. Translocations, the predominant cause of total sterility in sons of mice treated with mutagens. *Genetics* 76:73–91.

Ehling, U. H. 1971. Comparison of radiation- and chemically-induced dominant lethal mutations in male mice. *Mutat. Res.* 11:35–44.

Ehling, U. H., Doherty, D. G. and Malling, H. V. 1972. Differential spermatogenic response of mice to the induction of dominant-lethal mutations by *n*-propyl methanesulfonate and isopropyl methanesulfonate. *Mutat. Res.* 15:175–184.

Ford, C. E., Searle, A. G., Evans, E. P. and West, B. J. 1969. Differential transmission of translocations induced in spermatogonia of mice by irradiation. *Cytogenetics* 8:447–470.

Generoso, W. M. 1973. Evaluation of chromosome aberration effects of chemicals on mouse germ cells. *Environ. Health Perspect.* 6:13–22.

Generoso, W. M. and Cosgrove, G. E. 1973. Total reproductive capacity in female mice: Chemical effects and their analysis. In *Chemical mutagens: Principles and methods for their detection*, ed. A. Hollaender, vol. 3, pp. 241–258. New York: Plenum.

Generoso, W. M., Huff, S. W. and Stout, S. K. 1971a. Chemically induced dominant-lethal mutations and cell killing in mouse oocytes in the advanced stages of follicular development. *Mutat. Res.* 11:411–420.

Generoso, W. M., Stout, S. K. and Huff, S. W. 1971b. Effects of alkylating chemicals on reproductive capacity of adult female mice. *Mutat. Res.* 13:171–184.

Generoso, W. M., de Serres, F. J., Huff, S. W. and Cain, K. T. 1972. Studies on the induction of chromosomal aberrations in mice by hycanthone. *Biol. Div. Annu. Prog. Rep. June 30, 1972*, ORNL-4817, pp. 125–126.

Generoso, W. M. Russell, W. L. and Gosslee, D. G. 1973a. A sequential procedure for the detection of translocation heterozygotes in male mice. *Mutat. Res.* 21:220–221.

Generoso, W. M. Cain, K. T., Huff, S. W. and Rutledge, J. C. 1973b. Chemical induction of sex-chromosome loss in female mice. *Genetics* 74:s90–91.

Generoso, W. M., Russell, W. L., Huff, S. W., Stout, S. K. and Gosslee, D. G. 1974a. Effects of dose on the induction of dominant-lethal mutations and heritable translocations with ethyl methanesulfonate in male mice. *Genetics* 77:741–752.

Generoso, W. M., Cain, K. T. and Huff, S. W. 1974b. Dose effects of acute X-rays on induction of heritable reciprocal translocations in mouse spermatogonia. *Biol. Div. Annu. Prog. Rep. June 30, 1974*, ORNL-4993, pp. 136–138.

Generoso, W. M., Cain, K. T. and Huff, S. W. 1974c. Fertility of X-ray- or TEM-induced translocations in male mice. *Biol. Div. Annu. Prog. Rep. June 30, 1974*, ORNL-4993, pp. 133–134.

Generoso, W. M., Preston, R. J. and Brewen, J. G. 1977a. 6-Mercaptopurine, an inducer of cytogenetic and dominant-lethal effects in premeiotic and early meiotic germ cells of male mice. *Mutat. Res.*, in press.

Generoso, W. M., Huff, S. W. and Cain, K. T. 1977b. Comparative inducibility by 6-mercaptopurine of dominant-lethal mutations and heritable translocations in early meiotic male germ cells and differentiating spermatogonia of mice. *Mutat. Res.*, in press.

Gilliavod, N. and Leonard, A. 1973. Sensitivity of the mouse oocyte to the induction of translocations by ionizing radiations. *Can. J. Genet. Cytol.* 15:363–366.

Kratochvilova, J. 1973. Fertilization ability of male mice after treatment with tumor inhibitors. *Mutat. Res.* 21:192.

Matter, B. E. and Generoso, W. M. 1974. Effects of dose on the induction of dominant-lethal mutations with triethylenemelamine in male mice. *Genetics* 77:753–763.

Ray, V. A. and Hyneck, M. L. 1973. Some primary considerations in the interpretation of the dominant lethal assay. *Environ. Health Perspect.* 6:27–36.

Reddi, O. S. 1965. Radiation-induced translocations in mouse spermatogonia. *Mutat. Res.* 2:95.

Roderick, T. H. and Hawes, N. L. 1974. Nineteen paracentric chromosomal inversions in mice. *Genetics* 76:109–117.

Russell, W. L. and Hunsicker, P. R. 1975. The use of hycanthone to demonstrate the sensitivity of the X-chromosome loss method in mice. *Mutat. Res.* 31:343.

Russell, L. B. and Wickham, L. 1957. The incidence of disturbed fertility among male mice conceived at various intervals after irradiation of the mother. *Genetics* 142:392–393.

Russell, W. L., Hunsicker, P. R., Kelly, E. M., Vaughan, C. M. and Guinn, G. M. 1974. Preliminary test of the effect of hycanthone on X-chromosome loss in mice. *Biol. Div. Annu. Prog. Rep. June 30, 1974*, ORNL-4993, p. 116.

Searle, A. G. and Beechey, C. V. 1974. Cytogenetic effects of X-rays and fission neutrons in female mice. *Mutat. Res.* 24:171–186.

CHAPTER 7

CURRENT NEEDS FOR MUTAGENICITY TESTING IN MAMMALS

George L. Wolff

Department of Health, Education, and Welfare
Food and Drug Administration
National Center for Toxicological Research
Jefferson, Arkansas 72079

INTRODUCTION

Genetic disorders in humans result from mutations that were induced by unknown causes in the past and have been transmitted for many generations; for example, sickle-cell disease. Genetic disorders may also result from mutations induced by unknown causes in the germ cells of one of the parents and expressed in the offspring, but not passed on to succeeding generations because of partial or complete infertility or viability; examples are Turner's syndrome and Klinefelter's syndrome. The most recent compilation of genetic disorders in humans (McKusick, 1975) lists 1,142 entities where the mode of inheritance has been reasonably well defined and another 1,194 where the precise mode of inheritance has not been quite as well established.

The primary purpose of the testing of food additives, drugs, and other environmental chemicals for mutagenic potential is to identify substances that might contribute to an increased incidence of human disease syndromes with major genetic components in future generations by increasing the mutation rate in germ cells of human populations. Mutations are defined as changes in the sequence of nucleotides in the DNA of chromosomes and include those affecting only single gene loci as well as those affecting larger sections of chromosomes. Changes in chromosome number through breakage or through nondisjunction at meiosis are also included in the definition of mutations.

Screening of large numbers of chemical substances for the existence of mutagenic potential can be accomplished by using microbial (McCann and Ames, 1978) and mammalian (Fischer et al., 1974) cell culture systems. These assays only indicate whether the chemical agent is capable of inducing mutations and provide no information on the actual mutagenic potential of the agent in somatic cells or germ cells in situ in laboratory animals or humans.

Interactions between ultimate mutagens and chromosomal DNA that result in premutational lesions can occur in all germ cells. However, whether these interactions take place is determined by the metabolic and physiological processes involved in determining the concentration of ultimate mutagen that reaches the chromosomal DNA, as distinct from the dose of chemical administered to the animal. Whether the premutational lesion is actually translated into a heritable mutation depends on other metabolic processes that are involved in DNA repair, DNA replication, and meiosis. These physiological and metabolic processes, which act on the potentially mutagenic chemical from its initial administration to the induction of a heritable mutation, are so diversified and their interrelations are so complex that, at present, the whole animal is the only assay system available in which the risk of the induction of germ-cell mutations by a particular administered dose of agent can be assessed.

When a medically or economically important chemical is shown to be mutagenic in an *in vitro* test system, and satisfactory nonmutagenic substitutes are not available, it becomes necessary to establish whether exposure to environmental levels of the compound may induce transmissible genetic alterations in germ cells. To obtain relevant dose-response data for this purpose an animal system must be used.

Mutations induced by chemical agents may include recessive mutations, which may have deleterious effects only when homozygous (Green, 1971). Such mutations could spread through a human population without detection until their frequency became high enough to increase the probability of marriages between heterozygous carriers and the subsequent production of defective offspring, or offspring more prone to the development of particular disease syndromes.

The probability of the spread through a population of any single mutation is small; however, an increase in the total number of mutations induced by exposure of a human population to environmental mutagens increases the likelihood that deleterious mutations may be incorporated in the gene pool of that population. Since this possibility must be taken into account when making risk-benefit decisions, mammalian assays are needed to detect the induction of heritable microlesions by chemical mutagens and their subsequent spread through succeeding generations.

In this chapter I describe the conceptual basis and the experimental approaches used for the portion of the mutagenesis research program of the National Center for Toxicological Research that seeks to develop improved assay methodology to detect and quantify the induction of heritable germ-cell mutations in mammals. The aim of this program is to develop assay methods that are useful not only for determining the mutagenic potential per se of environmental substances in mammals, but also for developing dose-response information in relation to the mutagenic effects of long-term exposure to low dose levels of chemical mutagens.

MUTATIONS AND DISEASE SUSCEPTIBILITY

The responsiveness of mammals to the effects of environmental factors, be they organic or inorganic, living or inanimate, is based on a complex of physiological and metabolic reaction systems, all of which,. basically, are genetically determined. This is especially well illustrated by the strain- and tissue-specific differences in the incidence of spontaneous and chemically induced tumors (Heston, 1956; Murphy, 1966) and teratogenic malformations (Dagg, 1966) among different strains and genotypes of mice. What this might mean in terms of both the phenotypic end points that might be most relevant for mutagenic assay development and the mammalian whole animal assay systems themselves is worth considering.

Disease is defined as "an impairment of the normal state of the living animal . . . body or of any of its components that interrupts or modifies the performance of the vital functions, *being a response* to environmental factors (as malnutrition, industrial hazards, or climate), to specific infective agents (as worms, bacteria, or viruses), to inherent defects of the organism (as various genetic anomalies), or to combinations of these factors" (italics added) (Gove, 1971). For the present discussion, the concept that disease processes are responses is of fundamental importance because the function of the organism's genotype is to determine the range of qualitative and quantitative responses to any particular micro- or macroenvironmental stimulus.

It is important to realize that whether particular response patterns are elicited by environmental stimuli depends on a host of interactive physiological and metabolic responses of the organism, tissue, and cell involved. Each of these responses that directly or indirectly influence the overall response pattern is genetically controlled and, in turn, is modified by still other genetically controlled metabolic responses. The concepts here are that all physiological and metabolic responses in an organism are directly or indirectly influenced by each other through feedback mechanisms in the complex metabolic and physiological matrix of the organism, and that different steps in each of the myriad pathways involved are fundamentally determined and controlled by different gene loci. On the assumption that these concepts reasonably represent the actual functioning of an organism, it follows that a mutation affecting the structure and/or function of a polypeptide would alter all processes and metabolic pathways in which this polypeptide participated (Wolff, 1973) unless the effect of the mutation could be compensated for by homeostatic mechanisms.

The relative seriousness of the effect of the mutation on the organism depends not only on the importance of the most vital process affected by the mutation, but also on the relative positions in physiological and metabolic pathways occupied by the processes in which the affected polypeptide is involved. Mutations altering the functioning of polypeptides involved in very early steps of vital pathways may have serious consequences for the organism.

On the other hand, mutations affecting polypeptides involved in terminal steps of nonvital pathways will probably have less effect on the viability or fertility of the organism. Such mutations may still affect the survival of the organism if the so-called nonvital pathways affect characteristics of appearance or behavior that are of survival value in the environment.

The phenotypic expression of the genotype in terms of the range of specific qualitative and quantitative responses to physiological and environmental stimuli may be the basis not only for relative susceptibility to the development of specific disease syndromes, but also for the differential expression of particular aspects of specific syndromes in different individuals.

An example is the case of the contrasting responses of the inbred C57BL/6J and C57BL/KsJ mouse strains to the presence of the *ob* (obese) and *db* (diabetes) mutations (Hummel et al., 1972; Coleman and Hummel, 1973). These mutations are located on different chromosomes. Both mutations induce hyperphagia and obesity in both strains. In the C57BL/KsJ strain the presence of these mutations resulted in marked hyperglycemia and atrophy of the islets of Langerhans. Plasma insulin concentrations were elevated only in younger animals of this strain. In contrast, the C57BL/6J mice responded to the presence of the mutations by a mild and transitory hyperglycemia and marked hypertrophy of the islets of Langerhans, together with an increased proliferative capacity of the beta cells. Plasma insulin concentrations were markedly elevated at all ages in this strain. Mutant C57BL/KsJ mice stopped gaining weight at about 4 months of age, whereas mutant C57BL/6J mice continued gaining weight as long as they lived. This example emphasizes not only the profound and widespread effects mutations at single gene loci may have on the organism, but also the importance of the whole genetic constitution in determining the response of the organism to the defect induced by the mutation.

PHENOTYPIC EXPRESSION OF MUTATIONS

It should be realized that the classical genetic concepts of dominant and recessive mutations reflect only the degree to which homeostatic mechanisms can compensate for the phenotypic effects of a single mutation. If physiological and metabolic homeostatic mechanisms cannot fully compensate for the phenotypic effect of the single mutated allele in the presence of the original gene, the mutation appears to be dominant or codominant, since its presence can be easily detected in all carriers. In contrast, homeostatic mechanisms may compensate, at least partly, for the metabolic effects of a single mutation on the end point measured in the presence of the original allele. Then the presence of the mutated allele may not be obvious and it is regarded as recessive.

The nongenetic nature of dominance and recessiveness with respect to nonlethal alleles is well illustrated by the viable yellow (A^{vy}) mutation in the house mouse. Because it induces yellow coat color and obesity in the presence of all other alleles at the agouti locus, this mutation is regarded as dominant to them, except for lethal yellow (A^y) with which it is codominant. Most mice that carry only one A^{vy} gene and a recessive allele such as nonagouti (a) are yellow with various degrees of black and agouti mottling and also become fat. A certain proportion of such mice, however, appear to have the wild-type agouti coat color and do not become obese (Wolff, 1971). All A^{vy} heterozygotes, regardless of their phenotype, breed normally and produce the expected Mendelian proportions of yellow and nonyellow offspring. The gross physiological and metabolic responses of the pseudoagouti $A^{vy}a$ mice that have been examined so far resemble those of their black aa sibs rather than those of their mottled yellow $A^{vy}a$ sibs. Nevertheless, these mice are not completely normal since the regulation of the coat color pattern is quite aberrant although this is not apparent from their gross appearance (Galbraith and Wolff, 1974). This indicates that the detection of the presence of a mutant allele in an organism depends to a great extent on the phenotypic end point that is monitored.

Utilization of pleiotropic effects as phenotypic end points is the classic method for the detection of gene mutations induced in the germ cells of animals. The specific locus assay in the mouse (Searle, 1975) is an example. Mutations at the loci monitored are detected by changes in hair or eye color or ear size. The polypeptides altered by mutations at those loci have not been identified. The metabolic processes and pathways affected by mutations at these loci are also unknown. Thus, the fact that a mutation has occurred is revealed only by the change in the monitored pleiotropic end point, which may be far removed from the primary phenotypic expression of the muta-tion—that is, a specific polypeptide. As demonstrated by the phenomenon of the pseudoagouti phenotype of the $A^{vy}a$ genotype, the expression of different pleiotropic end points of specific mutations may be masked or altered by homeostatic effects related to the genetic background. This is also demon-strated by the differential expression of the ob and db mutations on different strain backgrounds (Hummel et al., 1972; Coleman and Hummel, 1973).

These complications resulting from the ramifications of the metabolic and physological effects of gene mutations suggest that it is desirable, if not essential, that the induction of mutations be monitored by using charac-teristics of specific polypeptides as phenotypic end points rather than morphological or physiological characteristics of the whole animal. The development of assays to detect mutations that alter the electrophoretic mobility of proteins is based on this desideratum.

Paigen (1971) has pointed out that half of the usual amount of enzyme activity is enough in most cases to allow normal functioning of the organism. In the case of mutations affecting enzyme proteins, both the original gene and the mutant allele are expressed in the heterozygote. Thus the presence of the mutant allele can be detected in the offspring of the animal in which the mutation arose.

While the structure of each polypeptide is controlled by a single gene locus, the realization of the enzymatic activity of that polypeptide is influenced and controlled by the direct and indirect effects of other loci (Paigen et al., 1975). Mutations at these other loci might alter the specific activity of the enzyme protein if their effects are not completely compensated for by homeostatic mechanisms. By measuring the specific activity of a single enzyme, therefore, it should be possible to detect mutations at several different loci.

ANIMAL SYSTEMS FOR MUTAGENIC ASSAYS

Ideally, the animal systems used to define mutagenic potential and dose-response characteristics of environmental chemicals should be similar to *Homo sapiens* in all metabolic and physiological characteristics that affect susceptibility to the induction in situ of heritable germ-cell mutations. On the basis of phylogenetic relationships it is reasonable to assume that the matrix of metabolic and physiological processes in humans, which determines not only whether, but also in what form, an exogenous agent may interact with nuclear DNA and induce a heritable mutation, is more closely akin to that of other mammals than to that of organisms belonging to other taxonomic categories. Primates are ruled out as experimental assay systems not only because of economic factors, but also because their generation time is too long to permit the timely determination of the heritability of detected variations. For pharmacokinetic studies directed toward determination of the effective dose of ultimate mutagen at the target cell and for metabolic transformation and detoxification studies, however, primates may be highly useful. Correlation of effective dose with induction of chromosomal aberrations in germ cells might be accomplished by cytogenetic examination of primate germ cells treated *in vivo*.

Because cf their short generation time, their large litter size, and the availability of inbred strains, rodents are the practical choice for mammalian whole animal assays to detect induced mutations. To meet the goal of relevance of the metabolic processing of test substances to the human situation, the pharmacokinetic characteristics and patterns of metabolic transformation and detoxification of compounds representing different chemical classes should be defined in different inbred strains or F_1 hybrids and offspring from multihybrid crosses. These patterns can then be compared with those characteristic of primate and human populations.

A large amount of work on the genetic control of the microsomal enzyme aryl hydrocarbon hydroxylase (Kouri et al., 1974; Nebert et al., 1975) has indicated the existence of differences between inbred mouse strains in the activity of this enzyme. This mixed-function oxidase enzyme system converts chemically inert lipid-soluble polycyclic hydrocarbons to water-soluble compounds. During this transformation chemically reactive intermediate metabolites are formed that are both cytotoxic and carcinogenic (Kouri et al., 1974); some of these compounds also appear to be mutagenic in Chinese hamster cells in tissue culture and in *Neurospora crassa* (Malling and Chu, 1974). It is reasonable to suggest that other enzymes, involved in the processing of compounds belonging to chemical classes other than polycyclic hydrocarbons, also may differ among mouse strains. Once such strains are identified, the synthesis of animal systems with humanoid patterns of metabolic transformation and detoxification of particular classes of chemical compounds may be feasible through the use of appropriate breeding techniques.

End Points in Mammalian Assay Systems

If the mutagenic assay system is to be used primarily for the generation of dose-response data that may be used in arriving at risk estimates for human populations, end points that are analogous to those found in humans might provide the most relevant information.

The primary gene product is mRNA, and the primary function of mRNA activity is specification of the amino acid sequence of a polypeptide. Therefore, the metabolic entity in which the phenotypic effect of a mutation is first expressed is a polypeptide. Except in the case of most visible mutations, a mutation is usually detected by its effect on the protein incorporating the mutant polypeptide. The existence of thousands of different proteins, each coded for by different genetic loci in the organism, provides the basis for monitoring a large number of loci for induced mutations. For the development of dose-response data this is of utmost importance because of the relative randomness of the induction of mutational events throughout the genome (Auerbach, 1969) and the marked variability with respect to mutability of different loci (Schlager and Dickie, 1971).

The relatively small number of individual germ cells that can be assayed in whole animal systems mandates that a large number of loci be monitored for induced mutations in each animal if reliable dose-response data are to be obtained. In a microbial or mammalian cell culture system, on the other hand, the mutagenic potential and dose response of a substance are measured by the number of mutations induced at a single locus in a large population of cells.

If dynamic end points, such as enzyme activity, are used to detect induced mutations, it is likely that mutations at loci other than the structural locus will also be detected. As mentioned before, enzyme activity is influenced by numerous factors, each of which is dependent on different genetic loci. Specific enzyme activity is also influenced by micro- and macroenvironmental fluctuations. Therefore, any change in enzyme activity that is detected in an animal must also be detected in subsequent generations before it can be designated as resulting from a heritable mutation.

Assays for the detection of induced mutations affecting the electrophoretic characteristics of proteins are available, and additional ones are under development (Malling and Valcovic, 1978). These assays detect mutations that alter the electrostatic charge on proteins by amino acid substitutions but do not necessarily alter the characteristics of their *in vitro* activity. To obtain as wide a sampling of the total genome as possible, assays that measure specific activity under various conditions as well as the electrophoretic mobility of enzymes should be employed to detect induced mutations.

Extrapolation of Animal Data to Humans

Metabolic processing is not the only parameter that must be taken into account when considering the relevance of animal data to the estimation of risk to human populations. Pharmacokinetic characteristics, transport of the mutagenic metabolite to the gonads and into the germ cells, binding to DNA and protein, and efficiency of DNA repair and misrepair in the different developmental stages of germ cells may also differ markedly between humans and rodents. Very little is known about these parameters in either species, so the first requirement is to develop comparative baseline data.

It should be emphasized that until the quantitative relations with respect to the induction of mutations by specific chemical agents in germ cells and somatic cells of laboratory mammals are compared with data obtained by assays utilizing human cells or tissue biopsies, estimates of potential mutagenic risk to human populations will be tenuous at best, even when mammalian assay systems are employed. This is the case because species differences in relevant metabolic processes such as activation, detoxification, and DNA repair preclude direct extrapolation to humans of the data on mutagenic potential obtained in nonhuman assay systems.

RELEVANCE OF ASSAYS TO DETERMINATION
OF MUTAGENIC RISK IN MAMMALS

In Vitro Assays

While heritable mutations in all organisms are induced by interaction of the ultimate mutagen with DNA, the series of metabolic and physiological processes through which potentially mutagenic chemicals must pass before such interactions can take place are very different, in both number and complexity, in microbial organisms, mammalian cells in culture, and whole mammals. As an example, one need only compare bacterial cells with mammals.

To a first approximation, mutagen molecules in the culture medium need only penetrate the bacterial cell wall before coming into contact with the chromosome. Contrast this pathway with that of a potential mutagen ingested by a mammal. Not only must the potential mutagen traverse the gastrointestinal tract with its microbial flora, but it must be absorbed into the bloodstream, pass through the metabolic detoxification, activation, and transformation systems of the liver, reach the ovary or testes through the bloodstream, be absorbed from the bloodstream and pass through the metabolizing gonadal tissue, reach the germ cells, pass through the germ-cell membrane, and thus enter the cytoplasm. Only then can the compound pass through the nuclear membrane and into the germ-cell nucleus and, in its ultimate mutagenic form, interact with the chromosomal DNA. Whether this interaction results in a heritable mutation depends on such factors as the developmental stage of the germ cell (Ehling, 1974b), the relative efficiency of DNA repair systems, and the physiological or metabolic effect of the induced mutation on the viability and fertility of the germ cell.

In view of the complex of pathways that a potential mutagen must traverse in a mammal before it can interact with the DNA of a germ cell in situ and induce a heritable mutation, *in vitro* assays, using microbial or mammalian cell systems, can at present provide only a qualitative indication of whether a specific chemical agent may be potentially mutagenic in mammals. A severe limitation on the utility of these *in vitro* assay systems is imposed by their lack of many of the enzymes required to transform nonmutagenic substances to their ultimate mutagenic metabolites.

Addition of mammalian tissue extracts to such *in vitro* systems in order to provide the enzymes necessary for transforming chemicals to their mutagenic metabolites (Malling and Frantz, 1973; Umeda and Saito, 1975) increases the usefulness of these assays for the detection of potential mutagens; however, even under these conditions, *in vitro* assays cannot provide information regarding mutagenic risk to mammalian germ cells in situ.

The detection in microbial systems of mutagenic metabolites in body fluids from animals treated with chemical agents (Commoner et al., 1974; Durston and Ames, 1974) provides more information on whether a substance may be a potential mutagen in mammals; however, it still remains to be determined whether the mutagenic metabolite detected in a body fluid such as blood or urine actually reaches and enters the germ cell in situ in unaltered form and in sufficient concentration to induce a mutation.

Induction of chromosomal aberrations or damage in response to exposure to chemical agents indicates that the agent interacts with and affects the genetic constitution of the cell. Chromosomal aberrations and aneuploidy are involved in numerous disease syndromes in humans, for instance, trisomy 21 and cri du chat (Vogel, 1970). Whole animal assays with end points such as dominant lethals, heritable translocations, and sex-chromosome loss can detect chromosomal effects of environmental chemicals but are not sufficient for making risk-benefit assessments with respect to mutagenicity.

These assays provide no information regarding the possible induction of subtle transmissible effects on the chromosomes by long-term exposure to the chemical substance at low dose levels. Perry and Evans (1975) have reported that chemical mutagens that induce chromosomal aberrations in mammalian cell cultures at high dose levels induce only increased frequencies of sister chromatid exchanges at low doses. Sister chromatid exchanges involve symmetrical exchanges of identical sections between sister chromatids and do not alter chromosome morphology.

By analogy, it is conceivable that dose levels of mutagenic chemicals that do not induce gross chromosome damage or alteration in germ cells may nevertheless induce transmissible effects on the chromosomes. From a regulatory point of view, assays are needed to determine exposure levels at which no detectable chromosomal effects, either gross or subtle, are induced.

Assays to Detect Effects of Low Doses of Chemical Mutagens on Chromosomes

An attempt to develop assay methodology to detect such subtle genetic effects is being made by our group. We are trying to determine whether exposure to chemical mutagens at dose levels that produce no effects in the dominant-lethal assay may alter the frequency of meiotic recombination in the house mouse.

Meiotic recombination results from reciprocal exchanges between homologous nonsister chromatids (Gardner, 1975). Therefore, by analogy with the increase in sister chromatid exchanges in somatic cells, it seems reasonable to postulate that chemical mutagens may increase the frequency of meiotic recombination at dose levels that do not induce gross chromosome damage or aberrations.

No information is available on the effects of chemicals on meiotic recombination in the mouse. Mitomycin C and formaldehyde have been reported to increase meiotic crossing-over in *Drosophila melanogaster* females (Schewe et al., 1971; Sobels, 1956). Formaldehyde also induces crossing-over in *D. melanogaster* males, in which spontaneous crossing-over is normally inhibited (Sobels and van Steenis, 1957).

The easy visual identification of recombinants among the offspring of treated mice is the practical basis for this proposed assay technique. In the mouse 8 of the 20 chromosomes carry visible mutations that are suited for detecting changes in the frequency of meiotic recombinations between known genetic loci on the chromosomes (M. C. Green and P. W. Lane, personal communication). These markers are easily identifiable and have no marked deleterious effects on fertility or viability.

If the development of such an assay technique is successful, it should be possible to utilize it for detecting effects on meiotic recombination induced by long-term exposure to mutagenic chemicals. Males heterozygous at the specific loci between which recombination is to be measured can be continuously exposed to the substance under test. At stated intervals these males would be mated to females homozygous at the specific loci, and the recombination frequency between these loci could be determined and compared with the spontaneous rate by examination of the offspring.

The absence of chromosomal effects at low dose levels would not necessarily indicate an absence of mutagenic potential since microlesions (any alterations in chromosomal DNA that are not detectable cytologically) might still be induced. Therefore, even though a substance may not induce any detectable chromosomal effects, it may still be a mutagen by virtue of inducing heritable microlesions.

Most chromosomal aberrations induced in premeiotic germ cells are lost before or during meiosis (Brewen and Preston, 1974; Adler, 1974) or induce complete or partial sterility in the offspring (Generoso et al., 1978). Therefore, they pose a relatively smaller danger from the point of view of multigeneration effects on the population than do heritable recessive gene mutations. This does not lessen their importance as a public health problem; however, since they are expressed in the individual carrying the chromosomal abnormality, chromosomal aberrations do not present as insidious a threat to human populations as do gene mutations or microlesions, which may be carried undetected in heterozygous carriers for many generations. On the basis of these considerations, a major effort of our group is focused on the development of assay methodology to detect and quantify the induction of microlesions.

Assays to Detect Induction of Heritable Microlesions

The detection of mutational microlesions (base-pair substitutions, frameshifts, duplications, and multilocus deletions) in mammals is presently limited to the loci monitored by the specific locus assay. Mutations induced at any of either seven or five different loci that influence coat color, eye color, or ear size of the house mouse, *Mus musculus*, can be detected by this assay (Searle, 1975).

At least part of the mutations induced at some of these loci by radiation appear to be very small chromosomal deletions or rearrangements covering more than one locus (Russell, 1971); however, there are no a priori reasons to assume that chemical mutagens may not also induce base-pair substitutions or frameshift mutations at these loci.

On the basis of the available information, which is admittedly inadequate, mutations appear to be induced at random throughout the genome (Auerbach, 1969). A further complication is that the spontaneous mutability of different loci differs severalfold (Schlager and Dickie, 1971; Schlager, 1972). This is also true for radiation- and chemically induced mutations monitored by the specific locus assay (Ehling, 1974a). Therefore, in order to obtain as meaningful an estimate of the mutagenic potency of a substance as possible, as large a proportion of the total genome of the organism as possible must be monitored. Toward this end, phenotypic end points other than visible effects must be utilized so that mutations at many loci that affect a wide range of metabolic and physiological processes may be detected.

The chemical mutagens tested so far have tended to induce mutations in spermatogonia more frequently at the agouti (*a*) and dilute (*d*) loci and less frequently at the albino (*c*) and spotting (*s*) loci than has gamma irradiation (Ehling, 1974a). In the absence of experimental data, the possibility that mutagens of different chemical structural classes may also preferentially induce mutations at different loci cannot be ruled out. To assess this possibility too, an assay method capable of detecting mutations at a large number of loci is a necessity.

Mutations may alter different characteristics of the enzyme molecule, such as thermal lability, which are involved in the determination of its specific activity under diverse environmental conditions. The phenotypic effects of such mutations can be detected by standard enzyme activity assays. Most mutations that directly affect the specific activity of enzymes have effects that are additive with those of the wild-type alleles. It is therefore possible to detect heterozygous individuals that carry a single mutant allele together with the wild-type gene by altered specific activity levels (Paigen, 1971).

Paigen et al. (1975) have suggested that several gene loci directly influence the activity of an enzyme in mammals: namely, a structural locus that dictates the amino acid sequence of the enzyme, regulatory loci that determine the rate of synthesis of the enzyme, temporal loci that determine the specific developmental stages during which the enzyme is synthesized, and processing loci that determine the cellular apparatus involved with the intracellular location, conjugation, and degradation of the enzyme molecules.

Mutations that change such factors as hormone synthesis, release, or degradation, hormone receptors, pH and cofactor availability may also affect the specific activity of numerous enzymes.

In view of the large number of enzymes for which activity assays are available, the inclusion in a test battery of assays to detect mutational changes in enzyme activity can potentially increase the number of loci monitored many times compared with the number of loci included in the specific locus assay (Searle, 1975). In many cases it will be difficult to identify the particular locus at which a detected mutation occurred. For the purpose of obtaining quantitative estimates of mutagenic potential, however, this need not necessarily be a problem. The primary requirement here is the ability to estimate rather accurately the total number of loci at which mutations have been induced and the total number of mutations that have been induced at particular loci by a particular level of mutagen. This can be done if the detectable phenotypic effects of the mutations segregate in Mendelian fashion so that they can be discerned in subsequent generations of test animals.

These considerations were the basis for a project undertaken in our group to develop an assay system for monitoring the induction of mutations affecting specific activity or electrophoretic mobility of 50-75 enzymes in liver, kidney, heart, brain, or erythrocytes of inbred mice (Mohrenweiser et al., 1976). For this purpose, male mice of an inbred strain are treated with a mutagen. After an appropriate time interval, depending on the sperm cell stage to be sampled, they are mated to untreated females of the same inbred strain. The young from these matings are designated F_1. These are sibmated to produce offspring, which are designated F_2. Blood and urine from F_1 mice are monitored to detect abnormal metabolite concentrations, which may indicate a storage disease or a decrease in activity of enzyme(s) that utilize the metabolite(s) in question. Only F_2 mice are sacrificed to obtain tissues for assays of enzyme activity and electrophoretic mobility.

Comparisons of enzyme activity data are carried out within litters to ascertain whether two presumptive populations—that is, normal homozygotes and mutant heterozygotes—can be identified within specific litters. The detection of such a presumptive difference within a litter will then be followed by similar assays on additional F_2 litters generated by the same parent for confirmatory evidence.

Since the heritable mutations induced in the germ cells of the mutagen-treated males are transmitted to the F_1 mice, the F_1 mice constitute the reservoir for these mutations. These mice are saved until all enzyme assays on the F_2 mice have been completed. Thus, it will be possible to generate additional F_2 mice, if necessary, to confirm assay data as indicated above, to carry out breeding tests to identify mutated loci, or to save and propagate mutations of value to biomedical research.

The twin problems of assaying the activities of large numbers of enzymes in single tissues of large numbers of individual mice were solved by the adaptation of enzyme assays for use with the miniature centrifugal fast analyzer (MCFA) (Burtis et al., 1973). By use of the MCFA, it is possible to carry out 100 enzyme assays per hour and to utilize only 1-2 μl of a $1 + 5$ tissue homogenate per assay (Mohrenweiser et al., 1976).

ASSESSMENT OF MUTAGENIC POTENTIAL IN GENETICALLY HETEROGENEOUS POPULATIONS OF MAMMALS

Whenever the extrapolation to human populations of the data obtained with toxicology bioassays in animals is considered, the question is raised whether several unrelated inbred strains or a genetically heterogeneous population would provide more relevant data.

If large numbers of loci are to be assayed for induced mutations that affect enzyme activity characteristics, inbred strains and F_1 hybrids provide the genetic homogeneity required to ascertain the heritability of detected variations. On the other hand, each inbred strain and F_1 hybrid possesses its own unique metabolic pattern, which will be expressed in the qualitative and quantitative characteristics of all the processes that determine whether a particular administered dose of test agent will induce a heritable mutation in the germ cells. Therefore, dose-response data obtained with any one or several inbred strains or F_1 hybrids will represent only one or a few of a myriad of possible metabolic patterns representative of the animal species employed.

The utilization of progeny of dihybrid or trihybrid crosses provides a great variety of metabolic patterns, especially if the parental inbred strains were chosen for their diversity in genetic background. A population of such experimental animals will provide a wide sampling of the patterns of metabolic processing of chemical mutagens and of the processes involved in the induction of mutations. It would thuse be more representative of a genetically heterogeneous human population. These genetically heterogeneous animals can be used for the detection of specific types of induced chromosomal aberrations if appropriate control populations are used. The disadvantage of using animals from such populations for mutagenicity assays is that the genetic heterogeneity of the animals makes the detection of induced microlesions that affect specific enzyme activities or other phenotypic end points of a quantitative nature highly problematic.

The metabolic heterogeneity of the population could conceivably result in the masking of the expression of induced mutations affecting enzyme activity within single litters and more especially among different litters from the parent animal carrying the mutation. The latter would be especially likely if the litters were produced by mating a mutant male to several different females, all of whom would be genetically and metabolically different. Therefore, it might be difficult to confirm the induction of a mutation.

The ultimate utility of a mutagenicity assay in which progeny of multihybrid crosses are used may depend on the results of a comparison of the dose-response relations between the induction of microlesions and the induction of specific types of chromosomal effects. These comparisons should be performed in the parental F_1 hybrids and possibly also in the grandparental inbred strains in order to ascertain the degree of uniformity of these relations. A high degree of uniformity might warrant an investigation of the validity of extrapolating to the genetically heterogeneous population the dose-response relations found between the induction of microlesions and the induction of chromosomal effects in the ancestral populations.

SUMMARY AND CONCLUSIONS

Although microbial and mammalian cell culture assays can be used to identify environmental chemicals that can interact with DNA and induce mutations, they are not suitable for ascertaining whether a particular substance will induce heritable germ-cell mutations in mammals or humans. Indeed, chemical agents that are not mutagenic themselves but are transformed to mutagenic metabolites by diverse enzyme systems in laboratory mammals and humans would not be identified as mutagens by these assay systems. This problem has been approached by the addition to these *in vitro* systems of mammalian tissue fractions that provide enzymes that transform some classes of chemicals to their mutagenic metabolites; however, chemical agents that are metabolically transformed to mutagenic substances by enzyme systems not present in the tissue fractions are still not identified as mutagens by these assays. At present, the only assay systems that are capable of identifying all environmental substances, regardless of chemical structure, that will induce heritable germ-cell mutations in mammals are whole animal systems.

Determining the frequency of induction of a particular genetic end point, such as a heritable microlesion or particular type of chromosomal effect, by administering a series of dose levels of the test substance to whole animals is at present the only way to determine the mutagenic potency of a chemical in terms that might provide a tenuous basis for estimating the magnitude of the risk incurred by exposure of human populations to particular environmental levels of the chemical. It must be emphasized that the extrapolation of mutagenic risk from test animal to humans is complicated by the manifold species- and strain-specific differences in the metabolic and physiological processes that determine whether the mutagenic form of a specific chemical will reach and enter the germ cells and subsequently induce heritable mutations.

Heritable mutations can induce serious disease syndromes. It is conceivable, however, that the most insidious long-term damage to human populations may result from the accumulation of chemically induced recessive mutations over many generations. Each of these mutations by itself, or even when homozygous, may not induce noticeably deleterious effects; however, in combination with different genetic backgrounds—that is, in different people—it might elicit serious disease syndromes. It is quite possible that susceptibility to different disease syndromes that tend to cluster in families but do not seem to be inherited in Mendelian fashion may be an example.

The presently utilized mammalian assays can detect only gross chromosomal damage or alterations induced by mutagenic substances. They are not suited for detecting subtle transmissible effects on mammalian chromosomes that may be induced by dose levels of chemicals that fail to cause major chromosomal changes. Assays for such subtle heritable chromosomal alterations are needed to detect possible effects on the genetic constitution of long-term exposure to low dose levels of environmental chemicals.

For determing the potential mutagenic risk of environmental substances, there is a critical need to develop assay systems that can generate quantitative data on the induction of heritable microlesions, such as base-pair substitutions, additions, or deletions, and multilocus deletions in mammalian germ cells in situ. Efforts to develop such assays are under way in several laboratories, using different characteristics of mammalian enzyme proteins as end points.

These assays are designed to detect mutations that alter the electrophoretic mobility or specific activity of different enzymes. Numerous gene loci, in addition to the structural locus, affect the realization of enzyme activity. This circumstance and the considerable number of enzymes that can be easily assayed for specific activity suggest that a sufficiently large number of loci can be monitored for the induction of mutations to allow the generation of statistically and biologically meaningful dose-response data.

Each inbred strain or F_1 hybrid population of test animals possesses an array of qualitative and quantitative capabilities for the metabolic processing of a diversity of environmental chemicals that is unique to the members of that population. Human populations, on the other hand, are genetically heterogeneous, and therefore are composed of individuals each of whom probably possesses a profile of such metabolic capabilities that is different from those of other members of the population.

The paucity of epidemiologic data with respect to chemically induced mutagenic events in human populations makes risk-benefit assessments of environmental dose levels of chemicals extremely difficult. The metabolic processing of environmental chemicals by the individual members of a population at risk is a major component in the mutagenic risk incurred by that population. Therefore, assay data obtained from genetically defined and controlled but metabolically heterogeneous populations of test mammals, such as offspring of multihybrid crosses, may be more relevant as an aid in making realistic risk-benefit assessments than data derived from single inbred or F_1 hybrid animal populations.

REFERENCES

Adler, I. 1974. *Mutat. Res.* 23:369–379.
Auerbach, C. 1969. *Trans. Kans. Acad. Sci.* 72:273–295.
Brewen, J. G. and Preston, R. J. 1974. *Mutat. Res.* 26:297–305.
Burtis, C. A., Johnson, W. F., Mailen, J. C., Overton, J. B., Tiffany, T. O. and Watsky, M. B. 1973. *Clin. Chem.* 19:895.
Coleman, D. L. and Hummel, K. P. 1973. *Diabetologia* 9:287–293.
Commoner, B., Vithayathil, A. J. and Henry, J. I. 1974. *Nature (Lond.)* 249: 850–852.
Dagg, C. P. 1966. In *Biology of the laboratory mouse*, ed. E. L. Green, 2nd ed., pp. 309–328. New York: Dover.
Durston, W. E. and Ames, B. N. 1974. *Proc. Natl. Acad. Sci. U.S.A.* 72: 737–741.
Ehling, U. 1974a. *Arch. Toxicol.* 32:19–25.
Ehling, U. 1974b. *Mutat. Res.* 26:285–295.
Fischer, G. A., Lee, S. Y. and Calabresi, P. 1974. *Mutat. Res.* 26:505–511.
Galbraith, D. B. and Wolff, G. L. 1974. *J. Hered.* 65:137–140.
Gardner, E. J. 1975. *Principles of genetics*, 5th ed., p. 141. New York: Wiley.
Generoso, W. M., Cain, K. T., Huff, S. W. and Gosslee, D. G. 1978. In *Advances in modern toxicology*, vol. 5, eds. W. G. Flamm and M. Mehlman, pp. 109–129. Washington, D.C.: Hemisphere.

Gove, P. B., ed. 1971. *Webster's third new international dictionary.* Springfield, Mass.: Merriam.

Green, E. L. 1971. *Mutat. Res.* 12:281–289.

Heston, W. E. 1956. *Cytologia (Tokyo) Suppl.*, pp. 219–224.

Hummel, K. P., Coleman, D. L. and Lane, P. W. 1972. *Biochem. Genet.* 7: 1–13.

Kouri, R. E., Ratrie, H. and Whitmire, C. E. 1974. *Int. J. Cancer* 13: 714–720.

Malling, H. V. and Chu, E. H. Y. 1974. In *Chemical carcinogenesis*, eds. P. O. P. Ts'o and J. A. DiPaolo, part B, pp. 545–563. New York: Dekker.

Malling, H. V. and Frantz, C. N. 1973. *Environ. Health Perspect. Exp. Issue* 6: 71–82.

Malling, H. V. and Valcovic, L. R. 1978. In *Advances in modern toxicology*, vol. 5, eds. W. G. Flamm and M. Mehlman, pp. 149–171. Washington, D.C.: Hemisphere.

McCann, J. and Ames, B. N. 1978. In *Advances in modern toxicology*, vol. 5, *Mutagenesis*, eds. W. G. Flamm and M. Mehlman, pp. 149–171. Washington, D.C.: Hemisphere.

McKusick, V. A. 1975. *Mendelian inheritance in man. Catalogs of autosomal dominant, autosomal recessive, and X-linked phenotypes*, 4th ed. Baltimore: Johns Hopkins.

Mohrenweiser, H. W., Burkhart, J. G., Feuers, R. J., Kane, A. C., Mays, J. B. and McAninch, J. E. 1976. *Proc. 7th Annu. Meet. Environ. Mutagen Soc. pp.* 32–33.

Murphy, E. D. 1966. In *Biology of the laboratory mouse*, ed. E. L. Green, 2nd ed., pp. 521–562. New York: Dover.

Nebert, D. W., Robinson, J. R., Niwa, A., Kumaki, K. and Poland, A. P. 1975. *J. Cell. Physiol.* 85:393–414.

Paigen, K. 1971. In *Enzyme synthesis and degradation in mammalian systems*, ed. M. Rechcigl, Jr., pp. 1–46. Basel: Karger.

Paigen, K., Swank, R. T., Tomino, S. and Ganschow, R. E. 1975. *J. Cell. Physiol.* 85:379–392.

Perry and Evans. 1975. *Nature (Lond.)* 258:121–125.

Russell, L. B. 1971. *Mutat. Res.* 11:107–123.

Schewe, M. J., Suzuki, D. T. and Erasmus, U. 1971. *Mutat. Res.* 12:269–279.

Schlager, G. 1972. *Mutat. Res.* 14:254–258.

Schlager, G. and Dickie, M. M. 1971. *Mutat. Res.* 11:89–96.

Searle, A. G. 1975. *Mutat. Res.* 31:277–290.

Sobels, F. H. 1956. *Z. Indukt. Abstamm. Vererbungsl.* 87:743–752.

Sobels, F. H. and van Steenis, H. 1957. *Nature (Lond.)* 179:29–31.

Umeda, M. and Saito, M. 1975. *Mutat. Res.* 30:249–254.

Vogel, F. 1970. In *Chemical mutagenesis in mammals and man*, eds. F. Vogel and G. Röhrborn, pp. 16–68. New York: Springer.

Wolff, G. L. 1971. *Am. Nat.* 105:241–252.

Wolff, G. L. 1973. *Environ. Health Perspect. Exp. Issue* 6:211–213.

CHAPTER 8

NEW APPROACHES TO DETECTING GENE MUTATIONS IN MAMMALS

Heinrich V. Malling and Lawrence R. Valcovic
Laboratory of Environmental Mutagenesis
National Institute of Environmental Health Sciences
Research Triangle Park, North Carolina

INTRODUCTION

The problems in the field of mutagenesis are much more complicated than simply identifying chemicals that possess mutagenic activity. For there are undoubtedly situations in which mutagenic chemicals may be of some benefit to society so that it may be either undesirable or in some cases impossible to remove them totally from the human environment. Therefore, we must have available methods for providing data in animal systems from which to estimate potential risks to the human population and thereby set so-called safe exposure limits, just as we have done historically with ionizing radiation. Model systems that will provide such data must approximate, as closely as is reasonably possible in a laboratory situation, the pharmacological and genetic situation as it exists in humans. In mutagenesis over the past number of years, the morphological specific locus test has provided a data base from which exposure limits for ionizing radiation have been set for the human population.

It is also important that systems be developed to monitor the human population to detect exposure to mutagenic agents. Some of the cytogenetic procedures are currently being employed to monitor workers in the industrial setting, and it is necessary to develop gene mutation systems to be incorporated into this program to provide the level of accuracy needed to identify low levels of genetic damage. For both practical and statistical reasons, these systems will utilize somatic cells to detect induced mutations.

Most of the systems described here have been published only in abstract form or the information has been obtained by personal communication. The review is as critical as it can be with the availability of sources. Some of the speculative concepts have been presented at the Second International Conference on Environmental Mutagens (Malling and Valcovic, 1977).

THEORETICAL CONSIDERATIONS

Repetitive DNA

The composition and architecture of the genetic material in mammals and other higher organisms are beginning to be understood and have unique features—for instance, a high content of repetitive DNA. These differences may influence the mutation rate and the spectrum of genetic alterations obtained in higher organisms in comparison to those obtained in microorganisms under similar treatment conditions.

During the evolution from microorganisms (excluding viruses) to higher animals, there has been an approximate 1,000-fold increase in the amount of DNA per haploid genome (Sparrow et al., 1971). Fungi such as *Saccharomyces cerevisiae* have the lowest haploid DNA content (4.5×10^7 nucleotides) found in any eukaryotic cell. The average size of a gene is estimated to consist of only 1,500 base pairs. The yeast cell contains enough DNA to code for 13,000 genes. Crow and Kimura (1970), on the other hand, have estimated the number of genes in a mammal to be about 30,000. The mammalian haploid genome contains 6×10^9 nucleotides. That means that only 6–9% of the available DNA functions as genes (Kimura and Ohta, 1971). Most of the remaining DNA is not transcribed. The genes that are translated are likely to have unique sequences. Melting-point analysis of mammalian DNA, however, indicated many different classes of repetitive DNA. In yeast the amount of repetitive DNA is low, indicating that the number of genes necessary to carry out the functions of a simple eukaryotic cell is close to 10^4. Presumably the evolution from yeast to humans has required only a threefold increase in the number of functional genes. The main increase in the amount of DNA has been in the different classes of repetitive DNA. The rate of X-ray induced specific locus mutations is positively correlated with the total amount of DNA per nucleus (Abrahamson et al., 1973; Schalet and Sankaranarayanan, 1976). Since the increase in the DNA is due to mainly an increase in the amount of repetitive DNA, it seems to indicate that the amount of repetitive DNA influences the yield of mutations after X-ray irradiation.

We have now seen how the repetitive DNA may influence the yield of mutations. Furthermore, there are indications in the literature that the amount of repetitive DNA in an organism also has an influence on the spectrum of the X-ray-induced mutations.

Let us again consider the specific locus mutations. These fall into two groups: (1) those that result from a physical removal of the gene and (2) those that result from point mutations in the gene. If the piece that was removed also uncovered a recessive lethal gene adjacent to the specific locus, then this mutation would be lethal in homozygotic conditions. Genetically, we can therefore distinguish between these deletions and nonlethal mutations. In the literature there are analyses of specific locus mutations in *Neurospora* by

Webber and de Serres (1965), in *Drosophila* by Alexander (1960), and in the mouse by Russell and Russell (1959), where such a comparison of the spectrum of genetic alterations could be made; mutation data exist for all three organisms after a total dose of 900–1,000 R at a dose rate of 90 R/min. As is clear from the data in Table 1, the more repetitive DNA, the higher the percentage of small deletions. However, correlative comparisons always contain oversimplifications. The amounts of repetitive DNA in Table 1 were not determined by the same methods; furthermore, there are several classes of repetitive DNA, and not all classes were included in some of the measurements. In addition, the type of repetitive DNA adjacent to a structural gene may influence the type of mutations recovered. So X-rays may induce a high percentage of deletions in certain genes and not in others (see Searle, 1974).

Many other types of correlations could be found, but the repetitive DNA has some unique characteristics that may explain why this type of DNA could influence the mutation spectrum after X-ray irradiation.

1. Annealing experiments indicate that the repetitive DNA, made single-stranded by heating, comes together much faster than the unique sequenced DNA.

2. X-rays induce double-strand breaks, which may be repaired by forming pieces of single-strand ends.

3. The probability of two single-strand ends sticking together depends on the complementarity of the bases in the single strand. Because of the similarity in the base sequence of the repetitive DNA, two independent breaks in this DNA would have similar ends and therefore would unite easily.

Although we have no direct proof that damage in repetitive DNA can result in deletions, the study of the deletion mutations in the β-hemoglobin

TABLE 1 Frequency of Lethality among the Specific Locus
Mutation Systems in Various Organisms after Exposure
to Acute X-rays

Organism	Homozygotic viable (%)	Homozygotic lethal (%)	Repetitive DNA (%)
Neurospora	99	1	10–15[a]
Drosophila	53	47	22[b]
Mouse	23	77	94

[a]Dutta, 1974.
[b]Peacock et al., 1973.

loci gives good indirect evidence for the importance of repetitiveness of the DNA in formation of interstitial deletions. In the β-hemoglobin complex several closely related genes are placed side by side on the DNA in the following sequence: ε, γG, γA, δ, β. There is so little difference between the amino acid compositions of these genes that it looks as if they arose through tandem duplications. Individuals carrying the mutant gene for hemoglobin Lepore produce a hemoglobin composed of δ and β instead of separated δ and β chains (Badr et al., 1973). Hemoglobin Lepore has been explained by uneven crossover but may also be explained by interstitial deletions, which may have been facilitated by the repetitive sequences in the duplicated genes.

There are good reasons for believing that repetitive sequences in the DNA play a role in the occurrence of small deletions. It is worthwhile to speculate about their role in the occurrence of bigger chromosome aberrations such as translocations and inversions. Both types of chromosome aberrations require reunion of two different broken ends, and it seems that this could be greatly facilitated through breaks in the repetitive DNA. One more point is that if 94% of the DNA in a mammalian nucleus is repetitive DNA, then 94% of all photons from X-ray irradiation are absorbed in this type of DNA. Naturally, therefore, most breakage and reunion phenomena will occur in the repetitive DNA, and it is also likely that the same is true for chemical mutagens.

Organization of the Gene

The organization of the mammalian gene may influence greatly the spectrum of genetic alterations induced by a certain mutagenic insult. A general but simple model for the mammalian gene is given in Fig. 1. The two important features of Fig. 1 are that the mRNA is approximately two to three times bigger than the piece translated into the protein, and that between each gene there seems to be a piece of repetitive DNA approximately 300–500 nucleotides long.

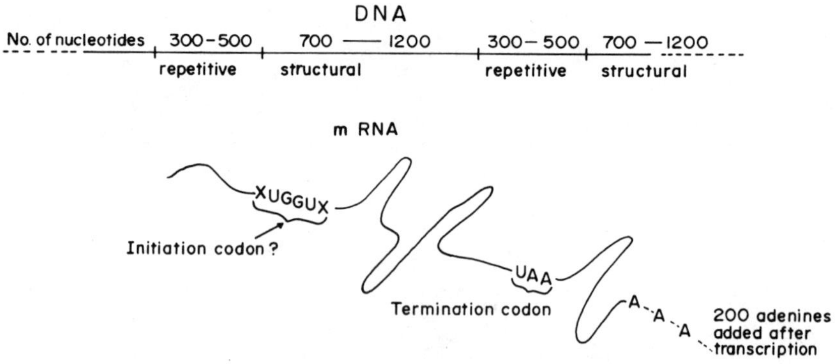

FIGURE 1 Model of the gene and the transcribed RNA.

If the natural terminator UAA is mutated by a base-pair substitution of, for example, CAA, the terminator will be read as glycine, and this amino acid will be added to the polypeptide chain; then the translation will probably continue until another nonsense codon is encountered. This type of mutation is probably what has resulted in the hemoglobinopathy Constant Spring, in which the normal hemoglobin has 31 more amino acids attached to the end (Milner et al., 1971; Clegg et al., 1971).

A similar type of alteration can result from a frameshift mutation that nullifies the natural terminator. Since the mRNA in higher organisms contains polynucleotides past the terminator, the polypeptide in such a mutant will be elongated until a code for a terminator occurs. This has probably happened in the hemoglobinopathy Wayne (Seid-Akhavan et al., 1976). In this α-hemoglobin variant the last three amino acids have been changed and five more have been added. This is definitely a different type of mutation spectrum than what could be expected from microorganisms.

Aside from the analysis of the hemoglobin mutants in humans, not many mutants have been characterized on the molecular level in mammals. One approach to this problem is to study mutations induced in loci that lend themselves to biochemical analysis. Several systems are not being developed that utilize various biochemical end points for the detection of gene mutations in mammals. The biochemical specific locus system is the only test that has yet been tried with mutagens.

IN VIVO GERMINAL GENE MUTATION SYSTEMS

Biochemical Specific Locus System

In this system electrophoresis is used to separate specific proteins and enzymes for the detection of the mutant phenotype (Valcovic and Malling, 1973). One of the main features of this procedure is that it is possible to detect mutations in which the enzyme is not functionally destroyed but merely has an altered charge and, hence, a shift in its electrophoretic mobility. However, the electrophoretic mobility mutation may give the smallest portion of mutants that affect the locus; as we have seen earlier, most of the mutations may be deletions and therefore produce no enzyme.

Because of technological problems, it is usually difficult to detect on a gel the loss of enzyme activity in an F_1; this requires seeing a band with half the intensity of the normal F_1. This problem is overcome by using two inbred strains of mice in which there are allelic differences at the loci under test (Fig. 2).

For a given enzyme, one strain (P_1) will show a band of fast mobility and the other strain (P_2) a slow band. If we assume that the enzyme is a dimer, then the interstrain hybrid will show three bands: a fast band and a slow band corresponding to the parental bands, and a third band in the middle representing the hybrid molecule.

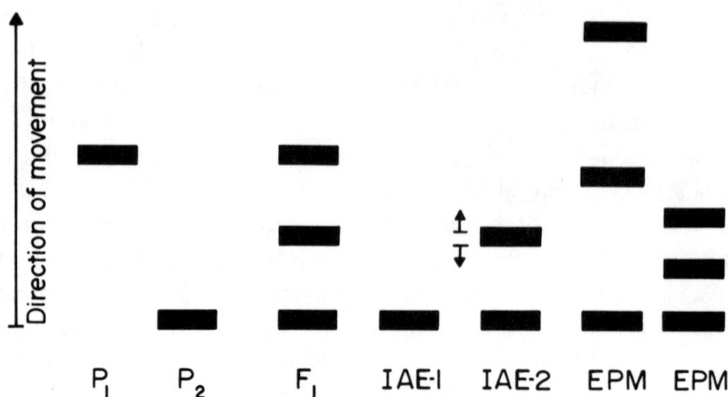

FIGURE 2 Electrophoretic pattern of parents, normal F_1, and possible mutant types in the biochemical specific locus mutation system. P_1, parents with fast-moving band; P_2, parent with slow-moving band; F_1, normal hybrid between P_1 and P_2; IAE-1, inactive polypeptide of P_1; IAE-2, inactive polypeptide of P_1 able to form complex with P_2 polypeptide; EPM, electrophoretic mobility mutants.

Now let us mutagenize the strain P_1 with the fast band and again look at the interstrain hybrid. If the mutation resulted in no enzyme produced or an inactive form, then the F_1 shows only the slow band and looks like the untreated parent, IAE-1; or if the produced polypeptide can interact with the active polypeptide, two bands may be formed, IAE-2. On the other hand, if the mutation was a base-pair substitution that merely altered the charge of the protein, the hybrid will still show three bands, but the fast and hybrid bands will be in an altered position (electrophoretic mobility mutants). It is therefore very easy to differentiate two types of mutations, only one of which is detected in the morphological specific locus test. In this example, we have considered only the types of mutations one sees if one parent is mutated. If the other parent was also treated, then an F_1 containing a mutation could look like the mirror image of any one of the mutant types in Fig. 2 and is easily differentiated from mutations in the other parent. In the F_1 it is possible to determine whether the gene from the male or the female has mutated. The F_1, therefore, can be the progeny of a cross where both parents are treated.

The first experiment was with X-rays as a mutagen. DBA/2J males were exposed to a total dose of 1,000 R, which was delivered as two 500-R doses with a 24-hr interfraction period. These males were then mated to females of the opposite strain (C57BL). The DBA males were sterile for approximately 3 months. All F_1 offspring were screened for mutations at nine different loci (Table 2).

We have tested more than 23,000 loci and have discovered 4 new mutations, which gives us an induced frequency of approximately 17.4×10^{-5} mutant per locus per generation. Using the same irradiation protocol and dose, Russell (1963) found 49.9×10^{-5} mutant per locus per generation; under similar irradiation conditions, but with a different set of markers in the specific locus test, Lyon and Morris (1969) got 13.9×10^{-5} mutant per locus per generation.

It is interesting that all four mutations that we have detected so far are mutations of the null activity or inactive enzyme type. This is not surprising since the mutants were induced by X-rays. Two of these mutations, which occurred at different times in totally different animals, were at the hemoglobin β locus, one was at the malic dehydrogenase locus, and one at the isocitrate dehydrogenase locus.

The frequency of dominant lethals induced by chemicals in males is highly dependent on the stage of spermatogenesis of the sperm at the time of treatment. Which stage is the most sensitive depends on the chemical; for instance, the most sensitive stages for ethyl methanesulfonate and methyl methanesulfonate are sperm and late spermatids (Ehling et al., 1968). Ehling (1974) has shown that induction of morphological specific locus mutations is positively correlated with the frequency of dominant lethals. The reasons for this correlation are not obvious.

Triethylenemelamine was the first chemical selected for use in the biochemical specific locus mutation system. Offspring were obtained from the treated late spermatid stage to maximize the yield of mutations, according to the correlation noted above. While the experiment is not yet complete, several presumptive mutants have been found (Soares and Malling, personal communication).

TABLE 2 Polymorphic Loci Presently Available
for Point Mutation Assay

	Alleles		
Locus	C57BL/6J	DBA/2J	Tissue
Es-1	a	b	Hemolysate
Es-3	a	a	Kidney
Gpd-1	a	b	Kidney
Gpi-1	b	a	Hemolysate
Id-1	a	b	Kidney
Mod-1	b	a	Kidney
Pgm-1	a	b	Hemolysate
Dip-1	a	b	Kidney
Hbb	s	d	Hemolysate

156   *H. V. Malling and L. R. Valcovic*

The efficiency of this system for evaluating the mutagenic risk of chemicals depends on the number of loci that can be screened simultaneously. It is clear that in terms of the number of progeny that have to be screened, this new system with its nine loci is not significantly better than previous specific locus systems. However, numerous other electrophoretic allelic differences have been identified in various inbred strains. Taylor (1972) has described the genetic relationship of the various mouse strains in a two-dimensional diagram. Most of the common inbred strains fall in a cluster to which DBA/2 belongs. C57BL/6 stands alone and quite far away from any of the other strains. C57BL/6J, therefore, was chosen to be the tester strain, and in collaboration with J. E. Womack and T. H. Roderick at the Jackson Laboratory (Bar Harbor, Maine), 14 other markers are being systematically backcrossed into the C57 strain (Fig. 3); the result will eventually be a new inbred strain with 25 allelic differences from DBA/2, including the two new differences uncovered recently between DBA/2 and C57BL/6. DBA/2 is closely related to a series of other strains, which nevertheless differ from DBA/2 and each other in many physiological traits such as resistance to radiation. The new strain will have a high number of electrophoretic differences from the strains closely related to DBA/2. By using this new strain as

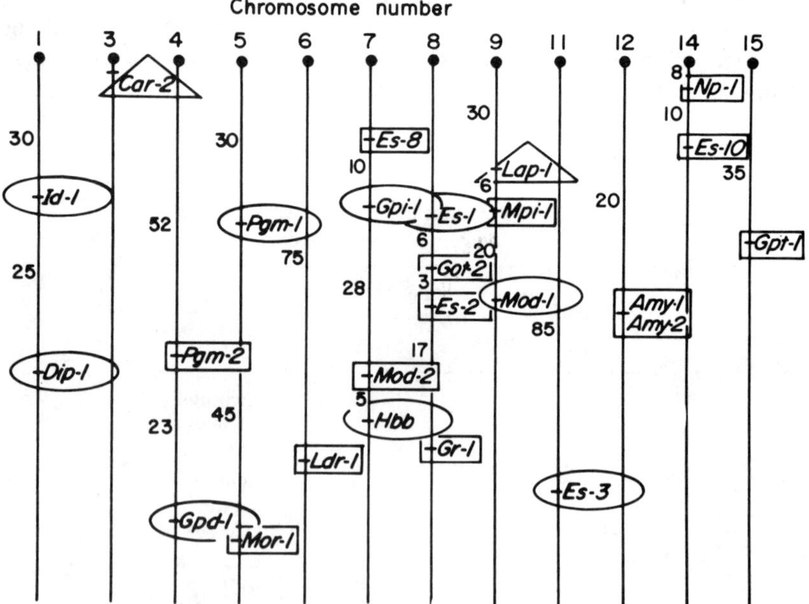

FIGURE 3 Location of present and future markers in the biochemicals specific locus mutation system on the mouse chromosomes. ◯ Original loci; ▢ newly detected differences between the two original strains; △ new loci.

a tester strain to which each treated strain is mated, it would also be possible to compare the effects of the physiological variations on the induced mutation rates.

Since these are normally occurring variants of enzymes that are fully functional, there should not be other than practical limits to the number of genes that can be accommodated in one strain. In addition, we are working to develop new electrophoretic methods for more enzymes that have not yet been adequately screened in the mouse to detect polymorphisms, and it is hoped that we will uncover more polymorphisms either within these strains or in other inbreds and further increase the number of loci that can be tested. Thus if, as we suppose, we can increase the number of polymorphic loci in the system to approximately 40, and remembering that we can treat both parents in a single experiment, then a single F_1 animal can be screened for mutations in 80 different loci. In this way a smaller number of animals will be required in the future to provide reliable data on which to base a risk estimation for the human population.

The electrophoretic mobility of enzymes and other proteins can be changed by attachment of charged side groups. Changes in the specificity of the enzymes that catalyze these attachment processes may result in changes in the enzymes that are screened for mutations and, thereby, changes in the electrophoretic mobility. Although these are not mutations that occur at the structural loci, they can be detected in the biochemical specific locus mutation system.

Many of the new alleles that are being added to the tests will be located on the same chromosome. There are seven chromosomes in which that is the case. In the morphological specific locus mutation experiment, some mutants were found in which two linked loci were apparently mutated independently and simultaneously, which is extremely improbable (Searle, 1974). These events have been explained as double nondisjunction. In the future the biochemical specific locus mutation system should be able to detect nondisjunction in seven different chromosomes, and it should be realized that certain chemicals are specifically active in inducing this type of mutation, such as hycanthone in mice and methyl mercury in *Drosophila.*

One further addition can be made to the biochemical specific locus mutation system. V. M. Chapman (personal communication) has found an electrophoretic variant of phosphoglycerylkinase-1; the gene is X-linked. If this system were polymorphic for an X-linked gene, it would be possible to detect X0 females. Electrophoretically, they would look like deletion of one of the *pgk* bands. The real nature of the mutant would have to be established cytologically. This last step could be avoided if we had two X-linked polymorphisms in the system.

Other Approaches

An assay is under development for detecting the induction of gene mutations that affect the specific activities of specific enzymes (Mays et al.,

1978). At present it is not known how many genes influence the specific activity of an enzyme. Conceptually, we can divide the genes controlling the activity of a single enzyme into five or more different classes.

1. The structural gene, which codes for the amino acid sequence in the protein.

2. The modifying gene, which modifies the protein structure after the primary polypeptide is formed.

3. The architectural gene, which determines in which organ the enzyme occurs (Paigen and Ganschow, 1965).

4. The temporal gene, which determines the time in development at which the gene is turned on and off (Paigen and Ganschow, 1965).

5. The regulatory gene, which modifies the production of the enzyme as a response to the internal and external environment.

This does not mean that there are that many genes controlling each enzyme activity. It is not known how many genes affect the specific activity of an enzyme in a certain tissue; therefore, in this system the mutation frequency cannot be expressed as a number per locus.

One of the features of this system is that a single inbred mouse strain is used and mutation induction is based on the detection of F_2 progeny with enzyme activity significantly different from normal. The F_2 generation is used to optimize mutant detection; that is, each mutant induced in the treated male will be expressed in half of the F_2 litter derived from that male. In addition, it is not necessary to keep the F_2 animal alive, which means that many different types of tissues can be sampled. If a mutation is found, the F_1 is still available for breeding.

One of the positive features of this approach is that computerized automatic enzyme analyzers (GEMSAEC) are being employed. This system is rapid and requires only a small amount of material (5 μl). Thus far, methods have been developed for the assay of approximately 30 enzymes.

Enzymes in which several isozymic forms are expressed in the same tissue and those whose activities vary with dietary conditions or hormonal levels are not readily amenable to this approach.

The two other systems are based on two-dimensional electrophoresis of enzyme groups in which there are many isozymes or a general denatured protein map (Klose, 1977; Narayanan and Rau, 1977). In both cases the assay is based on movement, disappearance, or appearance of a spot. Again, we have no idea how many genes are covered by a single spot, or how many spots are derived from an interaction between gene products (in the case of lactic dehydrogenase two genes give rise to five spots).

However, these criticisms should not be taken as an invalidation of these systems. They can be used together with a biochemical specific locus mutation system or the morphological specific locus mutation system in which the number of genes are known. The specific locus systems will form the basis for the calculation of the mutation rate. The more nonspecific systems are very important in the sense that they may give us information about mutation frequencies in classes of genes that are not detected in the biochemical specific locus mutation system, where we are mainly working with structural genes.

Mutation Rate in the Genes Private for Humans

All of these approaches use a series of very conservative genes, the household genes—genes that most cellular organisms have to have and that have been with us since the dawn of time. Is there a chance that these genes have mutated to a very stable form so that we are estimating the mutation rate in genes that are very stable? Look on it in a different way: What are the genetic differences between a chimpanzee and a human?—certainly not the household genes. β-Hemoglobin has exactly the same amino acid sequence in humans and chimpanzees. The genes that make up the difference must be comparably new in origin, and we have no idea about the mutation rate of those genes. If it is not new genes but the array in which they are put together, what is the mutation rate for disturbing this array?

On the other hand, the subspecies *castaneous* of the common laboratory mouse differs from most inbred strains at 30 of the analyzed biochemical loci (V. M. Chapman, personal communication). *Castaneous* is fully fertile when mated with several of the inbred mouse strains. This again points out that variation in the household genes may be rather unimportant for a Darwinian evolution within mammals.

IN VIVO SOMATIC GENE MUTATION SYSTEMS

A survey of the *in vivo* mutation systems in mammals will clearly indicate that there are plenty of systems for the detection of chromosome aberrations but a great lack of systems for the detection of point mutations in mammals *in vivo*. It is urgently necessary to develop such systems, because the point mutation systems in which the progeny of the treated animal are studied are extremely expensive. The benefit of developing *in vivo* somatic point mutation systems is that some of them can be used to monitor the human population for induction of mutations. Some of the animal tests will be nondestructive and can be performed on animals evaluated for other toxicologic effects. If somatic mutations and induction of cancer can be studied in the same tissue, we will be able to obtain badly needed data for the correlation between these two events.

Embryonic Spot Tests

The characters that can be used as markers for induction of mutations in a single cell have to be autonomous for that cell. They cannot be hormonal or diffusible characters. Formation of pigment in the melanocytes determines the color of the hair and skin and is autonomous. Two different types of pigment are produced, namely eumelanin (brown or black) or phaeomelanin (yellow). Both types of pigment can be present in granules in the melanocyte. Many different mutations affect the color, size, and distribution of these granules. The principle of the test is to produce embryos that are heterozygotic for several of these coat-color markers. A mutation in the wild-type allele will result in a melanocyte with this particular mutant phenotype. Many different mouse strains are available that are homozygotic for several recessive coat-color genes. For clear expression of the coat-color markers, it is advantageous for the embryo to be homozygotic for the nonagouti mutant gene. The first experiments utilizing such a system were done by Russell and Major (1957), who crossed C57BL and NB mice and used X-rays as the mutagen. After these initial experiments, the technique lay dormant for many years. Fahrig (1977) used a cross between C57BL/6 and the T stock. The embryos have the genotype $a/a; b/+; c^{ch}p/++; d\ se/++; s/+$. The progeny has a black coat and dark eyes like CB6. The homozygotic T stock has the genotype nonagouti (a/a); brown (b/b); linked chinchilla and pink-eyed dilution ($c^{ch}\ p/c^{ch}p$); linked dilute and short ear ($d\ se/d\ se$); and piebald spotting (s/s).

The development of the melanocytes has a great influence on the appearance of the spots. If only a few melanocytes are formed at the time of treatment, the mutant spots will be few and large; to obtain a sufficient number of treated cells, a greater number of animals has to be used. On the other hand, if treatment is performed late in the development at a time when many melanocytes are present, the mutant spot may be small and not easy to recognize. At 10½ days after conception there are approximately 200 melanocytes present, and this seems to be the optimal time for treatment with a mutagen.

Many different types of genetic events can give rise to a spot on the skin with a mutant phenotype. They are (1) a mutation in the wild-type gene, (2) a deletion of the wild-type gene, (3) a nondisjunction resulting in loss of the wild-type chromosome, (4) somatic crossover, and (5) gene conversion. The last two events have not been proved without doubt to occur in mammalian cells. As a preliminary screen for genetic activity of chemicals, it is an advantageous feature of the system that it detect as many genetic events as possible. Since the melanocytes are terminal cells, it is difficult at present to prove which genetic event led to the formation of the spot. Fahrig has demonstrated that the embryonic spot test responds positively to chemicals that are not mutagenic in the dominant lethal test and the host-mediated assay, and responds to lower doses of chemicals that are mutagenic in the two latter tests. The test has certain drawbacks such as the placenta barrier, which probably influences the concentration gradient of a chemical in a different way from the blood-testis barrier. The embryonic xenobiotic metabolism may be quite different from the same metabolism in adults. Also, nongenetic events such as cytotoxic effects on the malanocytes may give rise to spots, especially midventral white spots.

Eye Color Spot Test

The color of the retinal melanocytes is determined by many of the same genes as that of the skin melanocytes. Searle (1977) is developing a reverse mutation system using the unstable gene p^{un} (pink eye, dilution). The retinal melanocytes form a single-layered mosaic of hexogonal cells in the retinal pigment epithelium (RPE). After fixation of the eye in 2–3-day-old mice, the RPE can be dissected and cleared. The clones of darker-colored cells can easily be scored under a microscope. Searle found that a normal pigmented 3-day-old has approximately 10^5 retinal melanocytes. The spontaneous forward mutation frequency at the seven specific loci is about 10^{-5}. Even if the spontaneous reversion rate is considerably lower than 10^{-5}, relatively fewer animals must be prepared for determination of the mutation frequency, especially if the time between treatment and scoring can be kept short to increase the number of cells at risk.

There are no available data on the induction of reversion in this system by chemicals. Most reverse mutation systems are rather limited in the array of chemicals they respond to. No predictions can be made about this system before we know more about the nature of the genetic alteration that resulted in p^{un}.

Hemoglobin Antibody System in Mice

It is possible to produce antibodies that are so specific that they can recognize a difference of one amino acid between two proteins. In mice there exist three different alleles of the β chain in hemoglobin (Fig. 4). It should be possible to produce monospecific antibodies that recognize some of these differences. We have succeeded in making antibodies to hemoglobins d and s. Also, the α chain shows a polymorphism with several different alleles. The difference between two alleles is usually not more than one amino acid. Some of these may also be traceable and may be used to produce monospecific antibodies. The monospecific antibody will be marked with a fluorescent molecule. A smear of red blood cells will be fixed and stained with the antibody according to the following principle: anti-s absorbed with hemoglobin d will detect d to s mutations in red blood cells containing d. The antibodies are produced in Shetland ponies.

In Vivo Mutations Detected in Primary Cultures

The ability of chemicals to induce cancer in laboratory animals and their ability to induce mutations in lower organisms seem to be well correlated (Ames et al., 1973). If it were possible to study mutagenicity and carcino-

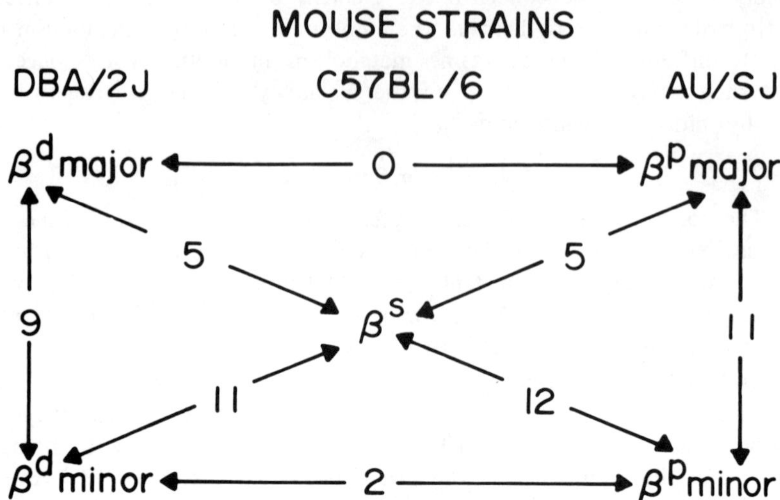

FIGURE 4 Type of variants in the β chain of hemoglobin in mice. The numbers between the arrows indicate the total numbers of amino acids that differ between the two chains (modified from Gilman, 1974).

genicity in cells from the same organ, correlative studies between these two biological events would be more relevant. Dean and Senner (1977) have developed such a system for lung cells from Chinese hamsters. Forward mutations were selected on media containing either 8-azaguanine or ouabain. The locus for azaguanine resistance is X-linked; ouabain resistance is codominant with the wild-type marker. Mutations were detected in primary cultures derived from lungs of 3-wk-old Chinese hamsters after treatment of the animals with the mutagen. The method will detect either direct-acting mutagens or mutagens formed by the mammalian metabolism in the lung or in other parts of the body if they are stable enough to affect the lung. The technique is limited to organs from whose cells primary cultures can be established.

SYSTEMS FOR MONITORING THE HUMAN POPULATION

The Problem

Monitoring of the human population for mutations can be done by screening offspring of exposed individuals or by screening the cells of exposed individuals. Mutation in a single gene is a rare event, and at present we can monitor only a few genes (< 50). This means that if we select the germinal method for monitoring, we will have to screen a great number of offspring. If the spontaneous mutation rate is 1×10^{-5} and we analyze 100,000 blood specimens from newborn for 20 proteins, then a 72.5% increase in the mutation rate could be detected at the 5% level (Neel, 1970). Instead of screening for electrophoretic variants, we could use dominant traits. Of all the dominant traits in the human population only four seem to have the qualities required for mutation studies (Vogel, 1970). Using these traits, Vogel calculated that detecting a 10% increase in the mutation frequency for 2 periods of 10 yr would require a population the size of Germany's. With these techniques, it may be possible to follow the general trend in the population. The required sample size is too large for these techniques to be used to pinpoint an exposure to a chemical in a factory that induces mutations in the individuals working there.

Another approach is to study the occurrence of mutations in single cells in an individual. In this case, the individual can be considered as a population, and to obtain significant data only a few persons will have to be monitored from any one exposed group. Blood and semen are probably the two types of samples containing single cells that are most readily available from the human population.

Hemoglobin Systems

Fluorescent antibody system. The red cells of an individual contain almost pure hemoglobin. In the human population there are many different germinal mutations that lead to the formation of individuals whose red blood cells contain a different hemoglobin. Some of these hemoglobins are sufficiently different from normal hemoglobin that it is possible to produce monospecific antibodies to them. Since mutations that give rise to a variant in the hemoglobin types can occur in the germ cells, we can also assume that they can occur in the stem cells for the red blood cells. By attaching a fluorescent molecule to the monospecific antibodies against a certain aberrant hemoglobin, we should be able to localize the few red blood cells that contain this different hemoglobin.

In the collaborative program of the National Institute of Environmental Health Sciences, scientists in Dr. George Stamatoyannopoulos' group at the University of Washington, Seattle, have made antibodies that react to one particular hemoglobin type. Their first success was the production of monospecific antibodies against hemoglobin S (Hb-S), which gives rise to sickle-cell anemia. The antibodies that react only with Hb-S were marked with a fluorescent molecule [fluorescent in isothiocyanate (FITC)]. The specificity of the Hb-S antibody was tested by counting the number of cells reacting with anti-S in artificial mixtures of Hb-S carriers and normal individuals. In these reconstruction experiments, the expected number of Hb-S cells was found. Monospecific antibody against Hb-C has also been produced, and this antibody seems to be as specific as the Hb-S one. Similar reconstruction experiments were done by making artificial mixtures of blood cells from normal individuals and from individuals heterozygotic for Hb-C, and again the expected number of Hb-C cells was found. Hemoglobin S has valine and Hb-C has lysine at the position 6 on the β chain; monospecific antibodies to Hb-S failed to bind to cells containing Hb-C. After these successful reconstruction experiments, red blood cells from normal individuals were screened for the presence of cells containing Hb-S, and it was found that they occurred with a frequency of 1 per 10 million normal cells.

The mutation that results in Hb-S is one particular type, namely a base-pair substitution. The nucleotide triplet that codes for glutamic acid is either GAA or GAG, and the nucleotide triplet that codes for valine is GUU, GUC, GUA, or GUG. The single base-pair change resulting in glutamine $\rightarrow$ valine is GAA $\rightarrow$ GUA or GAG $\rightarrow$ GUG. The nucleotide triplet that codes for lysine is either AAA or AAG, and the mutation resulting in glutamic acid $\rightarrow$ lysine need involve only one base-pair change, GAA $\rightarrow$ AAA or GAG $\rightarrow$ AAG. The genetic alterations that result in Hb-S and Hb-C are very specific, in a certain way analogous to a reverse mutation system, and may be expected to show a similar mutagen specificity. It is therefore very important to broaden our spectrum of mutants that can be screened in this system. In the human population there are many different hemoglobinopathies. Hemoglobin Cranston is produced by a frameshift mutation resulting in β-chain elongation. Hemoglobin Constant Spring (Hb-CS) is a variant with an abnormal α chain that has an additional 31 amino acid residues extending beyond the carboxyl terminal arginine of the normal α chain. The simplest explanation is that a mutation has occurred in the termination codon of the α chain. At present, Stamatoyannopoulos and his colleagues are proceeding to produce and isolate monospecific antibodies to 10 or so hemoglobinopathies. This will increase the spectrum of genetic alterations that can be scored in the system and also decrease the number of red blood cells that have to be screened to obtain accurate mutation frequencies. One could imagine mixing all 10 monospecific antibodies together and screening simultaneously for 10 different aberrant hemoglobins on the same slide, which should give an average background of 1 per 10^6 red blood cells.

However, not all amino acid differences can be recognized immunologically. Fetal hemoglobin contains two different γ chains, γA and γG. The only difference is that at position 136, γA contains an alanine and γG a glycine. Although antibodies can be isolated that react with γA and γG and not with β, it has not yet been possible to isolate antibodies that react only with γG and not with γA or vice versa.

At present, data are obtained by visually counting a spread of red blood cells. This is an extremely laborious process; to establish the spontaneous mutation frequency in one individual requires 1 human-month of work. This is the bottleneck of the system. In our laboratory we are developing automatic scanning techniques with the microscope, and we are collaborating with Lawrence Livermore Laboratories to adapt the red blood cells for use in the automatic cell sorter. This poses several technical difficulties. The hemoglobin is inside the red blood cell. The antibody must penetrate the cell wall in order to react with the hemoglobin. Holes big enough for the antibodies must, therefore, be made in the cell wall. However, the hemoglobin is smaller than the antibody, and will diffuse out of the red blood cell faster than the antibody can get in. Thus the hemoglobin must be made immobile inside the red blood cell. Another problem is that the mutant cell is so rare that the noise in the cell sorter will give more false positives than mutant cells at the present time.

Radioimmunoassay system. Another approach that can be used to detect mutant hemoglobin utilizes radioimmunoassay techniques. R. A. Doherty (personal communication) has utilized antibody that is very specific for Hb-S. This antibody was labelled with I^{125}. He performed the following experiment to show its specificity. In the presence of a standard amount of Hb-S the amount of hemoglobin from lysed cells was varied, and then for each concentration the level of Hb-S was determined. Below an Hb-S/Hb-A ratio of 10^{-7}, the added Hb-A did not interefere with the determination of Hb-S.

It is possible, however, that Hb-S can be produced by both a transcription error and a translation error. Both are rare events, and it can be assumed that the Hb-S molecules produced by either one of these mechanisms will be distributed evenly among all the red blood cells. In the system based on detection of Hb-S in the cells, the few molecules of Hb-S present in each cell will not be detectable, only the mutant cell with the high concentration of Hb-S. However, when the hemoglobin solution is screened by radioimmunoassay for Hb-S, both the Hb-S produced by mutation and that produced by translation and transcription errors will be detected. It is therefore surprising that Doherty did not find interference from the crude hemoglobin solution before the ratio of Hb-S to crude Hb-A was 10^{-7}. If the translation and transcription was a substantial factor in producing Hb-S, it could be expected that the interference would occur at lower ratios. One advantage of the radioimmunoassay is that it can be performed in 30 min per sample.

Aberrant amino acid incorporation system. Human hemoglobin has a peculiar biochemistry insofar as neither the α chain nor the β chain contains isoleucine. On the basis of this fact, Popp et al. (1976) have attempted to develop a somatic mutation system. Since isoleucine is not coded for, the only way it can occur in adult human hemoglobin is by mutation or by errors in the transcription or translation process. The hemoglobin has to be ultrapure to make accurate estimates of the isoleucine content. The red blood cells contain several nonhemoglobin proteins that contain isoleucine, fetal hemoglobin is present in various amounts in normal adults, and the γ chain of fetal hemoglobin contains four isoleucines per chain. Popp et al. have developed separation methods with which it is possible to assume that the contaminating isoleucine is only a small part of the total isoleucine. In the normal human the frequency of amino acid exchanges per amino acid in the α chain is 2×10^{-5}, and in the β chain 4.3×10^{-5}. It was possible for Popp et al. to obtain blood from irradiated victims from the Marshall Islands. The data are given in Table 3.

TABLE 3 Frequency of Incorporation of Isoleucine
into Human Hemoglobin from Exposed and
Nonexposed Individuals at the Marshall Islands[a]

Exposure (R)	Substitution frequency
0	$3.20 \pm 1.52 \times 10^{-5}$
69	$5.94 \pm 1.92 \times 10^{-5}$
175	$8.81 \pm 1.96 \times 10^{-5}$

[a]From Popp et al., 1976. Reprinted with permission of
S. Karger AG, Basel.

These data raise several questions. (1) The translation and transcription errors are not necessarily nongenetic, but could result from mutations in the enzymes catalyzing these processes. Stamatoyannopoulos found that the frequency of Hb-S containing red blood cells was 10^{-7}; the concentration of the mutant hemoglobin is therefore 0.5×10^{-7}, which is 600 times less than the amino acid substitution rate Popp et al. found. Is the surplus because of translation and transcription errors? In contrast, Doherty's data based on radioimmunoassays of Hb-S left no room for translation and transcription errors. (2) In general, base-pair substitutions are considered to be infrequent among X-ray-induced mutations in mammals. It is therefore surprising that the isoleucine system was able to detect an increase in the amino acid substitution rate after irradiation. If this is correct, it indicates that the system should be very sensitive for monitoring exposure to mutagens that predominantly induce point mutations. The control individuals varied with respect to age, and Popp et al. found that the substitution frequency increased with age to the rate of 2.96×10^{-7}/year.

Limitations of the systems. (1)The very specific type of mutations for which we are screening. As mentioned earlier, this can be helped by increasing the number of variant hemoglobins that show antigenic differences from the normal. In the system based on human hemoglobin it should be possible to score for lack of production of the α chain. In individuals with α-thalassemia we find a high frequency of β_4, which is antigenically different from $\alpha_2\beta_2$. In reconstruction experiments done with red blood cells from α-thalassemia patients and normal individuals, it is possible to detect the β_4-containing cells in the expected numbers (G. Stamatoyannopoulos, personal communication). The genetic alteration in α-thalassemia patients may be deletion of the α gene or some regulatory mutation. (2) How do we show that the cell that reacts with the monospecific antibody really contains the mutant proteins? The red blood cell is a terminal cell that cannot divide; we could probably use a cell sorter to enrich the sample of the mutant cells. At present there are technical difficulties. We have not yet developed a technique to react the red blood cells in suspension with the antibodies. For this reaction the cell membrane must open up and let the antibody get into the cell without the hemoglobin getting out of the cell. A light fixation is therefore performed on the slide.

Thioguanine-Resistant Lymphocytes

Peripheral blood lymphocytes can be stimulated to synthesize DNA by the addition of phytohemagglutinin (PHA). This stimulation can be inhibited by 8-azaguanine in normal individuals but not in boys with the Lesch-Nyhan (LN) syndrome. The LN syndrome is a deficiency in hypoxanthine guanine phosphoribosyltransferase (HGPRT). The DNA synthesis can be measured by addition of tritiated thymidine and scored in the nuclei by standard autoradiographic techniques. In females heterozygotic for LN, there is a drastic reduction in the frequency of thioguanine-resistant cells, which may indicate a strong selection against the LN cells (Strauss and Albertini, 1978). The frequency of resistant phenotypes depends on the concentration of thioguanine (TG). At a concentration of TG 2×10^{-4} M adult women heterozygotic for LN contain 10^{-3}–10^{-2} resistant cells, whereas normal young women contain on the average 8×10^{-5}. During chemotherapy treatment for cancer, the frequency of TG-resistant cells shows a significant increase.

Histochemical Techniques

Numerous techniques have been developed for localizing specific enzymes in cells (Pearse, 1968, 1972). Variants of enzymes have been found in the human population that differ from each other with respect to substrate specificity. In humans there is a rare variant of glucose-6-phosphate dehydrogenase (G6PD) that can utilize deoxyglucose 6-phosphate as substrate. Sutton (1974) attempted to develop a system based on detection of white blood cells that contain this variant G6PD because of a mutation in the stem cells. The system failed because a slight denaturation of the normal enzyme gives it an increased substrate specificity similar to that of the variants; this means that the stained cells in the reaction mixture containing deoxyglucose 6-phosphate should be considered as phenocopies. Histochemical techniques can be used to develop many other *in vivo* single cell mutation systems. We can write the general enzymatic histochemical reaction as follows: enzyme + coenzyme + cofactors + substrate + stain → stained cell. We can now think about detecting mutations by varying the coenzyme, substrate, or cofactor, or by adding an inhibitor.

In our laboratory we are developing such a system using mouse sperm. The midpiece of mammalian sperm contains a large number of mitochondria, which contain many different enzymes. Thus far, we have developed histochemical methods for lactate dehydrogenase, α-glycerolphosphate dehydrogenase, and succinic dehydrogenase. Enzymes located in cells do not behave like enzymes in suspension; for instance, succinic dehydrogenase is a flavin enzyme, and nitroblue tetrazolium should be reduced directly without phenazine methosulfate (PMS). Nevertheless, in order to stain for succinic dehydrogenase, the reaction requires PMS. α-Glycerolphosphate dehydrogenase should require NAD; however, coenzyme is not necessary for staining the sperm for this enzyme. On the other hand, the stain reaction in sperm for lactic dehydrogenase requires NAD and PMS, just like reaction mixtures used in electrophoresis.

We have elected to use enzyme inhibitors as the selective mechanism to detect mutational events. Malonic acid inhibits succinic dehydrogenase at a concentration of 0.1 mg/ml. Presumed mutant sperm would be those that exhibited a positive stain reaction with malonate present in the reaction mixture.

The experimental protocol for this system is simple. Sperm samples are obtained from control and treated mice; varying the time of sample collection after treatment will reflect the stages of the spermatogenic cycle. Both samples are subdivided and stained as follows:

Tube 1: Sperm (enzyme) + succinate + PMS

Tube 2: Sperm (enzyme) + succinate + PMS + malonate

The stained sperm in tube 1 represent the control population; this population will contain some fraction of defective (unstained) sperm. Only cells that are not inhibited by malonate will stain in tube 2. The mutant frequency is simply the stained cells in tube 2 divided by the stained cells in tube 1. The automatic scanning microscope mentioned previously is intended for use in this program to accelerate the scoring procedure.

Sperm cells, as they are used in this system, are terminal cells, and depending on the mutation frequency in sperm it may or may not be possible to compare it with a mutation frequency obtained in F_1 after treatment of the male parent. Furthermore, it is not even known that resistant mutations can occur. One way to get around this problem is to screen many different mouse strains and appropriate mutants to detect a resistant variant that can be determined by being controlled by a single gene. This work is now in progress in collaboration with Dr. Roderick at the Jackson Laboratory.

CONCLUSION

Several new mutation systems are being developed with the aim of preventing health hazards to the human population from deleterious changes in the human genome by exposure to environmental compounds. This task has barely started and developments are required in at least the following areas:

1. Increasing the data bank. There are very few data or no data at all for many of the new systems. The systems therefore need to be

verified and validated by accumulation of data from use or exposure to a broad spectrum of mutagens.

2. Relationship between indicator systems and adverse effect. For many systems the detection of mutations is based on characters where the mutation has no deleterious effect. A correlation has to be established between the mutation rate of the indicator character and the mutation rate in characters with deleterious effects.

3. Parallel systems in humans and other mammals. Data obtained with the monitoring systems for humans will be difficult to interpret without a parallel system in a laboratory mammal in which responses to the different classes of chemical mutagens can be studied.

4. Technical developments. Many of the new systems are laborious and require an intensive use of labor. Technical development of the cell sorter, microscopic scanning, and automatic electrophoresis is necessary before the systems can be implemented.

5. Molecular mechanisms of mutations in mammals. In many of the new systems that are being developed, the gene produced is known. That opens the possibility for elucidating the mutational mechanism, which is a prerequisite for rational decisions concerning the level of exposure to the human population.

6. Population genetics. To evaluate the cost to the human population of an increased frequency of mutations, it is necessary to know the fitness of newly induced mutations in the population. The relationship of the mutation rate in the stem cells for the red blood cells to the measured mutation frequency in the same cells must be understood.

7. Gene regulation. The molecular mechanism of gene regulation is barely understood in mammals. Therefore, it is not possible to create a mutation system in which mutations in regulator genes can be directly measured. The mutation rate in such genes may be different from the mutation rate in structural genes.

8. Private genes for humans. Humans have undergone a dramatic evolution during the last several million years. There are features of humans that separate them dramatically from other mammalian species. What are the inherited factors that lead to these differences, and do they behave differently from other genes in their response to mutagenic agents? Each species has such a private inheritance; what is the mutation rate in this inheritance?

The present generation is only a caretaker of the human genome of future generations. It is therefore our most precious possession. Our lack of understanding of the response of the genome to our technological society requires the investment of sufficient funds to ensure that an undamaged genome is passed on to future generations. The list above shows some areas where funds and development are needed.

REFERENCES

Abrahamson, S., Bender, M. A., Conger, A. D. and Wolff, S. 1973. *Nature (Lond.)* 245:460–462.

Alexander, M. L. 1960. *Genetics* 45:1019–1022.

Ames, B. N., Lee, F. D. and Durston, W. E. 1973. *Proc. Natl. Acad. Sci. U.S.A.* 70:782–786.

Badr, F. M., Lorkin, P. A. and Lehmann, H. 1973. *Nature New Biol.* 242: 107–110.

Clegg, J. B., Weatherall, D. J. and Milner, P. F. 1971. *Nature (Lond.)* 234: 337–340.

Crow, F. and Kimura, M. 1970. *An introduction to population genetic theory.* New York: Harper & Row.

Dean, B. J. and Senner, K. R. 1977. *Mutat. Res.* 46:403–407.

Dutta, S. K. 1974. *Nucleic Acid Res.* 1:1141–1149.

Ehling, U. H. 1974. *Arch. Toxicol.* 32:19–25.

Ehling, U. H., Cumming, R. B., and Malling, H. V. 1968. *Mutat. Res.* 5: 417–428.

Fahrig, R. 1977. In *Chemical mutagens, principles and methods for their detection*, ed. A. Hollaender, vol. 5. New York: Plenum. In press.

Gilman, 1974. *Ann. N.Y. Acad. Sci.* 241:416–433.

Kimura, M. and Ohta, T. 1971. *Nature (Lond.)* 229:467.

Klose, J. 1977. *Arch. Toxicol.* 38:53–60.

Malling, H. V. and Valcovic, L. R. (1977). In *Progress in genetic toxicology*, eds. D. Scott, B. A. Bridges, and F. H. Sobels, pp. 155–164. Amsterdam: Elsevier.

Mays, J., McAninch, J., Feurs, R. J., Burkhart, J., Mohrenweiser, H. and Casciano, D. A. 1978. *Mutat. Res.* 53:98–99.

Milner, P. F., Clegg, J. B. and Weatherall, D. J. 1971. *Lancet* 1:729–732.

Narayanan, K. R. and Rau, A. S. 1977. In *Electrofocusing and isotachophoresis: Proceedings of the fourth international symposium*, eds. B. J. Radola and D. Graesslin, pp. 221–231. Berlin: Walter deGruyter.

Neel, J. V. 1970. *Proc. Natl. Acad. Sci. U.S.A.* 67:908–915

Paigen, K. and Ganschow, R. 1965. *Brookhaven Symp. Biol.* 14:522–537.

Peacock, W. J., Brutlag, D., Goldring, E., Appels, R., Hinton, C. W. and Lindsley, D. L. 1973. *Cold Spring Harbor Symp. Quant. Biol.* 28: 405–416.

Pearse, A. G. E. 1968. *Histochemistry, theoretical and applied*, vol. 1. Baltimore: Williams & Wilkins.

Pearse, A. G. E. 1972. *Histochemistry, theoretical and applied*, vol. 2. Baltimore: Williams & Wilkins.

Popp, R. A., Bailiff, E. G., Hirsch, G. P. and Conrad, R. A. 1976. *Interdiscip. Top. Gerontol.* 9:209–218.

Russell, W. L. 1963. In *Repair of genetic radiation damage*, ed. F. H. Sobels, pp. 205–217. Oxford: Pergamon.

Russell, L. B. and Major, M. H. 1957. *Genetics* 42:161–175.

Russell, W. L. and Russell, L. B. (1959. *Radiat. Res. Suppl.* 1:296–305.

Schalet, A. P. and Sankaranarayanan, K. (1976). *Mutat. Res.* 35:341–370.

Searle, A. G. 1974. *Adv. Radiat. Biol.* 4:131–208.

Searle, A. G. 1977. *Arch. Toxicol.* 38:105–108.

Seid-Akhavan, M., Winker, W. P., Abramson, R. K. and Rucknaagel, D. L. 1976. *Proc. Natl. Acad. Sci. U.S.A.* 73:882–886.

Sparrow, A. H., Price, H. J. and Underbrink, A. G. 1972. *Brookhaven Symp. Biol.* 23:451–494.

Strauss, G. H. and Albertini, R. J. 1978. *Mutat. Res.* 53:119.

Sutton, H. E. 1974. *Proc. 4th Int. Conf. Birth Defects*, pp. 212–214.

Taylor, B. A. 1972. *J. Hered.* 63:83–86.

Valcovic, L. R. and Malling, H. V. 1973. *Environ. Health Perspect.* 6:201–205.

Vogel, F. 1970. In *Chemical mutagenesis in mammals and man*, eds. F. Vogel and G. Rohrborn, pp. 16–68. New York: Springer-Verlag.

Webber, B. B. and de Serres, F. J. 1965. *Proc. Natl. Acad. Sci. U.S.A.* 53:430–437.

Part 4

CHEMICAL MUTAGENS

CHAPTER 9

ENVIRONMENTAL SOURCES
OF CHEMICAL MUTAGENS
I. NATURALLY OCCURRING MUTAGENS

Lawrence Fishbein
National Center for Toxicological Research
Jefferson, Arkansas

INTRODUCTION

It is generally acknowledged that humans have always been exposed to a spectrum of naturally occurring potential toxicants of biological origin (e.g., mycotoxins, pyrrolizidine alkaloids, polycyclic aromatic hydrocarbons), as well as metals and metalloids and their derivatives (e.g., mercury, lead, arsenic, cadmium, selenium), radionuclides, and atmospheric gases (sulfur and nitrogen oxides, ozone).

The major objectives of this chapter are to bring into perspective comparative data on the amounts, residues, and transport in the environment of a number of representative mutagenic and potential mutagenic agents from diverse categories, including the naturally occurring mutagens of biological origin as well as the anthropogenic sources of air pollution. Admittedly, a number of the categories above overlap those that will be considered in Chapter 10, which focuses on industrial mutagens (e.g., metals and certain halogens, such as fluorine and chlorine, and their derivatives).

This assessment cannot be complete since in many instances the amounts of substances produced as well as distributed in the various environmental compartments are either unknown or not definitively known. However, these two chapters will attempt to illustrate, wherever possible, the major sources of naturally occurring and synthetic chemical mutagens and potential mutagens in the environment, their stability, transport, and mutagenic activity in various test systems, as well as possible aspects of their synergistic and health effects.

Rates of loss into the environment (National Academy of Sciences, 1975) can be classified according to the compartment into which the chemical is *originally* released, as follows: (1) *atmosphere*: direct release (volatile liquids, propellants, gases), evaporation (solvents, plasticizers), dispersive uses of liquids or solids (sprays, fire extinguishers), production losses of volatile materials (halogenated hydrocarbons) and gaseous by-products (SO_2, CO, HCl); (2) *land*: disposal of domestic and industrial wastes, pesticide usage; (3) *fresh waters*: production losses of materials, disposal of used liquids into drains, spills into river and lake transportation, sewage effluents; and (4) *ocean*: direct discharge via outfalls, industrial dumping, and marine and dredge spoils.

After the chemicals are released into the environment, a variety of mechanisms exists for their transport and transfer to other media. The most significant include: (1) *atmospheric processes*: transport of vapor-phase material per se (or on particles) by wind; vertical diffusion; fallout and/or rain-out of particles; chemical and photolytic changes; solution of vapor in the ocean; (2) *land processes*: diffusion into soil as vapor or in aqueous solution; volatilization from soil, burning dumps, incinerators, or reprocessing plants; leaching into groundwater; wind or water erosion of soil particles; adsorption and desorption from soil particles; metabolism by soil organisms and uptake; metabolism and elimination by plants and animals; (3) *fresh water*: adsorption and desorption from suspended particles or sediments; diffusion into and transport of sediments; distribution of water and its contaminants by irrigation; chemical transformations; uptake and metabolism by plants and animals; and (4) *ocean*: adsorption and desorption from suspended particles or sediments; diffusion into sediments; resuspension and transport of shallow-water sediments; chemical transformations; uptake and metabolism by plants and animals; concentration in surface films; evaporation or ejection in spray, vertical mixing and diffusion in upper layers, and transport in ocean currents.

For our purposes, the "dose-response" situation of the chemicals to be considered depends primarily on (1) their level in the biosphere as determined by interaction of factors including production, leakage during transport and storage, usage and disposal patterns, and biogeochemical redistributions and degradations (Goodman, 1974; National Academy of Sciences, 1975); and (2) trends in the biosphere as determined by changes in the relative activity of the above parameters.

The obvious major routes of human exposure to a potential toxicant are through food, drinking water, respired air, and direct contact exposure. More difficult to determine accurately are the effects of a rising trend from natural or background levels to an *effect* level at which a significant adverse response is recognized in humans from preset toxic levels or the percentage of affected organisms based on toxicological criteria (Goodman, 1974).

NATURALLY OCCURRING MUTAGENS

Mycotoxins

From genetic and toxicological considerations, it is generally believed that the most important group of naturally occurring chemicals is the mycotoxins (mold metabolites), which are found in a variety of food and feed materials such as meal, grain, and straw. The species and strains of fungi that produce these toxic substances are both large in number and complex.

The magnitude of this potential health hazard is thought to be considerable (Tazima, 1974; Arrhenius, 1973; Campbell and Stoloff, 1974). High humidity and temperature conditions, which favor the growth of molds, are normal in large agricultural areas. Harvesting and storage techniques for grain are not in the main considered to be totally adequate (even in developed countries) to counteract mold growth by decreasing the moisture content of the harvest in field and storage bins. The spectrum of grain species that have been shown to be infected with toxic molds is extraordinarily broad and encompasses the most common food and feed sources such as rice, wheat, barley, peanuts, copra, and sweet potatoes. Another very disturbing aspect is the appearance of mycotoxins in various food chains, as in meat and milk (Arrhenius, 1973).

Mycotoxins cause a variety of diseases, including disturbances of nerve function, liver damage, kidney malfunction, blood diseases, limb deformation during growth, high carcinogenic potency in several organs and damage to the growing fetus, and hormonal disturbances resulting in changed sexual behavior and decreased fertility.

Figure 1 illustrates some examples of mycotoxins, toxin-producing mold species, habitats of the molds, and diseases induced by the toxins. Table 1 summarizes a number of principal studies of mycotoxicosis in terms of the disease, date and location of the outbreak, affected organism, pathogenic organism, and mycotoxin implicated.

Aflatoxins. The aflatoxins are the best-known mycotoxins that may appear in the human diet and comprise eight major closely related toxins (see Fig. 1) produced by the genus *Aspergillus* (including primarily *A. flavus, A. parasitiens,* and *A. oryzae*). Aflatoxin production by strains of *A. niger, A. wentii, A. ruber, A. ochraceous, Penicillium puberulum, P. frequentas,* and *P. citrinum* has also been reported. Aflatoxin-producing fungal strains appear to be ubiquitously distributed, hence virtually every foodstuff or food product is *potentially* susceptible to contamination under conditions, particularly of moisture and temperature, favoring fungal growth, which can occur at any stage of food production or subsequent processing [International Agency for Research on Cancer (IARC), 1972]. Some samples of nearly every major dietary staple have been found to contain some aflatoxin at one time or another.

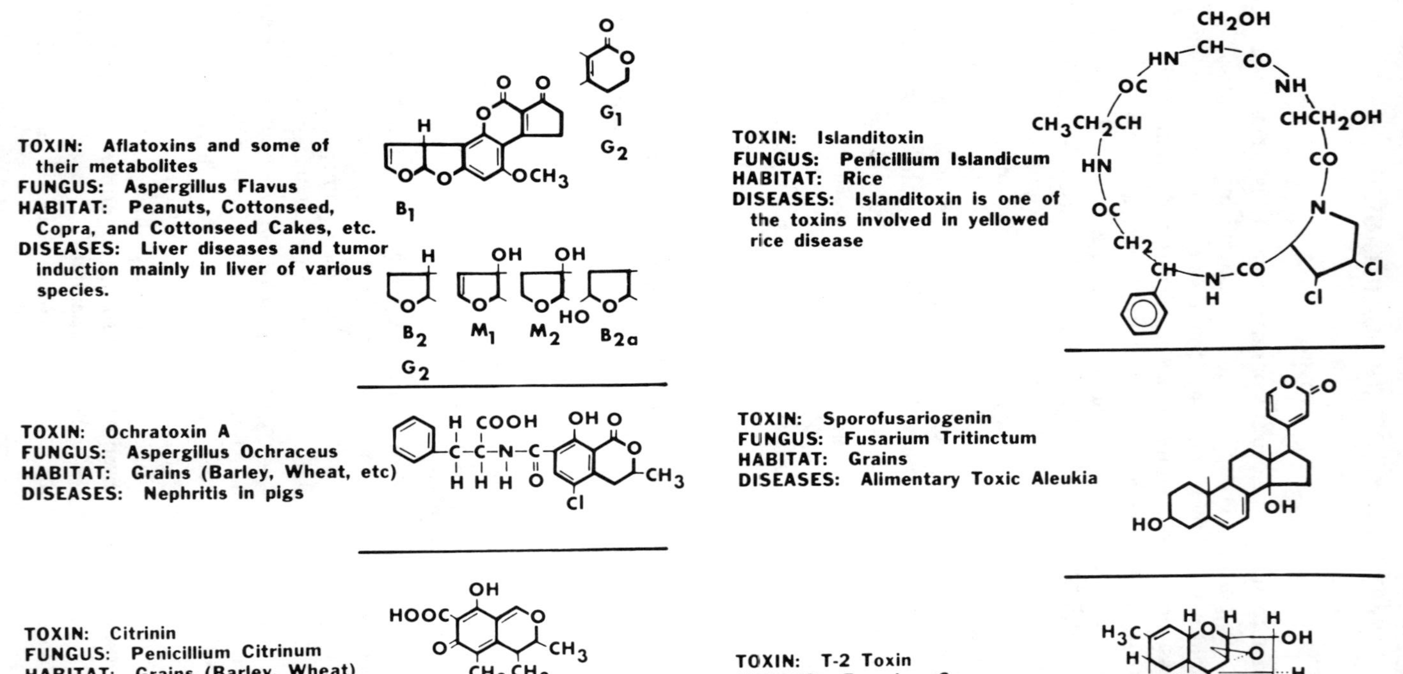

FIGURE 1   Some examples of mycotoxins, toxin-producing mold species, habitats of the molds, and diseases induced by the toxins.

TABLE 1 Summarized List of Studies of Mycotoxicosis

Disease and date of outbreak	Affected organism	Pathogenic organism	Mycotoxin	Location
Ergotism, 1762, 1966	Humans, cattle, sheep	*Claviceps purpurea*	Ergot alkaloid	Europe
Alimentary toxic aleukia, 1913, 1942	Humans, cattle, horse, pig, dog	*Fusarium sporotrichoides*	Sporofusarin	Soviet Union
Fusariotoxicosis, 1928	Swine, horse, humans, duckling	*Fusarium nivale*	Nivalenol; fusarenon-X	Japan
		Fusarium surpi	Diacetoxyscirpenol	United States, Europe
Yellowed rice toxicosis, 1940	Chicken	*Pencillium islandicum*	Luteoskyrin; cyclochlorotine	Japan
Turkey-X, 1960	Turkey, trout	*Aspergillus flavus*	Aflatoxins	Britain, United States
Hepatitis X, 1950	Dog	*Aspergillus nidulans*	Sterigmatocystin	South Africa
Hyperkeratosis, 1953, 1961	Calf	*Aspergillus clavatus*	Patulin	United States
		Penicillium urticae, etc.	Penicillic acid	United States
Hepatitis X, 1952	Dog, swine	*Penicillium rubrum*	Rubratoxin B	United States
	(Wheat, Katsuobushi)	*Aspergillus ochraceus*	Ochratoxin A	Japan, South Africa

It should be noted that under inadequate conditions, contamination can occur in a given locality with great variability with regard to types of food affected, frequency of contamination, and levels of aflatoxin present. The following generalizations are noted: aflatoxin B_1 is most frequently found in contaminated samples; aflatoxins B_2 and G_1 are present much less frequently and almost never in the absence of B_1 (IARC, 1972). Dietary surveys in Uganda, Thailand, and Swaziland have disclosed that peanuts, beans, and corn were the principal vectors of aflatoxins, with many samples (e.g., up to 50% of market samples of peanuts) containing 0.1–1 ppm of aflatoxin, while other grains such as rice were rarely contaminated (Alpert et al., 1971; Keen and Martin, 1971; Shank et al., 1972b). Mean aflatoxin levels of 0.121–0.351 $\mu g/kg$ of food and 0.05–0.167 $\mu g/l$ of beer have been reported in different regions of Kenya (IARC, 1972).

The chemical, physical, and biological properties and isolation of the aflatoxins occurring in foods and feeds have been extensively reviewed (Goldblatt, 1969; 1970; Kraybill, 1969; Miller, 1971; Bamburg et al., 1969; Marcuse et al., 1972; Borker et al., 1966; Wogan, 1966; 1968; Fishbein and Falk, 1970; Fishbein, 1972; IARC, 1972). The literature on the comparative metabolism and toxicity of the aflatoxins is equally extensive (Patterson, 1973; Barnes, 1970; Patterson and Allcroft, 1970; Patterson and Roberts, 1970; Kraybill and Shimkin, 1964; Wogan, 1969; Newberne and Butler, 1969; Campbell and Stoloff, 1974; IARC, 1972; Newberne, 1965; 1974; Wogan et al., 1971).

The carcinogenic effect of aflatoxin B_1 is subject to variation under the influence of genetic factors such as species, strain, and sex or of environmental factors such as diet. Sites of tumor induction by aflatoxins, other than the liver, include the stomach, kidney, salivary gland, and intestine. The diversity of responses suggests that metabolism may be an important factor in determining the toxic action of aflatoxin B_1 in different species (Patterson, 1973).

Aflatoxin B_1 (one of the most powerful hepatotoxins known) and aflatoxin G_1 are carcinogenic in four animal species, inducing tumors of the liver and some other organs following administration by several routes, including oral exposure. Aflatoxin M_1 produced liver tumors in the trout, and aflatoxin B_2 produced liver tumors in the rat, but only at doses more than 100 times higher than those of B_1 (IARC, 1972).

Evidence concerning the carcinogenicity of aflatoxin B_1 in nonhuman primates is both meager and conflicting (Cuthbertson et al., 1967; Deo et al., 1970; Tilak, 1975). For example, a mixed aflatoxin preparation given orally to rhesus monkeys once per week at a level of 62 $\mu g/kg$ produced histological evidence of liver damage, but no tumors in five surviving animals after 2 yr (Deo et al., 1970). Tilak (1975) reported a metastasizing intrahepatic bile duct carcinoma in a rhesus monkey receiving a mixed aflatoxin preparation (B_1, 44%; G_1, 44%; and B_2 and G_2, 2%) for 5.0 yr. Cuthbertson et al. (1967)

found that aflatoxin at levels of 0.07–1.8 ppm failed to induce liver tumors in six male and two female monkeys that survived for 3 yr, although histological evidence of toxicity was observed in the livers of the survivors.

Krieger et al. (1975) reported the hydroxylation of aflatoxin B_1 to aflatoxin Q_1 (AFQ_1) and aflatoxin M_1 in the rhesus monkey, and further established that this species belongs to the "fast metabolizing" group and is hence probably vulnerable only to the acute toxicity of aflatoxin B_1 and relatively resistant to its carcinogenic effects. Moreover, it was recently found that AFQ_1 was only 5.5% as toxic as aflatoxin B_1 and was not mutagenic to *Salmonella typhimurium* auxotrophs (Ames et al., 1973; Hsieh et al., 1974). Thus it was postulated by Krieger et al. (1975) that the rhesus monkey, which possesses a high potential for hydroxylating aflatoxin B_1 to AFQ_1, is relatively resistant to carcinogenic effects.

Aflatoxin Q_1

Results of comparative biochemical studies suggest that the rhesus monkey may be more similar to humans than are other experimental animals (Smith, 1967). It was found that AFQ_1 was the prominent *in vitro* metabolite of aflatoxin B_1 in human liver preparations treated in the same manner as the monkey liver preparations (Krieger et al., 1975). If humans respond to aflatoxin B_1 exposure in the same way as the rhesus monkey, they would be *relatively* resistant to its chronic, carcinogenic effects (Krieger et al., 1975).

Available evidence indicates that aflatoxin B_1 requires metabolic activation to elicit its carcinogenic activity (Garner, 1973; Garner et al., 1972; Miller and Miller, 1971; Schoental, 1970). Figure 2 illustrates a number of metabolic transformations of the aflatoxins by liver enzymes.

The agency causing tissue injury in a particular animal species is dictated by the rate and pattern of aflatoxin metabolism (Patterson, 1973). When aflatoxin is metabolized slowly, untransformed toxin is believed to be the active molecular species, with chronic liver damage the probable result, whereas when it is metabolized rapidly, metabolites rather than the original toxin seem to be involved (Patterson, 1973). Schoental (1970) proposed that the isolated vinyl ether double bond of aflatoxin is susceptible to metabolic oxidation in much the same way as the K region of polycyclic aromatic

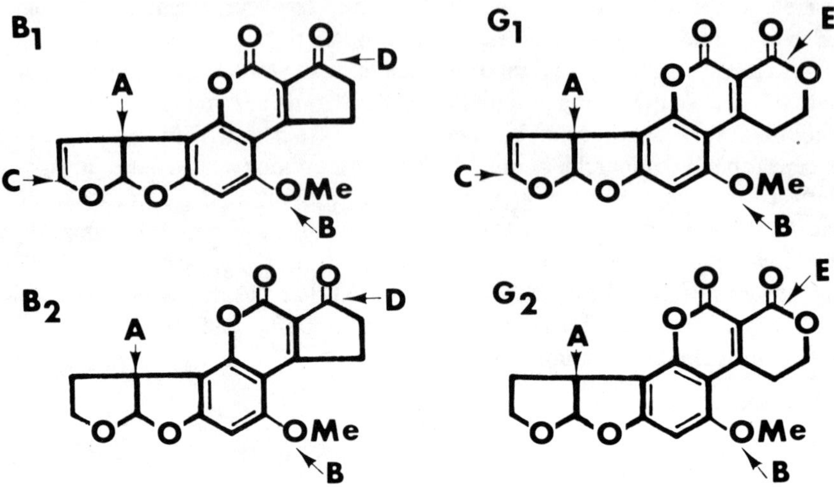

FIGURE 2 Metabolic transformation of the aflatoxins by liver enzymes: (A) 4-hydroxylation; (B) O-demethylation to a phenolic derivative; (C) hydration of the vinyl ether double bond to yield the 2-hydroxy derivative or hemiacetal; (D) cyclopentenone reduction (aflatoxins B) to form a secondary alcohol; (E) hydrolytic fission and decarboxylation of the δ-lactone ring of aflatoxins G (so far known only as a pathway of fungal metabolism). Known metabolites of aflatoxin B_1: aflatoxin M_1 (route A), aflatoxin P_1 (route B), aflatoxin B_{2a} or hemiacetal (route C), aflatoxicol or F_1 (route D). Known metabolites of B_2: aflatoxin M_2 (route A), dihydroaflatoxicol or F_2 (route D). Known metabolites of G_1: aflatoxin GM_1 (route A), aflatoxin G_{2a} (route C), aflatoxin B_3 or parasiticol (route E). Aflatoxin G_2 is probably hydroxylated to GM_2.

hydrocarbons and that this might account for the carcinogenic properties of the toxin. The suggested aflatoxin epoxide could also be an intermediate in the formation of aflatoxin B_{2a} (hemiacetal) by liver microsomal enzymes in certain avian and mammalian species (Patterson and Roberts, 1970, 1972).

It has been suggested that epidemiologic patterns of primary liver cancer incidence, together with what is known about the risks of aflatoxin contamination of foodstuffs and the potency of the compounds in animals, provide suggestive circumstantial evidence that aflatoxins (or other mold toxins) play a role in the etiology of the disease (Wogan, 1968, 1969), primarily in areas such as Swaziland (Keen and Martin, 1971), Thailand (Shank et al., 1972a, 1972b, 1972c), Kenya (IARC, 1972; Linsell and Peers, 1972), Uganda (Alpert et al., 1971), and Ethiopia (Coady, 1965). No causal relationship has been unambiguously established between an increased frequency of liver cancer and the consumption of diets contaminated by aflatoxins and possibly other mycotoxins.

A number of episodes have also occurred in which circumstantial evidence would appear to suggest the possible involvement of aflatoxin in *acute* toxicoses in humans (Kraybill and Shimkin, 1964), primarily in Thailand (Shank et al., 1971; Bourgeois et al., 1971; Amla et al., 1971), although in none of these cases was the information adequate for estimating effective doses for humans.

The carcinogenic action of aflatoxin is thought to depend on its binding to DNA (Patterson, 1973; Sporn et al., 1966), on inhibition of RNA synthesis (Wogan and Pong, 1970, and possibly on its interaction with sex-related binding sites on the endoplasmic reticulum (Williams and Rabin, 1971). Figure 3 is a schematic representation of the factors controlling the fate of an aflatoxin B_1 molecule in a typical liver cell.

In vivo, aflatoxin B_1 strongly inhibits DNA (Frayssenet et al., 1964), RNA (Clifford and Rees, 1966), and protein synthesis (Sarasin and Moulé, 1973). Its suppression of mitosis in human leukocyte cultures (Dolimpio et al., 1968) and human diploid and heteroploid embryonic lung cells (Legator, 1966; Legator et al., 1965; Legator and Withrow, 1964) and its inhibition of DNA synthesis and giant cell formation in tissue culture (Legator, 1969) in a manner similar to that of some of the alkylating agents (Gabliks et al., 1965) have all been reported. The cytogenic effects observed in human leukocyte cultures were found at concentrations of 1–50 μg/ml of aflatoxin B_1 and included gaps, breaks, fragments, deletions, and translocations, the majority of which affected only one chromatid (Dolimpio et al., 1968).

Aflatoxin B_1 has been shown to be mutagenic in the *Bacillus subtilis* transforming DNA assay *in vitro* (Maher and Summers, 1970) and in *Neurospora crassa* (Garner and Wright, 1973; Ong, 1970, 1971; Ong and de Serres, 1972) and to induce autosomal recessive-lethal mutations in

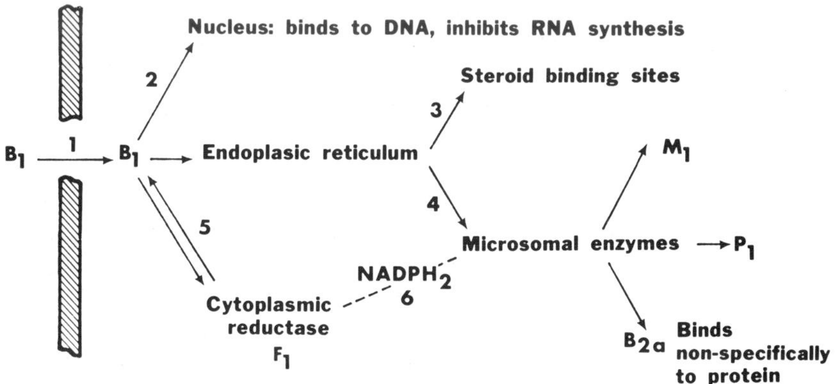

FIGURE 3 Schematic representation of the factors controlling the fate of an aflatoxin B_1 molecule in a typical liver cell. Following transport across the cell membrane (1) the aflatoxin molecule may bind to nuclear DNA (2) or to sex-determined sites on the endoplasmic reticulum (3). Alternatively, it may be metabolized by microsomal enzymes (4) or undergo reversible reduction by cytoplasmic enzymes (5). The cofactor $NADPH_2$ (6) is required for routes 4 and 5.

Drosophila melanogaster (Lamb and Lilly, 1971). The mutagenic effect of aflatoxin B_1 on nuclear and extranuclear DNA in a unicellular green alga, *Chlamydomonas reinhardii*, has been reported (Schimmer and Werner, 1974).

It has been demonstrated that, like most carcinogens, aflatoxin B_1 must be enzymatically converted into active metabolites to be effective. These derivatives inhibit RNA (Moulé and Frayssinet, 1968) and protein synthesis *in vitro* (Sarasin and Moulé, 1973) and they are toxic (Garner et al., 1972), mutagenic for *S. typhimurium* (Ames et al., 1973), and act as both inducers and mutagens of *Escherichia coli* K_{12} (λ) (Goze et al., 1975).

The active aflatoxin B_1 metabolite has been suggested to be a 2, 3-epoxide derivative (Garner, 1973; Swenson et al., 1973), although no direct mutagenic experiments with this epoxide have supported this hypothesis.

Lillehoj and Ciegler (1970) and Legator (1966) have reported that aflatoxin B_1 itself induces lysogenic *B. megaterium, Staphylococcus aureus,* and *E. coli* K_{12} (λ). However, these findings may have resulted from impure aflatoxin preparations (Goze et al., 1975). A mixture of aflatoxins (B_1 and G_1), when examined in the dominant lethal test in mice, yielded an increase in early postimplantation loss, and this effect occurred during both the post- and premeiotic divisions (Epstein and Shafner, 1968).

Leonard et al. (1975) reported that aflatoxin B_1 given at a dose of 5 mg/kg body weight does not produce gross structural chromosome changes in male mouse germ cells. Since aflatoxin B_1 had been previously demonstrated to be mutagenic in different systems (Maher and Summers, 1970; Ong, 1971; Lamb and Lilly, 1971), and to produce chromosome aberrations in plant material (Lilly, 1965; Reiss, 1971) and in mammalian chromosomes *in vitro* (Dolimpio et al., 1968; Green et al., 1967; Promchainant et al., 1972; Withers, 1965), the absence of mutagenic effects *in vivo* (Leonard et al., 1975) could be explained by low penetration in the testes or by its metabolic degradation (Steyn et al., 1971).

The ip administration to hamsters of 4 mg/kg of aflatoxin B_1 on day 8 of pregnancy has been reported by Ellis and DiPaolo (1967) to result in teratogenic effects in the central nervous system. In the rat, ip administration of aflatoxin B_1 caused hemorrhagic lesions at the uteroplacental junction, with subsequent embryonic death (Platt et al., 1962), while repeated injection of small doses retarded fetal growth (Le Breton et al., 1964). Feeding aflatoxin B_1 to rats on day 16 of pregnancy caused growth retardation of the fetus but failed to induce embryonic death (Butler and Wigglesworth, 1966).

Ochratoxins. The widespread distribution of ochratoxin A (Fig. 1), one of six closely related metabolites of *A. ochraceus* (Steyn and Holzapfel, 1967), as well as other species of *Aspergillus* and *P. viridicatum* (Van Walbeek et al., 1968), has given rise to increasing concern since the toxin has been shown to possess a high acute toxicity to ducklings, rats, chicks, and rainbow trout and to cause kidney and liver damage (Doster et al., 1971; Peckham et al., 1971; Purchase and Theron, 1968) in farm stock including pigs (Szczech,

1973). It has also been implicated in cases of bovine abortion (Food and Cosmetics Toxicology, 1975; Munro, 1973). Subacute toxicity of ochratoxin A to chickens and rats is evident at levels as low as 0.2 ppm in the feed (Tucker and Hamilton, 1971). Although ochratoxin A was not found carcinogenic to rats (Purchase and Van Der Watt, 1970), it produced liver tumors in rainbow trout when fed together with sterculic acid (Doster et al., 1971).

Intraperitoneal administration of ochratoxin A to mice in a single dose of 5 mg/kg on one of days 7–12 of pregnancy increased prenatal mortality, decreased fetal weight, and caused various fetal malformations including exencephaly and malformations of the eyes, face, and digits. While these findings involved injection of the toxin rather than oral administration, which is of more obvious relevance for a food or feed contaminant, it does demonstrate that the mouse placenta does not act as an effective barrier to this mycotoxin.

Samples of moldy grains, beans, and peanuts collected in Canada have been found to contain 0.02–27 ppm of ochratoxin A (Scott et al., 1972). Steyn and Holzapfel (1967) have isolated and identified the methyl and ethyl esters of ochratoxins A and B from fungal cultures of *A. ochraceus* in a number of cereal and legume crops in South Africa. Ochratoxin A has been also detected in occasional samples of U.S. corn and barley (Nesheim, 1971; Shotwell et al., 1971).

Sterigmatocystin. Sterigmatocystin [3*a*,12*c*-dihydro-8-hydroxy-6-methoxy-7*H*-furo[3′ 2′:4,5] furo[2,3-*c*] xanthen-7-one] (I) is a carcinogenic metabolite of *A. versicola, A. nidulans, A. ugulosus, P. luteum,* and a *Bipolaris* species (Ballantine et al., 1965; Holzapfel et al., 1966; Purchase and Van Der Watt, 1970) that has also been detected in grains (Scott et al., 1972).

Sterigmatocystin produced hepatomas in Wistar rats when administered in doses of 0.15–2.25 mg/day by gavage, or in the diet for 52 wk. Male rats were more susceptible to hepatoma development than females, and histologically, the tumors bore a marked resemblance to those occurring in humans (Purchase and Van Der Watt, 1970). In the original experiments of Dickens et al. (1966), aflatoxin appeared to be approximately 200 times more carcinogenic in the rat than sterigmatocystin when administered. The studies of Purchase and Van Der Watt (1970) indicated that with oral administration, aflatoxin was no

(I) Sterigmatocystin

more than ten times as potent or carcinogenic as sterigmatocystin in Wistar rats.

A comparison was made between sterigmatocystin-produced lesions in the rat and the pathology of hepatitis in Africans of Mozambique. Although many similarities were observed, it was difficult to attribute liver disease in the Bantu to any single agent in their environment (Torres et al., 1970).

Penicillium *toxins.* Species of *Penicillium* have been identified as frequent contaminants of grain and feeds. *P. puberubum* Banier, for example, has yielded among its metabolic products aflatoxin, tropolone, puberulic and puberulonic acids, and penicillic acid. *P. cyclopium*, which is ubiquitously distributed, has been frequently isolated from stored grain and cereals. Cyclopiazonic acid (II), isolated from *P. cyclopium*, has caused acute toxicoses in ducklings and rats (Holzapfel, 1968).

Citrinin (4,6-dihydro-8-hydroxy-3,4,5-trimethyl-6-oxo-3*H*-2-benzopyran-7-carboxylic acid) (Fig. 1) and penicillic acid (3-methoxy-5-methyl-4-oxo-2,5-hexadienoic acid) (III) are toxic antibiotics produced by several species of both *Penicillium* and *Aspergillus* (Korzybski et al., 1967). Citrinin causes kidney damage in experimental animals (Ambrose and Deeds, 1946; Krogh et al., 1970), while penicillic acid has been found to cause local tumors on injection in rats and mice (Dickens and Jones, 1965). Both citrinin and penicillic acid have been isolated from grain and feed samples (Scott et al., 1972).

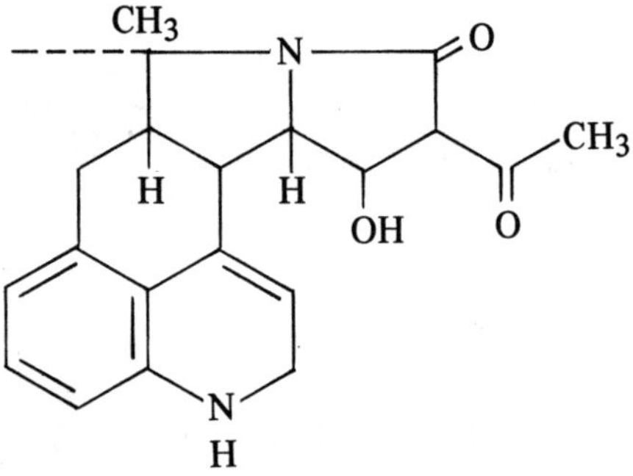

(II) Cyclopiazonic acid

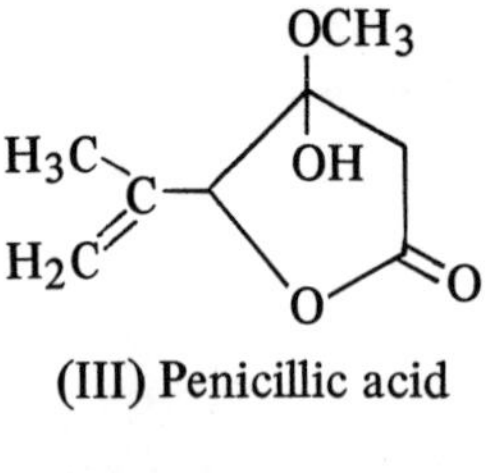

(III) Penicillic acid

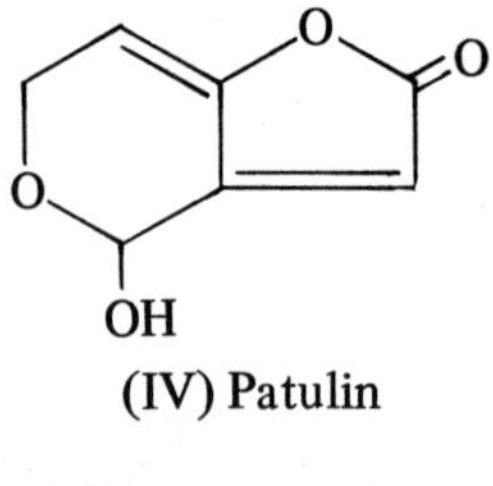

(IV) Patulin

Patulin [4-hydroxy-4*H*-furo[3,2-*c*]pyran-2(6*H*)-one] (IV) is an α,β-unsaturated lactone antibiotic derived from the metabolism of several species of *Penicillium* and *Aspergillus* (e.g., *P. patulum, P. expansum, P. melinsis, P.*

leucopus, A. clavatus, and *A. claviforme*). Some of these fungal species are probably contaminants of foods. For example, *P. expansum*, the common storage rot of fruit; *A. clavatus, A. terreus, P. cyclopium,* and *P. urticae*, isolated from flour (Graves and Hesseltine, 1966); and *Byssochlamys nivea* and the heat-resistant fruit juice contaminant identified by Keuhn (1958) as the *Gymnoascus* species of Karow and Foster (1944) have all been shown to produce patulin (Abraham and Florey, 1949). Patulin is also produced by fungi in apples (Brian et al., 1956) and by field crops (Norstadt and McCalla, 1963) and has been isolated by Ukai et al. (1954) from a *Penicillium* that infected a malt feed responsible for the death of cattle.

Patulin is carcinogenic in the rat (Dickens and Jones, 1961) and has also been shown to induce petite mutations in *Saccharomyces cerivisiae* (Mayer and Legator, 1969) and chromosome aberrations in avian eggs during mitosis (Sentein, 1955) and in human leukocyte cell culture (Withers, 1965).

It has been shown that moldy rice can induce bile duct proliferation, hepatic necrosis, and hepatoma in the rat (Uraguchi, 1961). The principal toxic fungus in moldy rice, *P. islandicum*, can produce identical lesions and is believed to be the responsible agent (Kobayashi, 1959).

Two toxic substances have been isolated from *P. islandicum*: islanditoxin (Fig. 1) and luteoskyrin (V).

(V) Luteoskyrin

The former is a chlorine-containing peptide and is a potent and fast-acting hepatotoxin, while the latter is carcinogenic and produces chromosomal aberrations in cultured Ehrlich ascites tumor cells (Schachtschabel et al., 1969).

Fusarium *toxins.* The trichothecenes are a family of closely related tetracyclic sesquiterpenoid metabolites of various strains of *Fusarium, Trichoderma, Trichothecium, Myrothecium,* and other species of fungi commonly found in soil and on grains and other feeds (Bamburg et al., 1968). Twenty-two naturally occurring trichothecenes have been isolated from grains and characterized. Circumstantial evidence has incriminated these compounds in outbreaks of moldy grain toxicosis involving poultry, swine, and cattle in the United States and other countries. Symptoms include severe inflammation of the gastrointestinal tract, hemorrhaging, edema, leukopenia, and degeneration of bone marrow.

Zearalenone [6-(10-hydroxy-6-oxo-*trans*-1-undecenyl)-β-resorcylic acid lactone; estrogenic factor F-2] (VI) is produced by *F. graminareum* (Mirocha et al., 1968).

The fusaria often attack wheat, barley, and maize, many species being actively toxigenic. Zearalenone is anabolic and is teratrophic in rats, mice, and guinea pigs and is suspected of contributing to infertility in dairy cattle and swine (Mirocha et al., 1968).

OH   O   CH₃

C—O—CH—(CH$_2$)$_3$

C=O

HO   CH=CH—(CH$_2$)$_3$

(VI) Zearalenone

The fungus *F. nivale* has been extensively studied in Japan because of its damage to the wheat crop and the subsequent findings of human and animal poisonings related to "scabby grains" resulting from its infestation. A number of sesquiterpenoids have been isolated from wheat and rice, including the scirpenol derivatives nivalenol ($3\alpha,4\beta,7\alpha,15$-tetrahydroxy-scirp-9-en-8-one) (VII), fusarenon-X (3,15,17-trihydroxy-scirp-4-acetoxy-9-en-8-one) (VIII), and T-2 toxin [4,15-diacetoxy-8-(3-methylbutyryloxy)-scirp-9-en-3-ol] (Fig. 1).

Nivalenol has been found to cause cell degeneration of bone marrow, lymph nodes, intestine, testes, and thymus following ip administration to mice (Tatsumo, 1968), to induce radiomimetic damage in animal cells (Ueno and Fukushima, 1968), and to inhibit protein and DNA synthesis of HeLa cells and ascites tumor cells (Ueno and Fukushima, 1968; Ohtsubo et al., 1968).

The mold *F. nivale* is found on tall fescue and important foliage crops that occasionally become toxic to ruminants. Yates et al. (1967) isolated DL-4-acetamido-4-hydroxy-2-butyric acid-γ-lactone (butenolide) (IX) from *F. nivale* Fries cesati. Grove et al. (1970) identified this butenolide (produced by

F. tricinctum isolated from corn and fescue) as the possible cause of fescue foot syndrome in cattle.

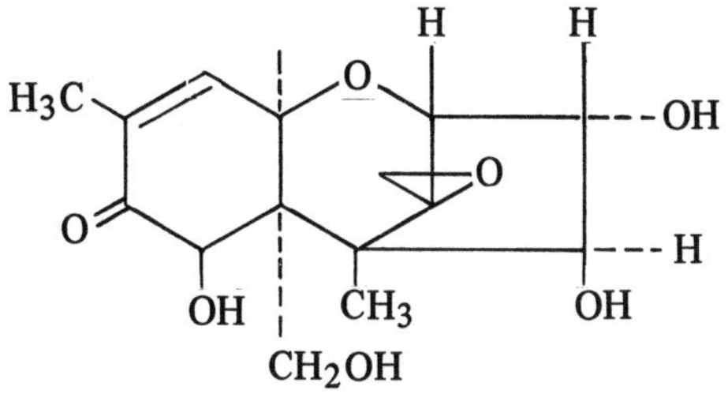

(VII) Nivalenol

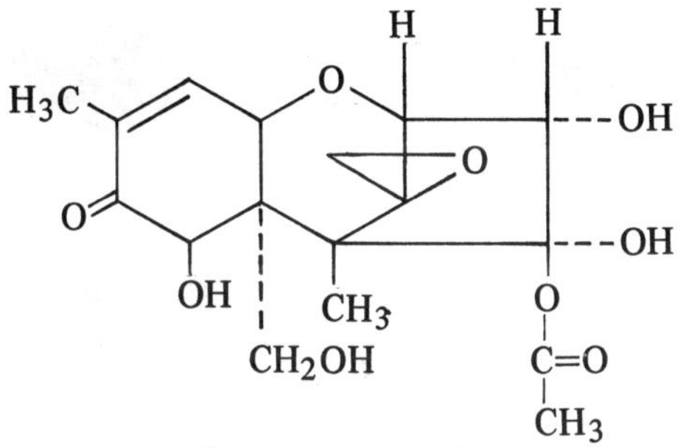

(VIII) Fusarenon-X

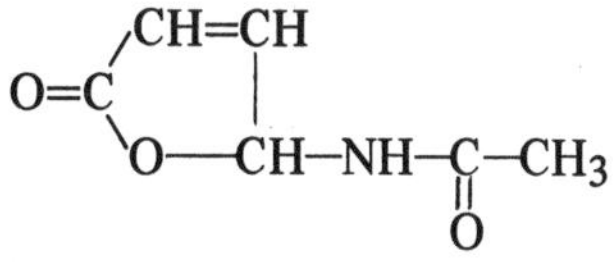

(IX) DL-4-Acetamido-4-hydroxy-2-butyric acid-γ-lactone

Information as to the mutagenicity of mycotoxins other than aflatoxin B_1 is very scant indeed. Table 2 (Tazima, 1974) summarizes the mutagenic effects of a number of the mycotoxins discussed above.

Pyrrolizidine Alkaloids

Alkaloids of the pyrrolizidine class occur with a wide distribution in several plant genera, principally *Amsinilsia, Crotalaria,* and *Senecio* (Kingsbury,

TABLE 2   Mutagenic Effects of Mycotoxins

Mycotoxin	Mitotic injury	DNA double strand break	Chromosome aberration	Mutation
Aflatoxin B$_1$	+	+[a]	+[b,c]	+[d,e]
Sterigmatocystin	+	−	+	+[e]
Luteoskyrin		−[a]	+	+[e]
Patulin	+[f]	+[a]	+[c]	+[e,g]
Penicillic acid	+	+[a]		±[e]
Fusarenon-X	+	−[a]		−[e]
Nivalenol	+			

[a] Umeda et al., 1972.
[b] Lilly, 1965; Dolimpio et al., 1968.
[c] Withers, 1965.
[d] Epstein and Shafner, 1968; Lamb and Lilly, 1971; Ong, 1970.
[e] Kada, 1973.
[f] Sentein, 1955.
[g] Mayer and Legator, 1969.

1964; Mattocks, 1972a; Muenscher, 1951). At least eight species of *Crotalaria* are used as food in East Africa, where the leaves are usually cooked and eaten as a vegetable, but in some cases flowers or fruits are also used (Schoental and Coady, 1968). A number of common plants containing pyrrolizidine alkaloids are found in many parts of the world; for many years they have been consumed as bush teas or herbal remedies in considerable quantity in Asia, Africa, and South America (Schoental, 1968; Schoental and Coady, 1968). In Guinea, these plants are used for yaws and ulcers, and infusions of flowers are used for menorrhagia. They are used both to induce and to prevent abortion, and are also used in many diseases of childhood (Schoental, 1968). At least seven species of *Senecio* are used medicinally in eastern Africa (Schoental, 1968), including use by women in pregnancy and parturition. Utilization of such plants in pregnancy and lactation would appear to present a particular hazard to the fetus or the suckling baby (Schoental, 1968).

The common plants are also hepatotoxic to livestock (Sippel, 1964; Mattocks, 1972a; Bulk et al., 1968), and the alkaloids they contain have been established as the responsible compounds (Schoental, 1963, 1968; Culvenor and Smith, 1965; Warren, 1966; Fowler, 1968). Figure 4 shows the structures of a number of the most important pyrrolizidine alkaloids. The most hepatotoxic alkaloids are cyclic diesters—for example, monocrotaline and senecionine. The double bond present in the pyrrolizidine moiety of the alkaloids is considered essential for their hepatotoxic action (Schoental, 1957), and the principal reaction appears to result from alkylation (Culvenor et al., 1962), possibly resulting from an alkyl-oxygen fission of the ester linkage. It has also been suggested that the pyrrolizidine alkaloids themselves are not

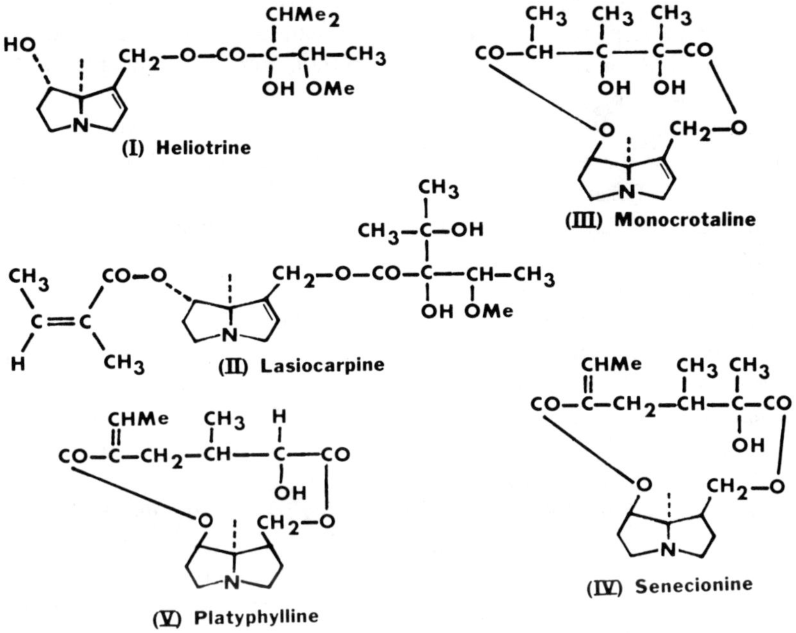

FIGURE 4 Pyrrolizidine alkaloids.

hepatotoxic but are converted by mixed-function oxidases in the liver to highly reactive pyrrolic derivatives (X), which can act as bifunctional alkylating agents and can cross-link DNA *in vitro* (Mattocks, 1972b; White and Mattocks, 1972).

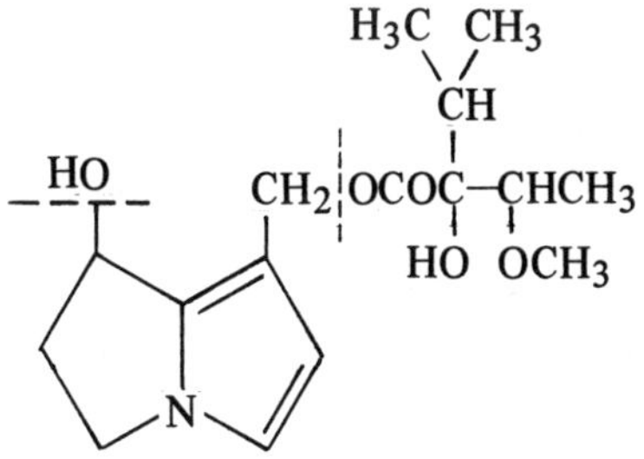

(X) Pyrrolic derivative of heliotrine

As illustrated above (X), either of the bands indicated by dashed lines may be broken, especially under acidic conditions, giving rise to a carbonium ion that will alkylate DNA (Culvenor et al., 1970), while the presence of two such sites on a molecule permits the possible formation of cross-links in DNA (White and Mattocks, 1972).

A number of pyrrolizidine alkaloids have been shown to produce liver cancer in experimental animals. Liver damage is manifested in several ways, depending on dose, duration of action, and the diet fed or other compounds administered with the alkaloids (Newberne and Rodgers, 1973; Harris and Chen, 1970; McLean, 1970). Acute and chronic lesions and hepatomas have been produced in rats after a single dose of retrosine (Schoental and Bensted, 1963) or lasiocarpine (Harris and Chen, 1970) at levels of 100 mg/kg. (However, the liver lesions or hepatomas may not be apparent for 1.5–2.5 yr.)

Heliotrine, lasiocarpine, and monocrotaline produce mitotic inhibition and chromosomal damage in plant and animal cells, for example, in *Vicia faba* and *Allium cepa* (Avanzi, 1963; Mariani and Mannucci, 1969) and *A. nidulans* (Alderson and Clark, 1966). These pyrrolizidine alkaloids were strongly mutagenic in *Drosophila* (Brink, 1965; Clark, 1959, 1963), the *N*-oxides were less so, and the necic acids and bases were completely inactive (Sullman, 1971; Brink, 1965, 1969; Clark, 1959, 1963).

Green and Muriel (1975a) treated *E. coli* WP2 and its repair-deficient derivatives with heliotrine and monocrotaline in the presence of a liver microsomal fraction. The doubly repair-deficient strains WP 100 *uvrA recA* and CM-611 *uvrA exrA* showed considerable killing. The singly repair-deficient strains WP2 *uvrA*, CM561 *exrA*, and CM57 *recA* showed slight killing. In strains WO2 and WP2 *uvrA*, induced reversion to TRP$^+$ was not detected with either monocrotaline or mitomycin C. These results are considered to be consistent with liver activation converting pyrrolizidine alkaloids into bifunctional alkylating agents. It is of interest to note that, like mitomycin C, pyrrolizidine alkaloids per se are ineffective mutagens in bacteria (e.g., on survival or mutation of *E. coli* or *S. typhimurium*) in the absence of liver microsomes.

The teratogenicity of pyrrolizidine alkaloids in rats has also been noted by Green and Cristie (1961).

Pyrrolizidine alkaloids have been suggested as possible etiologic factors in the high incidence of liver diseases, such as kwashiorkor and liver cirrhosis, and of primary kidney tumors in parts of the tropics and subtropics (Schoental, 1963). Alkaloid-containing plants may be grazed by domestic animals that are used for milk production or human consumption.

A number of reports of human poisoning have been ascribed to the pyrrolizidine alkaloids in Central Asia (Savvina, 1952; Khanin, 1956), and cases of bread poisoning have been described in South Africa that appeared to be related to the consumption of bread made from flour contaminated with parts of *Senecio* plants (Nealme and Pillay, 1964; Selzer and Parker, 1951).

There are over 100 pyrrolizidine alkaloids, which have the basic structure shown in XI. The hepatotoxic alkaloids are all esters of 1-hydroxy-methyl-1,2-dehydro-7-hydroxypyrrolizidine with branched-chain necic acids (XII).

(XI)

(XII)

Cycasin

Cycasin (methylazoxymethanol β-D-glucoside) (XIII) and its aglycone methylazoxymethanol (MAM) (XIV) are naturally occurring alkylating agents, which are found in the seeds, roots, and leaves of cycad plants, primarily from the very widespread species *Cycas circinalis* and *C. revolata* (IARC, 1972). The cycad nuts are a source of starch and are often used as food after appropriate preparation.

$$CH_3-N=N-CH_2O-C_6H_{11}O_5$$

(XIII) Cycasin

$$CH_3-\overset{+}{N}-N-CH_2OH$$

(XIV) MAM

There is a high incidence of human neurological diseases in areas of the world where cycads are utilized as food and medicines (principally in the tropics and subtropics), implicating the principal constituents of cycads (cycasin and MAM) (Whiting, 1963).

Cycasin is carcinogenic in five animal species, inducing tumors in various organs (IARC, 1972). Following oral exposure, it is carcinogenic in the rat, hamster, guinea pig, and fish (the data on the mouse are of borderline significance). The hepatotoxic and carcinogenic properties of cycasin have been shown to require prior deglucosylation to MAM provided by the β-glucosidase activity of the intestinal flora (Spatz et al., 1966, Kobayashi and Matsumoto, 1965; Laquer and Spatz, 1968). Enzymatic hydrolysis to MAM is also possible in the subcutaneous tissue of newborn rats (Spatz, 1968).

MAM caused hepatomas in rats (Matsumoto and Strong, 1963) following oral administration and neoplasms of the liver, kidney, and intestinal tract in rats following repeated sc administration (Laquer and Matsumoto, 1966). In hamsters, MAM administered iv produced multiple cystadenomas and other tumors of the liver and adenomas and adenocarcinomas of the colon (Spatz et al., 1969). Mickelsen et al. (1964) reported that hepatotoxic factors were excreted in the milk when lactating females rats were given cycasin.

It has been shown that MAM methylates nucleic acids *in vitro*

(Matsumoto and Higa, 1966), at the N-7 position of guanine, and the same methylated base has been identified in the nucleic acids of some rat tissues following cycasin or MAM acetate administration (Shank and Magee, 1967). Single, nonlethal doses of MAM acetate induced early inhibition of DNA synthesis in tissues of the rat susceptible to the carcinogenicity of this agent (Zedeck et al., 1970).

MAM has been found to be teratogenic in the golden hamster (Spatz et al., 1966, 1967; Laquer and Matsumoto, 1966). It is mutagenic in *S. typhimurium* (Smith, 1966) and *Drosophila* (Teas and Dyson, 1967) and induces chromosome aberrations in onion root tip cells (Teas et al., 1965). In repeated *in vitro* studies, cycasin per se was found to be nonmutagenic (Tazima, 1974), but *in vivo* (following transformation to MAM) it has been shown to be mutagenic (Gabridge et al., 1969).

Vandenberg and Ball (1972) studied the effects of MAM acetate on DNA synthesis and cell proliferation of synchronous HeLa cells. The maximum effect on DNA synthesis was not expressed until the alkylated template had undergone one round of replication. DNA synthesis in the following cycle was then severely inhibited, with an extension of the S phase and mitotic delay. During this delay there was a contamination of gross RNA and protein synthesis, resulting in the appearance of enlarged cells. These results were analogous to those found by Plant and Roberts (1971) for the action of MNU (*N*-methyl-*N*-nitrosourea) on synchronized HeLa cells and for MMS (methyl methanesulfonate) on synchronized HEp-2 cells (Myers and Strauss, 1971).

The nature of the original DNA lesion arising from MAM acetate treatment and of the subsequent postreplicative lesion is not yet known. A possibility exists that, as with MNU, alkylation by MAM acetate may yield the minor alkylation product *O*-6-methylguanine, which may be responsible for the subsequent effects on DNA synthesis. This product has been detected following alkylation of deoxyguanosine *in vitro* (Loveless, 1969) and of DNA *in vivo* (Lawley and Thatcher, 1970) by some alkylnitrosamides and nitrosamides, and it may be an important factor in mutagenesis (Loveless, 1969).

The similarity in biological effects between cycasin and dimethylnitrosamine has also been described (Shank and Magee, 1967; Miller, 1964). Figure 5 illustrates the proposed degradation and metabolic pathway for dimethylnitrosamine and cycasin, as proposed by Miller (1964).

POLYNUCLEAR AROMATIC HYDROCARBONS

The environmental polynuclear aromatic hydrocarbons that are of major concern because of their potential carcinogenicity and mutagenicity are illustrated in Fig. 6. They include benzo[*a*]pyrene (I), benzo[*e*]pyrene (II), benz[*a*]anthracene (III), dibenz[*a,h*]anthracene (IV), benzo[*j*]fluoranthene (V), and benzo[*b*]fluoranthene (VI).

The general aspects of polynuclear aromatic hydrocarbons (PAH) that

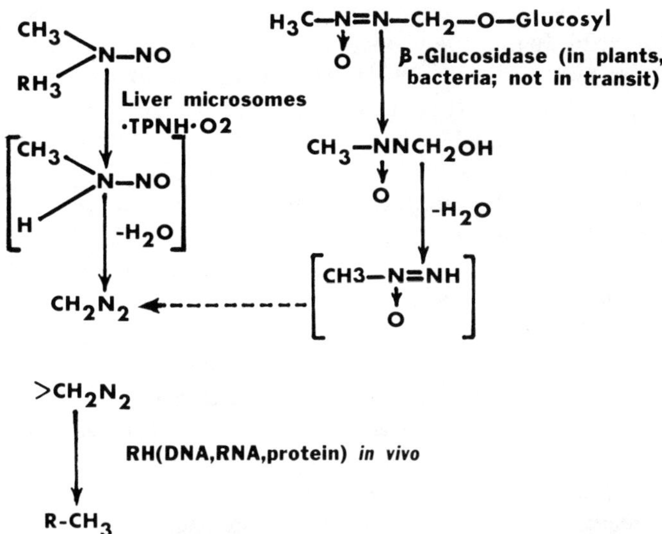

FIGURE 5 Proposed degradation and metabolic pathways for dimethylnitrosamine and cycasin.

are germane for our consideration and have been reviewed include the following: occurrence, isolation, and identification in the human environment (air, water, soil) [IARC, 1973; Fishbein, 1975, National Academy of Sciences (NAS), 1972, Shabad et al., 1971; Gunther and Buzzetti, 1965; Sawicki, 1967; Andelman and Suess, 1970] and in foodstuffs (Haenni, 1968; Gunther

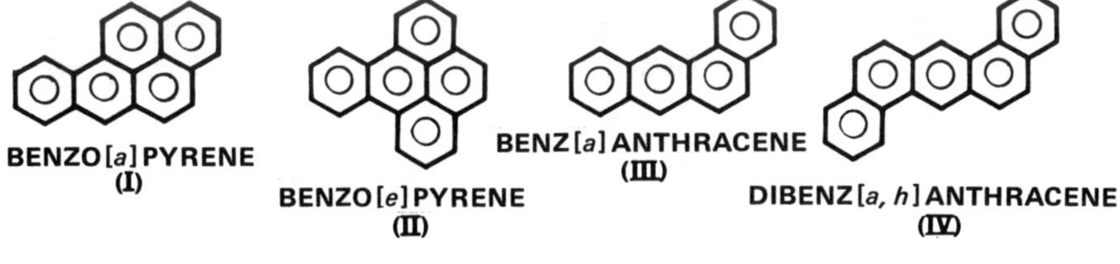

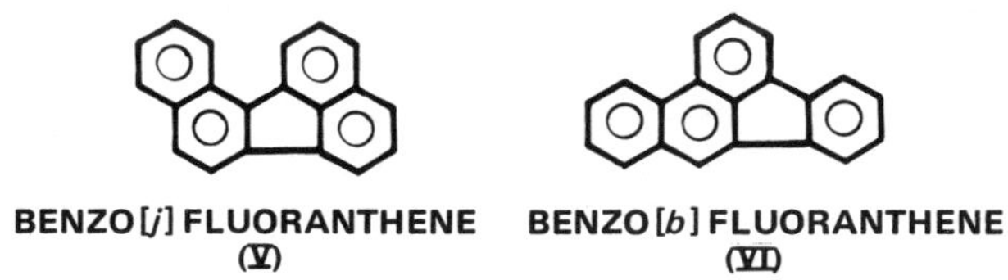

FIGURE 6 Structures of some carcinogenic and mutagenic polynuclear aromatic hydrocarbons.

et al., 1967; Tilgner and Daun, 1969; metabolism (Boyland and Weigert, 1947; Heidelberger and Jones, 1948; Van Duuren, 1958); and carcinogenic aspects and mode of action (IARC, 1973; NAS, 1972; Hueper and Conway, 1964; Brookes and Lawley, 1964; Arcos et al., 1968; Gelboin, 1969; Gelboin et al., 1972; Heidelberger, 1973; Miller, 1970; Weisburger and Williams, 1975).

Incomplete solid fuel combustion products, as produced by various industrial processes, space heating, and vehicle exhaust fumes contain a small but measurable amount of PAH. For example, industrial operations in the pyrolytic processing of organic raw materials (e.g., coal and petroleum) form PAH when they are carried out at high temperatures (e.g., 700°C), whereas they form paraffins, cycloparaffins, olefins, and phenols at lower temperatures (300–450°C). Utilization of these pyrolytic products (coal tar, coal tar pitch, gasoline) can also produce PAH (Anderman and Snodgrass, 1974).

Some of the industrial operations that produce PAH are the preparation of acetylene from natural gas and from other organic solvents, pyrolysis of wood, coke production, gas production from petroleum, oil refinery operations, production of synthetic alcohol, and manufacture of electrolytic aluminum using graphite electrodes (NAS, 1972; Fishbein, 1975).

The PAH are all fairly nonvolatile, high-melting solids, and as such they exist in the air as pollutants in the form of crystals adhering to particulate matter, rather than in gaseous form. They are chemically inert and hence are removed from the air only by rain or slow sedimentation of particulates; eventually they can be deposited into surface waters or onto plants and soil, thence carried by runoff into surface waters (Anderman and Snodgrass, 1974). Because of the endogenous formation of PAH, a "background" level of PAH is present in most soils.

A large body of widely varying data exists on the quantities of PAH present in air at many localities under various conditions, such as season, traffic density, industries, general pollution level, geographic location and so on, determined by utilizing various methodologies and sampling techniques (IARC, 1973; NAS, 1972).

The concentration of the polynuclear aromatics in urban air varies widely from place to place but appears to be greatest in industrial urban areas; it is also substantially higher in the winter, when space heating is at a maximum, and during periods of increased smoke in the atmosphere (Berry and Lehman, 1971). The concentration ranges from ~ 0.1–60 μg/1,000 m^3 in urban areas to ~ 0.01–2 μg/1,000 m^3 in rural areas (Sawicki, 1967).

It is well recognized that vehicle exhaust fumes are a significant source of PAH (IARC, 1973; NAS, 1972), the composition and levels of which depend on such factors as type and compression of engine, fuel variables (e.g., tetraethyl lead, fuel aromaticity, type of aromatic at constant total level of aromatics), work loads, and presence or absence of a catalytic afterburner (Candeli et al., 1974).

Of the polynuclear aromatics, benzo[*a*]pyrene (BP) is the most ubiquitous toxicant of environmental significance. Table 3 lists a number of the most important sources of BP. Benzo[*a*]pyrene is quantitatively the most important compound present in soot and the most potent carcinogenic agent in polluted air, where its presence has been reported for decades (IARC, 1973; NAS, 1972). Detailed studies of air pollution have been made in a variety of cities in the United States (Sawicki et al., 1962), Europe (Commins and Waller, 1967; Grimmer, 1966), Australia (Cleary and Sullivan, 1965), and South Africa (Louw, 1965) and the levels of BP delineated.

The concentrations of BP in the atmosphere depend on geographic location, presence of nearby sources of pollution (such as industries and vehicular traffic), and season. In general, concentrations of BP are greater during periods of increased smoke in the atmosphere, greater in urban areas (e.g., up to 100 times more) than in nonurban areas, and about 100 times greater in winter than in summer (e.g., 0.6-104 μg/1,000 m^3 compared with 0.03-4 μg/1,000 m^3) because of the greater number of polluting BP sources (heating systems and what appears to be a higher rate of decomposition by UV irradiation in summer) (IARC, 1973; Shabad et al., 1971).

TABLE 3 Occurrence of Benzo[*a*]pyrene
in Environmental Sources

Source	References
Soil	Shabad, 1968; Shabad et al., 1971; Blumer, 1961; NAS 1972
Air	IARC, 1973; Fishbein, 1975; Katz and Monkman, 1964; Sawicki, 1967; Kotin and Falk, 1963; NAS, 1972
Water	Andelman and Suess, 1970; NAS, 1972; Anderman and Snodgrass, 1974
Occupational exposure	IARC, 1973; Fishbein, 1975; NAS, 1972; Hangebrauck et al., 1964; Sawicki et al., 1965b
Exhaust from gasoline engines	Begeman and Colucci, 1968; Kotin et al., 1954; IARC, 1973
Exhaust from jet engines	Shabad and Smirnov, 1969; Shabad, 1971
Gasoline	Begeman and Colucci, 1968
Rubber-tire dust	Falk et al., 1951
Cigarette smoke	Surgeon General's Report, 1964; IARC, 1973
Food (general)	IARC, 1973; Haenni, 1968; Gunther et al., 1967
Smoked fish	Masuda and Kuratsune, 1971
Roasting coffee and coffee substitutes	Fritz, 1968a
Baking bread and biscuits	Fritz, 1968b
Margarine and mayonnaise	Fritz, 1968c
Oranges	Gunther et al., 1967
Refined oils (mineral oil)	Haenni and Hall, 1960
Commercial wax	Howard and Haenni, 1963
Freshly mined asbestos	Harrington, 1962

The amount of BP emitted annually into the atmosphere of a large industrial city can be substantial— 30–40 kg (Shabad et al., 1971). In London, during a period in which smoke condensation was high (December, 1957), a concentration as high as 2,220 μg/1,000 m^3 was recorded, but after that winter values did not exceed 54 μg/1,000 m^3 (Commins and Waller, 1967).

The contribution of automobiles to levels of atmospheric BP has been found by Sawicki (1967) to vary between 5 and 42%, the percentage being influenced by seasonal factors. Aviation has also proved to be a significant cause of environmental contamination by carcinogenic hydrocarbons (Shabad and Smirnov, 1969; Shabad, 1971). Aircraft engines eject considerable amounts of BP, estimated in milligrams per minute, which can cause an increase in the BP content of 10- to 100-fold in air, soil, and airfield vegetation (Shabad et al., 1971).

Aspects of occupational exposure to BP, as well as other polynuclear aromatic hydrocarbons, are well documented (IARC, 1973). The isolation of BP from coal tar was first reported by Cook et al. (1933). Levels of BP of 0.4 mg/1,000 m^3 in domestic (U.S.) coal combustion stack effluents have been noted by Sawicki et al. (1965b). In the workers' atmosphere in coal and pitch coking plants, average concentrations of BP ranging from 0.3 to 35 mg/1,000 m^3 have been found (Masek, 1971). Lawther et al. (1965) measured mean concentrations of BP ranging from 1.4–4.8 mg/1,000 m^3 in gas works retort houses.

Emission levels from incineration and open burning of municipal refuse, automobile tires, and the like have ranged from 0.016 to 7.3 mg/kg of particulate matter from a municipal incinerator, 58 to 180 mg/kg of particulate matter for a commercial incinerator, and 11 to 1,100 mg/kg of particulate matter in open burning (Hangebrauck et al., 1964). The emission levels of BP from heat generation sources ranged from 19 to 400 μg/10^6 Btu heat input (coal) and 20 to 200 μg/10^6 Btu heat input (gas) (IARC, 1973).

Badger et al. (1960, 1962) have proposed that the formation of BP during pyrolysis proceeds as depicted in Fig. 7. In this scheme, possible intermediate compounds would be ethylene or acetylene for I, butadiene or vinyl acetylene for II, styrene or ethylbenzene for III, and phenylbutadiene, *n*-butylbenzene, or tetralin for IV and V.

Benzo[*a*]pyrene has been reported, in a large number of studies from all over the world, to be present in cigarette smoke in amounts ranging from 0.2 to 12.2 μg per 100 cigarettes (Surgeon General's Report, 1964). The average of ten values based on adequacy of the analytical procedure has been found to be 1.6 μg per 100 cigarettes (IARC, 1973); however, it should be noted that loss of BP during the process of fractionation and purification was considered likely. An average concentration of 1.31 mg/kg of BP in cigarette smoke concentrate has also been reported (Elmenhorst and Grimmer, 1968).

Air pollution is considered to be the main source of BP in soil and

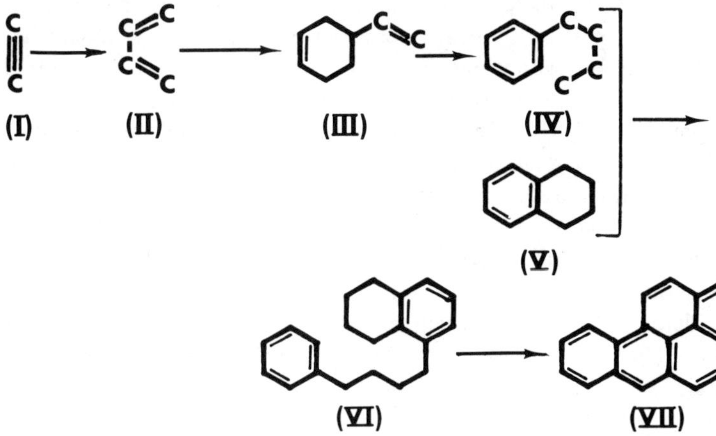

(I)   (II)   (III)   (IV)

(V)

(VI)   (VII)

FIGURE 7   Hypothesis of benzopyrene formation during pyrolysis. (Badger et al., 1962).

water (IARC, 1973); however, microorganisms in the soil may either metabolize or accumulate BP (Shabad, 1968). BP has been found in soil near highways (up to 2,000 μg/kg) (Zdrazil and Picha, 1966) and in the soil of oil refinery plants (200 mg/kg) (Shabad, 1968).

Considerable quantities of PAH can be carried into surface waters by industrial effluents, domestic sewage, and storm water runoff from roads and contaminated land (Anderman and Snodgrass, 1974). The maximum amount determined in any of these sources has been 134 μg/liter (Borneff and Kunte, 1965).

Benzo[a]pyrene has been found in a wide range of concentrations (1-1,840 μg/m^3) in samples of surface waters; its presence may be related to industrial effluents or to bituminous contamination (Borneff and Kunte, 1965).

The literature on the carcinogenicity of PAH is extensive and the most relevant aspects have been summarized by IARC (1973). No epidemiologic studies on the significance of BP exposure to humans are available, and no conclusive evidence exists at the present time to prove that BP is carcinogenic for humans, although coal tar and other materials that are known to be carcinogenic to humans may contain BP.

Benzo[a]pyrene has been found to be mutagenic in *Drosophila* (Demerec, 1948b; Fahmy and Fahmy, 1973), *E. coli* (Scherr et al., 1954), and mice (dominant lethal test). Fahmy and Fahmy (1973) found the mutagenic activity of BP to require crucial conditions for its metabolic activation. In a comparison of the genetic and carcinogenic activities of BP and its methylated derivatives, Fahmy and Fahmy (1973) suggested that these compounds were metabolically converted into complex ionic species with multiple reactive centers, which could differentially attack the cellular macromolecules. The carcinogenically significant events appeared to involve reactions with DNA analogous to those responsible for alkylation mutagenesis. An outstanding feature of the mutagenicity of BP was that it was expressed not only on the heterochromatic loci (bb's and M's) but also on the euchromatic genes (X-recessive lethals and visibles). In this way these compounds differed from the intrinsically nonreactive aromatic carcinogens and resembled the oncogenic alkylating and arylating agents (Fahmy and Fahmy, 1971, 1973). This was particularly evident with respect to the mutagenic selectivity for the rRNA genes, as indicated by the bb/X mutation ratios. [The values for BP were virtually identical to those obtained with typical alkylating agents such as mustard gas (Fahmy and Fahmy, 1971).] It was suggested that BP carcinogenesis might be related to alkylation mutagenesis, being consequential to alterations in genic DNA as a result of electrophilic attack on some of its bases, particularly the N-7 position of guanine moieties.

The mutagenic activities of seven PAH—benzo[a]pyrene; benzo[e]-pyrene, dibenzo[a,i]pyrene, dibenzo[a,e]pyrene, benz[a,h]anthracene, and 3-methylcholanthrene—with different grades of carcinogenic activity (judged by the Iball test in the mouse) (Iball, 1939) were investigated with *S. typhimurium* LT2 mutants to examine the quantitative correlation with the mutagenic potential (Teranishi et al., 1975). In TA1537 or TA1538 tester strains, BP, 3-methylcholanthrene, and dibenzo[a,i]pyrene, which are known to exhibit the highest carcinogenicities, gave rise to significant number of *his*[+] revertants. Benzo[e]pyrene, dibenz[a,h]anthracene, and benz[a]anthracene metabolites, which have relatively low carcinogenicities, did not do so in any of these strains. All the compounds tested were converted to frameshift mutagens (in accord with Ames et al., 1973) when they were metabolized by rat liver homogenate. There was a clear quantitative correlation between carcinogenicity and mutagenicity of the PAH tested in strain TA1538 using the rat liver enzyme induced with both dibenz[a,h]anthracene and phenobarbital. Ames et al. (1972) previously noted the difference between TA1537 and TA1538 in the mutability response to PAH.

In evaluating the TA1538 tester strain for determining the mutagenic potential of air pollutants, Teranishi et al. (1975) found that benzene-extracted materials (50 μg per plate) from about 25 m^3 of air in the vicinity of Kobe gave significant revertant colonies in TA1538 compared with the control in the phenobarbital plus dibenz[a,h]anthracene-induced enzyme system.

It is also important to consider the occurrence and activities of other PAH, such as benz[a]anthracene, benzo[b]fluoranthene, benzo[j]fluoranthene, and dibenz[a,h]anthracene. Detailed studies of air pollution in various cities in Europe, the United States, and Australia have shown that, as with BP, the concentrations of these PAH depended on geographic location, presence of nearby sources of pollution (e.g., highways or industries), and season (IARC, 1973). Summer concentrations of benz[a]anthracene ranged from 1.6 μg/1,000 m^3 in Siena to 136 μg/1,000 m^3 in Pittsburgh, while winter values ranged from 94 μg/1,000 m^3 in Siena to 361 μg/1,000 m^3 in Bochum. In Sydney, Cincinnati, and Detroit, concentrations of benz[a]anthracene ranging from 0.6 to 13.7 μg/1,000 m^3 were found, depending on the traffic situation.

Benzo[j]fluoranthene concentrations of 62-205 mg/kg were found in tar samples in the Detroit area (Colucci and Begeman, 1965), 0.62 mg/kg in dust from air, and 6-97 mg/kg in road dust (Borneff and Kunte, 1965).

Benzo[b]fluoranthene has been found in the air of Sydney in concentrations ranging from 0.5 to 1.5 μg/1,000 m^3 (Cleary, 1963), the highest value being found in December. Levels of 15-62 mg/kg in dust from roads and 0.16 mg/kg in dust from air have also been reported (Colucci and Begeman, 1965; Borneff and Kunte, 1965).

Dibenz[a,h]anthracene was not detected among the PAH found in polluted air (Kotin and Falk, 1963; Sawicki, 1967). However, the dust of 12 German cities during February was found to contain 3.2-32 μg/1,000 m^3, and tunnel dust contained 4-39 μg/kg (Grimmer and Hildebrandt, 1965).

Occupational exposure studies of benz[a]anthracene showed concentrations of 800-14,000 μg/1,000 m^3 in the air of two gas works and one electrical plant (Kreyberg, 1959), 0.7 mg/1,000 m^3 in air polluted by coal tar pitch, and up to 1,300 mg/1,000 m^3 in industrial effluents (Sawicki, 1965a). Benz[a]anthracene was found in flue gases from various coal-fired installations at 44-5,700 μg/1,000 m^3 (Diehl et al., 1970), and its emission levels from heat generation sources (coal) ranged from 19 to 3,900 μg/10^6 Btu of heat input. The emission levels of benz[a]anthracene from incineration and open burning of municipal refuse, automobile tires, and so on ranged from 0.09 to 0.26 μg/g of particulate matter for a municipal incinerator, 5 to 210 μg/g for a commercial incinerator, and 25 to 560 μg/g in open burning (Hangebrauck et al., 1964).

Benzo[b]fluoranthene and benzo[j]fluoranthene have been reported to average 8.4 and 7.3 mg/kg, respectively, in soot samples (Fischer, 1970). Stefanescu and Stanescu (1968) found 300-3,000 mg/1,000 m^3 of dibenz[a,h]anthracene in different kinds of soot.

Cigarette smoke has been found to contain a variety of PAH including the previously discussed BP. For example, concentrations of benz[a]anthracene ranging from 1.2 to 14 μg have been found in the smoke condensate of 100 cigarettes, while levels of 0.03 and 4.6 μg/g have been reported in cigarette smoke condensate (IARC, 1973).

Smoke condensates of 100 cigarettes have yielded benzo[b]fluoranthene and benzo[j]fluoranthene at levels of 0.1-2 μg and 0.6 μg, respectively. In addition. 0.15-0.2 mg of benzo[j]fluoranthene has been isolated from smoke condensate (IARC, 1973).

Dibenz[*a,h*]anthracene has been found at levels ranging from 0.05 to 0.4 μg in the smoke condensate of 100 cigarettes (Wynder and Hoffmann, 1959; Van Duuren, 1958) and 0.1 to 0.15 mg/kg in cigarette smoke condensate (Elmenhorst and Grimmer, 1968; Wynder and Hoffmann, 1959).

The carcinogenicity of benz[*a*]anthracene, benzo[*b*]fluoranthene, benzo[*j*]fluoranthene, and dibenz[*a,h*]anthracene has been reviewed by IARC (1973). As in the case of BP, no case reports or epidemiologic studies of the significance of exposure to these PAH are available.

Dibenzanthracene has been found to be mutagenic in *Drosophila* (Demerec, 1947, 1948a, 1948b), *Neurospora* (Barrett and Tatum, 1951, 1958), *E. coli* (Scherr et al., 1954), *S. typhimurium* (TA1538) (Teranishi et al., 1975), and the mouse (Carr, 1947). Its nonmutagenicity in the mouse has also been reported (Auerbach, 1940).

Huberman et al. (1971) studied the mutagenicity to Chinese hamster cells of epoxides and other derivatives of a number of polycyclic hydrocarbons including benzo[*a*]anthracene and demonstrated that metabolic activation of polycyclic hydrocarbons was required for mutagenic activity in mammalian cells.

Ames et al. (1972) reported that K-region epoxides of carcinogenic PAH such as benz[*a*]anthracene, dibenz[*a,b*]anthracene, and 7-methylbenz[*a*]-anthracene were frameshift mutagens. It was postulated that PAH may be carcinogenic because of the mutagenicity of epoxides in intermediates formed during metabolism, and that the mechanism of action may involve intercalation followed by covalent reaction.

NITROSAMINES

In recent years, there has been increasing concern about the possibility that nitrosamines might constitute an environmental hazard for humans (Lijinsky and Epstein, 1970; Magee, 1971; Newberne and Shank, 1973).

The carcinogenicity of preformed nitrosamines (and nitrosamides) has been well documented in many animals and many species. At least 80 different nitroso compounds have been reported to be carcinogenic in at least one animal species, and there is evidence that 15 organs are susceptible to the carcinogenic action of these compounds (Druckrey et al., 1967; IARC, 1972; Magee and Barnes, 1967).

The sources of human exposure to nitrosamines, either preformed or formed *in vitro* and/or *in vivo*, are diverse. Patent applications (primarily for diethyl- and dimethylnitrosamines) cover use in the manufacture of rubber, dyestuffs, lubricating oils, plasticizers, polymers, explosives, rocket fuels, insecticides, and fungicides (Fishbein et al., 1970; Magee, 1972a; Wolff and Wasserman, 1972). There is increasing concern about nitrosation of dietary amines by sodium nitrite, a common food additive, and the possible relationship of this reaction to cancer in humans (Druckrey et al., 1967; *Food and*

Cosmetics Toxicology, 1968; *Lancet*, 1968; Lijinsky and Epstein, 1970). Nitrosamines have been found in tobacco smoke, alcoholic beverages (McGlashan et al., 1968), mushrooms (Ender and Ceh, 1968), and, more significantly, foods such as grains, pasteurized milk, and cheese (Hedler and Marquardt, 1968; Freimuth and Glaser, 1970; Kroeller, 1967) and nitrite-treated cheese, fish, smoked fish, and meat (Ender and Ceh, 1968; *Food and Cosmetics Toxicology*, 1968; Howard et al., 1970; Sen et al., 1970; Freimuth and Glaser, 1970; Crosby et al., 1972; Wasserman et al., 1972; Fiddler et al., 1972). The concentrations of nitrosamines that have been reported in foods are generally less than 5 ppm (Lijinsky and Epstein, 1970). For example, samples of cod, hake, and haddock have been shown to contain 1–4 ppm of dimethylnitrosamine (DMN) (Crosby et al., 1972); herring meal, 0.15–0.45 ppm (Sakshaug et al., 1965); samples of sable, shad, and salmon, 4–26 ppb (Fazio et al., 1971); salami and sausage, approximately 10–80 ppb; and bacon, from 0 to 16–40 ppb (Fazio et al., 1971). The formation of nitrosopyrrolidine during the frying of bacon is cited as an additional source of concern (Sen et al., 1973a; Fazio et al., 1973).

The occurrence of fairly high levels of nitrosamines in certain types of meat-curing mixtures containing spices and nitrite indicates that some of the nitrosamines in cured meat products may originate from these curing mixtures (Sen et al., 1973b). Nitrosamines in these premixes are apparently formed under dry conditions, because of the interaction of amines in spices and nitrite, both of which are major components of these formulations (Sen et al., 1974).

It is important to note that the accuracy of many of the earlier studies involving the identification of nitrosamines in various foodstuffs is questionable, as specific methods for confirming the identification (primarily mass spectrometric) were not employed and a number of other food components are known to appear as artifacts in the analyses (Pensabene et al., 1972; IARC, 1973).

It is generally acknowledged that nitrite, which is added as a preservative, reacts with amines present in meats during processing, storage, or cooking to form these nitroso compounds.

There is increasing evidence that nitrosamines may be formed from nitrite and secondary amines under the acidic conditions of the human stomach (Druckrey et al., 1963; Sander, 1967). As experimental models for this hypothesis, numerous animal studies were carried out involving the chronic feeding of sodium nitrite with a variety of secondary amines. For example, feeding of sodium nitrite with morpholine or *N*-methylbenzylamine induced various tumors in the rat (Newberne and Shank, 1973; Sander et al, 1968; Sander and Bürkle, 1969); lung adenomas were induced in Swiss mice chronically fed nitrite plus morpholine, piperazine, or *N*-methylaniline (Greenblatt et al., 1971), but not dimethylamine. This sensitive test system (Shimkin et al, 1969) was also used to estimate the extent to which each amine was nitrosated *in vivo* (Greenblatt et al., 1971).

The formation of nitrosamines by the interaction of nitrites or oxides of nitrogen and secondary amines under acidic conditions also occurs *in vitro* in the gastric juice of various species, including humans (Sander, 1967; Alam et al., 1971a, 1971b), and also *in vitro* at near-neutral pH in the presence of enteric bacteria (Sander, 1968).

The rate of formation of nitrosamines from amines and nitrite is dependent on many factors such as the nature of the amines, concentration of the reactants, pH, and temperature of the reaction medium (Mirvish, 1973). There is also evidence that nitrates can be reduced to nitrites in the gastrointestinal tract (Sander, 1967; Sander and Seif, 1969).

$$\begin{array}{c} R_1 \\ {\diagdown} \\ {}NH + HNO_2 \rightleftharpoons \\ R_2{\diagup} \end{array} \quad \begin{array}{c} R_1 \\ {\diagdown} \\ {}N-NO + H_2O \\ R_2{\diagup} \end{array}$$

It is important to consider the potential sources in the environment of precursors of nitrosamines. Nitrates are widely distributed in nature, particularly in plants, forage, and water, and nitrites are readily formed from them. Nitrates are widely found as natural components of many foods (Phillips, 1968). Levels as high as 4,850 ppm of NO_3 and 233 ppm of NO_2 have been found in spinach, and samples of beets, cauliflower, cabbage, rhubarb, and radishes have been found to contain over 1,000 ppm of NO_3 (Eisenberg et al., 1970).

Excessive use of nitrate fertilizers, use of the herbicide 2,4-D[(2,4-dichlorophenoxy)acetic acid], and molybdenum deficiency in soil can result in the accumulation of nitrates in plants and forage (Vlitos, 1962; Lijinsky and Epstein, 1970). Nitrates can occur in significant concentrations in water, particularly in agricultural areas, but also from contamination resulting from sewage discharges, intensive use of nitrate fertilizers, and rising water tables, which leach subsoil nitrates into well waters.

Nitrate in drinking water has been associated with approximately 2,000 cases of methemoglobinemia in infants in North America and Europe from about 1945 to 1971 (Winton et al., 1971), with chemical and subclinical cases of the disease in infants consuming water having less than 45 mg/l of NO_3 (Knotek and Schmidt, 1964).

Nitrites are intermediates in the reduction of nitrates in plants and other sources by nitroreductases which are present in a wide range of saprophytic and parasitic bacteria (Nason, 1962; Lam and Nicholas, 1969). Nitrite might also accumulate during the oxidation of ammonia under alkaline conditions.

Relatively large concentrations of nitrites are found in stored green vegetables, especially spinach, as a result of bacterial reduction of nitrate (Sinios and Wodsak, 1965).

Nitrates and nitrites are broadly used as preservatives in meat and fish, with permissible concentrations in the United States of 500 and 200 ppm, respectively (*Federal Register*, 1968). The average daily intake of nitrite has been estimated as 22 μmol (Sander, 1967), equivalent to 1.5 mg of $NaNO_2$.

Phillips (1968) calculated that in a typical Canadian meal, adults may consume about 313 mg of nitrate from various fresh foods or about 4.5 mg/kg under normal circumstances; this would not be considered detrimental. However, if all of this nitrate, or a major portion, was converted to nitrites before eating, or by stomach flora after eating, the effect might be toxic (Shuval and Gruener, 1972).

It is generally believed that the limiting factor in the formation of nitrosamines in an environmental context is the availability of nitrosatable secondary amines (Lijinsky and Epstein, 1970). Secondary amines occur, particularly as dimethylamine and diethylamine in cereals, tea, fish meal, and fish products (Miyahara, 1966; Preusser, 1966) and in tobacco and tobacco smoke (Neurath et al., 1966a, 1966b). Dimethylamine is also found in urine (Brooks et al., 1972), feces (Van Rheenen, 1962), higher plants (Smith, 1971), and algae (Rolle et al., 1971).

Because dimethylamine may also be formed by demethylation of trimethylamine (TMA), the tertiary amine is also a possible DMN precursor and TMA occurs in plants, fish, and algae (Cromwell and Richardson, 1966; Sasajima, 1968). Dimethylamine can also be formed from the pesticide thiram (tetramethylthiuram disulfide) (Maeda and Tonomura, 1971).

Formation of a number of carcinogenic nitroso compounds from nitrite and some types of agricultural chemicals including thiram and carbaryl (1-naphthyl *N*-methylcarbamate) has been reported by Elespuru and Lijinsky (1973).

Eisenbrand et al. (1974) found that the carcinogenic nitrosamine DMN could be formed rapidly by interaction of nitrite with ziram and ferbam *in vitro* under simulated gastric conditions and *in vivo* in rat stomach, which adds another dimension to the toxicological potential of this class of fungicides. Residual levels of such fungicides in the human diet represent potential precursors for the formation of carcinogenic nitrosamines when they are ingested with nitrite. Under the selected conditions, the optimum pH for the formation of DMN was 1.5–2.0. At pH 2.0, more than 1 mg DMN was produced after a 10-min incubation of 10^{-4} M ziram with a 20-fold molar excess of nitrite. This corresponded to about 8% of the theoretical yield, assuming that two molecules of the carcinogen were formed from one molecule of ziram.

Ayanaba and Alexander (1974) reported a number of transformations of methylamines and formation of DMN in samples of treated sewage and lake water in New York and New Hampshire. Added trimethylamine was converted to dimethylamine in samples of raw sewage and lake water; the rates of formation and disappearance of dimethylamine were governed by the pH and the type and amount of inorganic nitrogen present. DMN was also found in sewage and lake water samples receiving trimethylamine. Thiram was converted to dimethylamine in sterilized sewage at pH 4.0, and small amounts of DMN were also produced in the presence of nitrite; the yields of both products were far greater in nonsterile, thiram-amended sewage. Micro-organisms were involved in some stage of the conversion of trimethylamine to the secondary amine and DMN in nonsterilized sewage, since these products were not formed in sterilized sewage.

Other sources of secondary or tertiary amines that may be encountered in the environment and are potentially nitrosatable are nitrilotriacetic acid, proposed as a component of detergent formulations (Ayanaba and Alexander, 1974), and pesticides such as derivatives of alkylureas and alkylcarbamic acids, which can yield dialkylnitrosamine or an *N*-nitroso derivative or both on reaction with nitrite under mildly acidic conditions (Elespuru and Lijinsky, 1973).

Other sources of secondary amines are formed as a consequence of cooking (Lijinsky and Epstein, 1970). For example, pyrolysis of protein and cooking of protein food might produce free amino acids such as proline, arginine, and hydroxyproline and nitrosatable secondary amines such as pyrrolidine and piperidine. Lijinsky and Epstein (1970) cite the possibility that proline ingested in food could be converted into nitrosoproline by nitrite present in the stomach. The nitrosoproline could then be decarboxylated (possibly bacterially) in the alkaline conditions prevailing in the duodenum and small intestine, yielding the highly carcinogenic nitrosopyrrolidine.

It is not known whether nitrosamine acids occur in nitrite-containing foods, since the requisite analytic methods have not yet been developed (Mirvish et al., 1973). However, nitrosopyrrolidine occurs at levels of 1–80 ppm in fried but not uncooked bacon (Crosby et al., 1972; Sen et al., 1973b) and may form during frying by decarboxylation of nitrosoproline. Similarly, DMN in nitrite-preserved foods (Crosby et al., 1972; Sen et al., 1973b; Wasserman et al., 1972) may arise through decarboxylation of nitrososarcosine.

Hence, nitrosamino acid formation during food storage or preparation may be a significant consideration, since these compounds may be decarboxylated to yield highly carcinogenic nitrosamines when the food is cooked (Mirvish et al, 1973).

Secondary and other amines are formed during alcoholic fermentation; for example, nitrogenous bases have been found in spirits, and several amines, including pyrrolidine, have been found in wine (Stastny, 1942; Drawert, 1965). The high incidence of esophageal cancer associated with the consumption of crude beers and other liquors in Zambia is believed by some to be related to both secondary amines and nitrosamines (Neurath, 1967; Marquardt and Hedler, 1966; McGlashan et al., 1968).

DuPlessis et al. (1969) reported the presence of DMN in the fruit of a solanaceous bush (*Solanum incanum*), the juice of which is used to curdle milk. The resulting curds are a major source of sustenance of the Bantu people in localized areas of the Transkei, where there is also a high incidence of esophageal cancer.

A number of commonly used drugs that are taken either in large doses or for long periods of time contain secondary amine groups or structures that may be amine precursors (Wolff and Wasserman, 1972; Lijinsky and Epstein, 1970). There is obvious interest in the internal nitrosation of such drugs, if ingested with nitrite or water containing high levels of nitrate. Model studies of Lijinsky (1971) indicate that both oxytetracycline and antipyrine yielded DMN when reacted with nitrite, while diethylnitrosamine was obtained when disulfiram was reacted with nitrite.

Mirvish (1972), conducting a large number of kinetic studies on *N*-nitrosation reactions, recently reported on the types of nitrogen compounds that are likely to be *readily* nitrosatable. These include weakly basic secondary amines (e.g., morpholine, piperazine, *N*-methylaniline), some *free* amino acids with secondary amino groups (hydroxyproline, sarcosine), and alkylureas and *N*-alkyl carbamates. The presence in food of even small concentrations of these compounds is of obvious concern if the nitroso derivatives are carcinogenic and/or mutagenic and if sufficient nitrite is present, because of the possibility of intragastric nitrosation and also of nitrosation during food storage, especially under acidic conditions. Less readily nitrosatable compounds, such as strongly basic secondary amines (piperidine, dimethylamine), free proline, and alkylguanidines (e.g., arginine and methylguanidine), are less likely to be significantly nitrosated *unless* relatively large concentrations occur in food (Mirvish, 1972).

It is generally acknowledged that nitrosamines require metabolic conversion to an active form to produce their cellular and biochemical effects (Magee and Barnes, 1967; Magee, 1972b; Kruger, 1972). Although a number of nitrosamines have been shown to alkylate nucleic acids (especially the base guanine at position N-7) and proteins of animals and bacterial cells *in vivo* (Magee, 1972b; Swann and Magee, 1968), the significance of these alkylation reactions is not entirely clear.

According to a proposed mechanism (Fig. 8) (Magee and Hultin, 1962; Rose, 1958; Druckrey et al., 1967), the initial step should be an enzymatic α-hydroxylation of one of the aliphatic chains, which is followed by its hydrolytic cleavage, leading to the formation of the corresponding aldehyde and a monoalkylnitrosamine. The monoalkylnitrosamine rearranges to the corresponding diazohydroxide, from which a diazoalkane is formed that then decomposes to the corresponding alkyl cation by removal of a nitrogen molecule.

However, the nature of the reactive intermediates in the formation of the alkyl cation has not been unambiguously elaborated (Kruger, 1972; Lee and Lijinsky, 1966; Lijinsky and Ross, 1969). For example, reactive products expected from cyclic nitrosamines would be formed by α-oxidation, followed

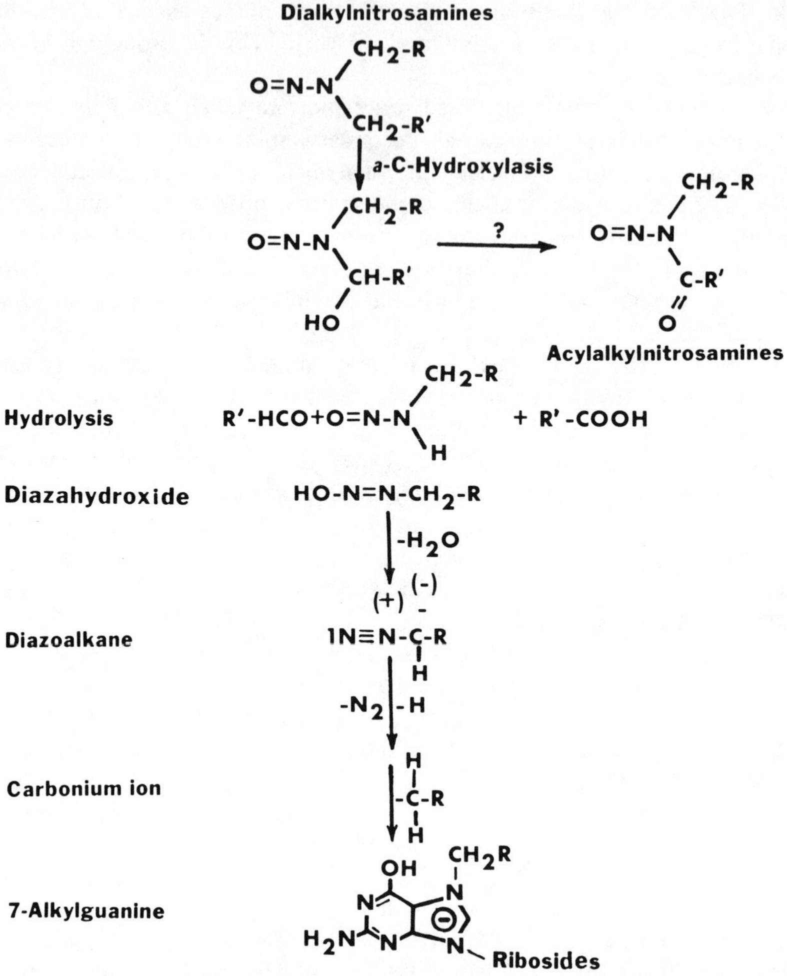

FIGURE 8 Proposed mechanism for the alkylating intermediates from
dialkylnitrosamines and dialkylnitrosamides.

by hydrolytic cleavage of the heterocyclic ring system, and finally transfer of
the corresponding aldehyde or of carboxylic acid to the genetic material,
which should contain all the carbon atoms of the heterocyclic system (Fig. 9).

Another mechanism can be invoked (Fig. 10) that would account for
cyclic and higher di-*n*-alkylnitrosamines being metabolically degraded to
methylalkylnitrosamines or DMN, which would then act as methylating agents
(Magee and Lee, 1964; Kruger, 1972). This appears possible if nitrosamine
metabolism is considered to be analogous to the established metabolic
pathway of fatty acid degradation (Fig. 10).

The mutagenic activity of some carcinogenic nitrosamines has been demonstrated in *Drosophila* (Fahmy et al., 1966; Pasternak, 1962, 1963, 1964) and in a tyrosineless strain of *E. coli* (Pogodina, 1966). In other strains of *E. coli*, all tested nitrosamines were found to be nonmutagenic (Geissler, 1962; Pogodina, 1966; Trams and Künkel, 1964, 1965).

The mutagenic activity of nitrosamines was also absent in *Serratia* (Geissler, 1962) and yeast (Marquardt et al., 1964). Veleminsky and Gichner (1968) described the mutagenic activity of nitrosamines in a higher plant, *Arabidopsis thaliana*; of 12 nitrosamines tested, only dimethyl-, methylethyl-, methylbenzyl-, and ethylvinylnitrosamine were found to possess mutagenic activity and induce high sterility. With the exception of ethylvinylnitrosamine, all of these mutagenic nitrosamines possessed at least one methyl group. It was postulated (in accord with the theory of specific enzymes decomposing the nitrosamines) that a hydroxylase or hydroxylases in seeds of *Arabidopsis* are specific for these methyl groups. Ethylvinylnitrosamine is known to be unstable (Druckrey et al., 1967), and hence no enzymes were required for its decomposition.

Until recently, DMN was believed to be nonmutagenic in *Neurospora* (Marquardt et al., 1963). All suggested metabolic routes for DMN involve an initial oxidative dealkylation of nitrosamine, and the previously observed lack of mutagenicity in both bacteria and *Neurospora* may have resulted from their inability to carry out this dealkylation reaction (Malling, 1971). The dealkylation process is probably initated by hydroxylation of the carbon atom in

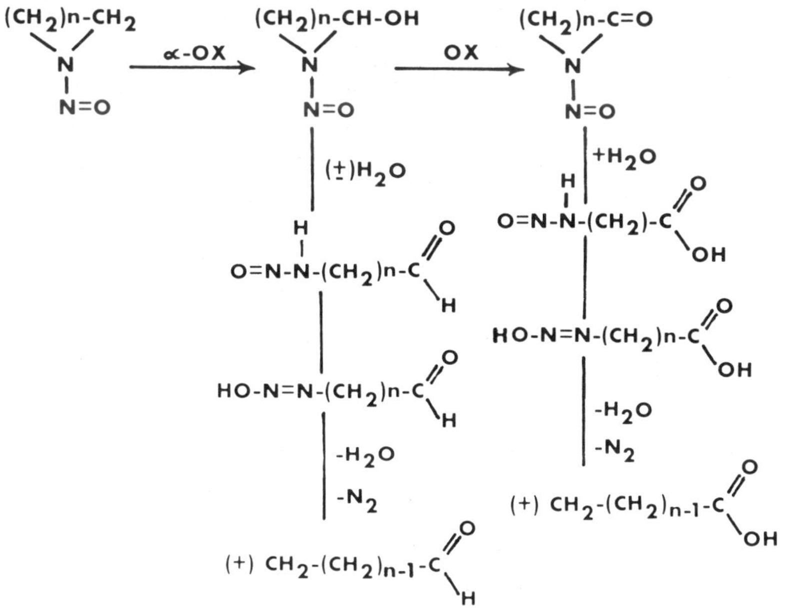

FIGURE 9 Reactive products expected to be formed from cyclic nitrosamines after α-oxidation and the following steps (see Fig. 8).

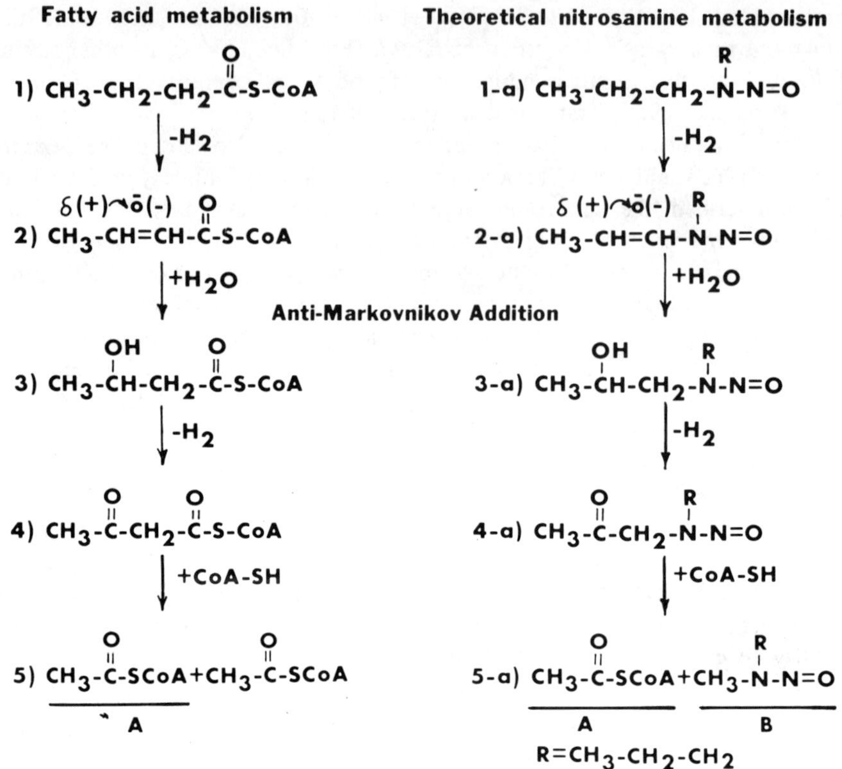

FIGURE 10 Theoretical pathway of nitrosamine degradation in analogy to fatty acid metabolism: (A) activated acetic acid, and (B) methylalkylnitrosamine or dimethylnitrosamine if $R = CH_3$.

direct proximity to the amine nitrogen (Malling, 1971), as demonstrated in chemical systems (Preussman, 1964; Udenfriend et al, 1954). A much higher frequency of *ad*-3 mutation is found among *Neurospora conidia* treated with DMN in such a chemical system under an O_2 atmosphere than among those treated under similar conditions without DMN (Malling, 1966).

Malling (1971) found that in *S. typhimurium* tester strains TA1530, G46, C207, and C3076, only TA1530 and G46, which revert by base-pair substitutions, do so after treatment with DMN and liver enzymes. It was shown by Malling (1971) that liver enzymes are ablt to form mutagenic compounds from DMN, and that they are stable enough to enter the bacterial cell and induce mutations. This conclusion is supported by the studies of Gabridge and Legator (1969) in the host-mediated assay system, using strain G46 as an indicator organism and the mouse as host; *S. typhimurium* lacks the enzymes to activate DMN, but activation is performed by the host mouse.

Recently, Couch and Friedman (1974) reported that doses of sodium nitrite as low as 25 mg/kg lowered the frequency of observed mutants produced by DMN in *S. typhimurium* G46 in the host-mediated assay. The failure of sodium nitrites to suppress the mutagenicity of BCNU [1,3-bis-(β-chloroethyl)-1-nitrosourea], which does not require biotransformation by the host to an active form, supports the hypothesis that $NaNO_2$ effects DMN metabolism directly, and not some other parameter such as absorption of the compound. The ability of $NaNO_2$ to suppress the mutagenicity of DMN would appear to confuse the assessment of the danger of human exposure to this agent.

Fahrig (1974) described a differential response of yeast cells injected into testes of rats and peritoneum of mice and rats to six mutagens, which included the *indirect* mutagens 1-(pyridyl-3)-3,3-dimethyltriazene, 2-[bis-(chloroethyl)amino] tetrahydro-2*H*-1,3,2-oxazaphosphorine 2-oxide (Endoxan), and DMN and the *direct* ones triethylenemelamine, 1-phenyl-3,3-dimethyl-triazene, and methyl methanesulfonate (MMS). Induction of mitotic gene conversion in *S. cerevisiae* was chosen as the indicator of genetic activity, except for DMN. All substances were genetically more active in the testes than in the peritoneum of rats, and, with the exception of MMS, all substances were genetically more active in rats than in mice. The sensitivity to DMN can be summarized as: rat peritoneum > mouse peritoneum > rat testes. The technique employed by Fahrig (1974), injection of yeast cells into the testes, makes it possible to determine whether a mutagen or mutagenic metabolite reaches the testes and hence is potentially able to induce mutations in germ cells.

Green and Muriel (1975b) described studies utilizing repair-deficient *E. coli* strains and liver microsomes to characterize mutagenesis by DMN. Strains WP_2 and its derivatives WP_2 *μvrA* and CM 611 *μvrA xrA* were mutated to about the same extent with *activated* DMN, similarly to MNNG (*N*-methyl-*N'*-nitro-*N*-nitrosoguanidine) or MNU (*N*-methyl-*N*-nitrosourea). No mutagenicity was found in the presence of soft agar and the absence of the liver fraction. MNNG and MNU cause mutation by misreplication as well as misrepair [e.g., they mutate *exrA* strains of *E. coli* nearly as efficiently as they mutate *exrA*$^+$ strains (Hince and Neale, 1974; Witkin, 1967)]. The mutagenic lesions are not subject to excision by *μvr* endonuclease (e.g., mutation is equal in *μvr* and a *μvr*$^+$ strain) (Hince and Neale, 1974; Witkin, 1967).

Additional mutagenicity studies have been reported utilizing the cyclic nitrosamine *N*-nitrosomorpholine. This nitrosamine failed to induce dominant lethal mutations in mice at dose levels of 50 and 100 mg/kg because of an adverse effect on mating activity; no increase in the incidence of dominant lethal mutations was observed between the weeks 5 and 8. At a dose of 35 mg/kg, mating activity was normal during the initial 3-wk period studied, but there was no evidence of increased mutations (Park et al., 1973). This result is of interest because the same compound, which is a potent carcinogen, was found to be positive in the host-mediated assay using *S. typhimurium* in Swiss mice, (optimal effects at a dose of about 100 mg/kg) but negative for the bacterium alone (Zeiger and Legator, 1971).

The teratogenic effects of both nitrosamines and nitrosamides have been compared (Magee, 1971; Magee and Barnes, 1967). As with the transplacental carcinogenic action, it appears that the nitrosamides are more effective teratogens than the nitrosamines. This may well be related to the relative chemical stability of the two types of compound and the most likely requirement for metabolic activation of the nitrosamines (Magee, 1971). Napalkov and Alexandrov (1968) failed to observe teratogenic effects in the rat with dialkylnitrosamines.

ATMOSPHERIC MUTAGENS

It is generally agreed that knowledge of the worldwide atmosphere is quite incomplete. However, despite the geographic differences in topography, climatology, and civilization, the worldwide atmosphere has been found to be reasonably similar at moderate distances—a few kilometers in the vertical direction or a few tens of kilometers in the horizontal direction—from particular sources (Fischer, 1972).

The terrestial atmosphere may be divided in several ways—for instance, into the troposphere, stratosphere, mesosphere, and thermosphere. Between the "spheres" there are short regions called the tropopause, the stratopause, and the mesopause. Each altitude has an exact temperature and density that do not depend on latitude, solar activity, or time of the year (Hendel, 1973).

The two major areas for our consideration of atmospheric mutagens are the troposphere and the stratosphere. The troposphere (where most of the clouds are located) extends up to an average of 7 mi (12 km). Although the chemical composition of the normal dry, unpolluted air remains essentially unchanged at the different altitudes, the concentration of minor gases such as O_3, SO_2, and NO_2 varies slightly while the content of water vapor and aerosols varies greatly, especially between the tropics and the polar regions.

The stratosphere, which is the next major layer, extends to about 30 mi up and has a chemical composition similar to that of the troposphere, except that CO_2 is greatly reduced, O_3 is greatly increased (up to $\sim$ 10 ppm), and the amounts of aerosol (including water droplets) and pollutants are practically nil (Hendel, 1973).

Substances deposited in the biosphere and the troposphere can often be eventually transported great distances from their original site of application or introduction—for instance, chlorinated hydrocarbon pesticides (Miller and Berg, 1969), polychlorinated biphenyls (PCBs) (Hammond, 1972), and SO_2 (Blokker, 1973; Swedish Secretariat, 1972).

It is important to note that most air contaminants are removed from the atmosphere by a variety of scavenging processes (e.g., precipitation, gravitational settling, impaction of particulates on vegetation or the ground, absorption of pollutants by vegetation, soil, and water surfaces). All of these processes transfer the pollutant from the atmosphere to both terrestrial and aquatic environments (Babich and Stotzky, 1973).

Pollutants that, in the form of trace constituents or elements (CO, CO_2, SO_2, NO_2, NH_3, H_2S), can arise from natural sources (e.g., soil erosion of rock material, sea spray, emission of volcanic gases, entrainment of biological products, smoke produced in natural fires) are *generally* present in air in very small quantities, the gaseous components representing less than 0.1% of the total volume, and only in extremely exceptional cases do aerosols attain a total mass of 10^{-3} g/m^3 of air (Israel and Israel, 1974).

However, the development of human civilization has greatly added to the same types of gases and aerosols produced by natural sources, and in some cases the artificial or anthropogenic sources have significantly exceeded the natural abundance. The use of fossil fuels for home heating, energy generation, motor vehicle traffic, manufacturing, mining, smelting and refining processes, and incineration makes the major contribution to the pollutant trace constituents. In a large part of the world today, the pollutants produced by fossil fuels are the main contributors to air pollution caused by human activity (Israel and Israel, 1974).

Sulfur Oxides

The global atmospheric sulfur budget is illustrated in Fig. 11 which shows that anthropogenic emissions are only a portion of the total global emissions. Sulfur enters the atmosphere worldwide as air pollutants in the form of H_2S, SO_2, H_2SO_4, and particulate sulfate and as natural emissions in the form of H_2S and sulfates; approximately one-third arises from air pollution (mostly in the form of SO_2), the remainder from natural processes. Hydrogen sulfide from natural processes accounts for approximately half of the total released to the atmosphere (Israel and Israel, 1974).

The approximate average tropospheric concentrations in uncontaminated

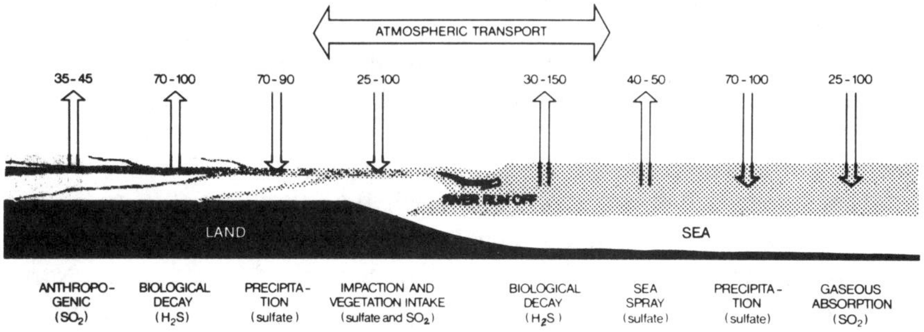

FIGURE 11 Global atmospheric sulfur budget, showing sulfur (in millions of tons) that passes through the sulfur cycle annually. Quantities emitted by anthropogenic sources are given on the far left.

atmosphere are SO_2, 0.5 ppb; sulfate aerosols, 2 $\mu g/m^3$; and H_2S, 0.2 ppb, while in polluted atmospheres the approximate concentrations are SO_2, 2,000 ppb and H_2S, 500 ppb (Corn and DeMaio, 1964; Robinson and Robbins, 1970a, 1970b; Waller, 1963).

Sulfur dioxide enters the atmosphere mainly by the combustion of coal and oil, while natural emissions from volcanoes are only a minor source of atmospheric SO_2.

Depending on origin, coal and fuel oil contain $\sim$ 0.3–5% elemental sulfur by weight. Coal containing 2–4% sulfur has been used traditionally for space heating and power generation, while a much lower sulfur content is required of coal intended for steel production (Berry and Lehman, 1971). For every ton of sulfur in the fuel, 2 tons of SO_2 is produced. Typically, the concentration of effluent SO_3 is about $\frac{1}{40}$ to $\frac{1}{80}$ of the concentration of SO_2. Approximately 80% of anthropogenic SO_2 pollution results from burning fossil fuels containing sulfur compounds; $\sim$ 45% results from burning fossil fuels in electric power plant operations [National Industrial Pollution Control Council (NIPCC), 1971]. The estimated U.S. emissions of sulfur oxides in 1968 were 33 million tons (mostly from stationary fuel combustion and industrial processes) and accounted for $\sim$ 15% by weight of the total of more than 200 million tons of pollutants entering the air per year (NIPCC, 1971).

The approximate percentages of total anthropogenic emissions of sulfur oxides in the United States in 1965 were: electric power generation (coal), 42; electric power generation (oil), 4; other coal combustion, 17; other petroleum combustion (other petroleum), 3; refinery operations, 5; smelting of ores, 12; coke processing, 2; sulfuric acid manufacture, 2; and other, 1 [National Air Pollution Control Association (NAPCA), 1968; U.S. Department of Health, Education, and Welfare, 1969].

The annual worldwide emission of SO_2 (for 1965) was estimated by Robinson and Robbins (1967) at 146.4 million tons, of which 102 million tons came from coal burning, 23 million from petroleum combustion, 5.7 million from petroleum refining, and 15.7 million from smelting of nonferrous metals, principally copper. These emissions, based on figures for 1965, are approximately twice those of 1940 (Berry and Lehman, 1971).

The estimated amount of SO_2 emitted by pollutant sources in the Northern Hemisphere in this period was 136 million tons, equivalent to 68 million tons of sulfur, whereas the natural sulfur emission (from H_2S) was estimated at 62 million tons (Robinson and Robbins, 1967).

The following figures for sulfur emission [in millions of tons, from 1968 Office of Economic Cooperation and Development (OECD) data] illustrate the annual emission distribution among a number of countries in Northwestern Europe (Swedish Secreatariat, 1972): Belgium, France, Germany, Netherlands, and Luxembourg, 3.7; Austria and Switzerland, 0.2; Scandinavia, 0.6; United Kingdom and Ireland, 3.1; and neighboring Eastern European countries, 1–3.

The form of the pollutant during its initial entry into the atmosphere may not be the form that is eventually deposited in the biosphere. In summarizing the atmospheric chemistry of sulfur oxides, it should be noted that the rate of oxidation of SO_2 to sulfuric acid and its conversion to suspended sulfates are greatly accelerated in polluted air compared with pure air, although the interactions between sulfur oxides and common pollutants (e.g., nitrogen oxides, hydrocarbons, particulate matter) and the contribution of each to the effects of air pollution have not been fully resolved (Cox and Penkett, 1971; *Ambio,* 1972; Atkins et al., 1972; McKay, 1971; Smith et al., 1969).

For example, SO_2 undergoes a variety of photochemical and catalytic reactions in the atmosphere, with the subsequent formation of sulfuric acid mist or sulfate (SO_4^{2-}) salts, so that the concentration of SO_2 high in the atmosphere or far from sources is close to the natural level of about 0.2 ppb (Berry and Lehman, 1971). During the daytime and under conditions of low humidity, the predominant reaction is the oxidation of SO_2 in mixtures of hydrocarbons and nitrogen dioxide, with the resultant formation of H_2SO_4 aerosols. At night, or in foggy, rainy, or high relative humidity conditions, the major reaction involves the absorption of SO_2 onto water droplets, a reaction accelerated by NH_4^+, and the subsequent oxidation of SO_2 to SO_4^{2-}. Hence some of the initial SO_2 molecules may finally interact within the biosphere in the form of excess hydrogen ions and/or SO_4^{2-} ions (Babich and Stotzky, 1973).

Berry and Lehman (1971) reported a worldwide layer between 17 and 24 km above sea level in which the sulfate concentration is about four times that in the lower troposphere. This layer contains only a small fraction of the total amount of atmospheric sulfur (only about 30,000 tons/yr pass through it) (Berry and Lehman, 1971).

The ambient distribution of sulfur in the atmosphere is considered to be about 65% in the form of sulfate or sulfuric acid aerosol, about 23% as gaseous SO_2, and 12% as H_2S. By comparing emissions of sulfur within different regions with the deposited amounts, it has been estimated that the sulfur remains in the air for an average of 2-4 days (Swedish Secretariat, 1972; Robinson and Robbins, 1967) and is usually transported more than 1,000 km before being deposited on the ground (Swedish Secretariat, 1972).

The principal mechanism for removal of SO_2 appears to be oxidation to SO_3 and direct absorption at the earth's surface. Sulfur trioxide reacts with atmospheric water to form sulfuric acid, which forms aerosols whose individual droplets grow over a period of a few days to 0.1-1 μm. These particles are eventually removed from the atmosphere by rain, snow, or gravitational settling (Berry and Lehman, 1971).

The SO_2 molecule may also be directly absorbed in or adsorbed on the moist surfaces of the biota or soil, or in the surface waters of the aqueous environment. Sulfur dioxide is highly soluble in water; for example, 11.28

g/100 ml at 20°C. On contact with water, SO_2 forms sulfurous acid (H_2SO_3), which, depending on the pH, can dissociate into the bisulfite (HSO_3^-) or the sulfite (SO_3^{2-}) ion.

$$SO_2 + H_2O \rightarrow H_2SO_3$$

$$H_2SO_3 \rightarrow H^+ + HSO_3^- \quad pK = 1.76$$

$$HSO_3^- \rightarrow H^+ + SO_3^{2-} \quad pK_2' = 7.21$$

The specific concentrations of SO_3^{2-}, HSO_3^-, and H_2SO_3 are pH-dependent. Hence, at pH 1 H_2SO_3 is the dominant species, while between pH 2 and pH 7 HSO_3^- is dominant and above pH 7 SO_3^{2-} is dominant. It should be noted that, on oxidation, the solubility products are transformed to sulfuric acid, and consequently the final effect of SO_2 on the biosphere may be an acidic effect (e.g., H_2SO_3 or H_2SO_4), an ionic effect (e.g., SO_3^{2-}, SO_4^{2-}, or HSO_3^-), or a combination of acidic and ionic effects (Babich and Stotzky, 1973).

In urban regions emitting large quantities of SO_2, the subsequent adsorption of SO_2 by water droplets lowers the pH of rain. The increasing anthropogenic emissions in Europe and the United States have been correlated with the decreasing pH of precipitation (Blokker, 1973; Swedish Secretariat, 1972; Babich and Stotzky, 1973).

It is generally acknowledged that the chemical form of sulfur oxides in the ambient air that is associated in epidemiologic studies with morbidity and mortality has yet to be clearly identified (Rall, 1974). The sulfur-containing products that have been implicated include SO_2, sulfuric acid, and inorganic sulfates. Health effects may range from discomfort through physiological deviations from the norm, prevalence of symptoms, appearance of illness, lost working time and premature retirement to complete incapacity and death. The implications of daily levels of SO_2 and particulates have been studied in particularly vulnerable groups such as patients with chronic bronchitis and emphysema. Although it has not been possible to state a concentration of SO_2 and particulates below which health effects (acute respiratory infections in children, chronic respiratory diseases in adults, and decreased levels of ventilatory lung function in both children and adults) will not occur, it has been concluded that health effects are found when annual levels of particulates or SO_2 exceed 100 $\mu g/m^3$ and that of SO_4^{2-}, 13.5 $\mu g/m^3$; in Western urban areas the corresponding values are particulates, 3.4; SO_2, 22; and SO_4^{2-}, 6.4 $\mu g/m^3$.

It should also be stressed that additional burdens of sulfates and sulfuric acid mist can arise in various sections of the United States through the use of catalytic converters, which were being installed on automobiles in 1975 to control pollution (Rall, 1974). The exhaust from equipped cars is expected to contribute only a small portion of the atmospheric sulfate. However, this may be disproportionately significant, since it can occur in the breathing zone of a large portion of the urban population (Rall, 1974).

Both oxides of sulfur and particulate matter have been implicated in a number of acute air pollution episodes (Rall, 1974; Amdur, 1974) in the United States, Great Britain, Belgium, and Japan. In London, a rise in the death rate was detected when the concentration of SO_2 rose abruptly to levels at or about 0.25 ppm in the presence of smoke at 750 $\mu g/m^3$ (NIPCC, 1971). The elderly and patients with heart or lung disease were predominantly affected. Concentrations of SO_2 in excess of 0.52 ppm for 1 day in conjunction with levels of suspended particles exceeding 2,000 $\mu g/m^3$ have resulted in an increase in the death rate of 20% or more above baseline (NIPCC, 1971).

Although synergism between SO_2 and soluble aerosols (NaCl) has been observed in experimental animals (guinea pigs) (NAPCA, 1970), analogous effects in humans have not been consistently observed (NAPCA, 1970; Amdur, 1969). Human exposures to mixtures of SO_2 and metallic aerosols that produce irritant sulfates have not been reported, and there are apparently no human exposure data on the combined effects of sulfur oxides and other commonly occurring pollutants such as mutagenic oxides, ozone, or hydrocarbons (Rall, 1974).

Bisulfite ion (one of the reaction products of SO_2 in water) has been shown to have mutagenic effects on viruses, bacteria, and plants. For example, Mukai et al. (1970) reported reversion studies with *E. coli* mutants (K12 and K15) indicating that sodium bisulfite (1 M in 0.2 M phosphate buffer at pH 5.2 for 30 min) induced mutations in only mutants that had cytosine-guanine at the mutant site.

Hayatsu and Miura (1970) described the mutagenic activity of sodium bisulfite toward lambda phage and proposed that this activity resulted from C-G to T-A transitions. The frequency of the *c* gene was increased about ten times as much as that of spontaneous mutation by treatment of the phage with 3 M $NaHSO_3$ solution at pH 5.6 and 37°C for 1.5 hr. In the studies of Mukai et al. (1970) and Hayatsu and Miura (1970), a maximum response was observed within very short treatment intervals, no further mutagenicity being observed thereafter.

Summers and Drake (1971) reported that treatment of bacteriophage T4rII mutants with 0.9 M bisulfite for 4 hr resulted in mutations at G-C reverting sites very specifically, but also probably produced G-C $\rightarrow$ A-T transitions. In terms of mutations per mole per hour, bisulfite was judged to be about as effective as nitrous acid applied at pH 5.3 (Freese, 1959), but about 100 times weaker than nitrous acid applied at pH 3.7 (Tessman, 1962).

Conversion of cytosine to uracil *in vitro* and modification of cytosine-containing nucleic acids by high concentrations of bisulfite have also been reported by Shapiro et al. (1970, 1973), Furichi et al. (1970), and Hayatsu et al. (1970a, 1970b).

Bisulfite at a high concentration (e.g., 1 M) adds to the 5,6 double bond of cytidine and uridine by ionic reaction, forming 5,6-dihydrocytidine 6-sulfonate and 5,6-dihydrouridine 6-sulfonate, respectively. The cytidine derivative is readily deaminated to the uridine derivative, which is thence convertible to uridine under slightly alkaline conditions (Shapiro et al., 1970; Hayatsu et al., 1970a, 1970b). This reactivity of bisulfite has been utilized for the chemical modification of tRNA (Furichi et al., 1970; Singhal, 1971).

At a lower concentration of bisulfite (e.g., 0.01–0.1 M), 4-thiouridine (Hayatsu, 1969) and isopentenyl adenosine (Furichi et al., 1970; Hayatsu et al., 1972), which are known to be the minor components of tRNA (Zachau, 1969), can react with bisulfite by a radical mechanism requiring oxygen.

Recently, Inoue et al. (1972) described enhanced effects of low bisulfite concentrations (1 $M \to 2 \times 10^{-2}$ M) on inactivation of the transforming activity of *Bacillus subtilis* DNA *in vitro*. The reactive species in this reaction was suggested to involve free radicals generated by the aerobic oxidation of sulfite, such as the sulfite anion radical ($\cdot SO_3^-$) and/or the superoxide anion radical ($\cdot O_2^-$). The resulting DNA alterations were different from UV-induced DNA damage because they could not be repaired by the excision repair mechanism, which can operate for thymine dimer-type damage. The failure of efficient protection of DNA by nucleic acid constitutents against bisulfite action further suggests that the DNA molecule is a far more sensitive target than mononucleotides or the RNA molecule (Inoue et al., 1972). Inoue et al. (1972), on the basis of these studies, speculated on what could occur *in vivo* when cells are exposed to exogenous sulfite. It has been shown (Pryor, 1971) that the membrane is highly sensitive to small amounts of radicals, which can produce cell ruptures. Membrane contains a high proportion of unsaturated lipid, to which the sulfite ion radical could add quite readily. Alcohols, thiols, and amines, which can act as the radical scavengers, would be present in abundance in a cell. Enzymes are also present that can convert sulfite into sulfate under anaerobic conditions (Cohen and Fridovich, 1971; Mudd et al., 1967). Further, DNA in the eukaryotic cell is sealed in the nucleus. However, in spite of all of these defense mechanisms with which the cells are equipped, the potential for bisulfite damage exists in hereditary materials (Inoue et al., 1972). It should be further noted that, in addition to the possibility that bisulfite is present in small amounts in polluting environments, bisulfite salts (as well as SO_2) are used as food preservatives.

Sparrow and Schairer (1974) reported that SO_2 (as well as O_3 and N_2O) was a weak mutagen when tested in the *Tradescantia* stamen hair test system. (The maximum response obtained was little more than twice the spontaneous rate.)

Ma et al. (1973) recently reported on the low level of SO_2-enhanced chromatid aberrations in *T. paludosa* pollen tubes and the seasonal variation of the aberration rates. In these studies, SO_2 enhanced the chromatid aberration rates (average, 46 breaks per 100 cells) in cultures grown from field or hothouse plants during three consecutive summers (1970–1972), while there was a gradual decrease in the fall and a gradual increase in the spring in both background and enhanced aberration rates.

While the biochemical reaction between cellular components, especially chromosomes, and a low level of SO_2 has not been unambiguously elaborated, evidence of SO_2 damage to vegetation (Middleton et al., 1958) as well as SO_2-enhanced chromatid aberration in *Tradescantia* (Sparrow and Schairer, 1974; Ma et al., 1973) indicates the potential effect of SO_2 in plant systems.

Schneider and Calkins (1971) reported that SO_2 at a relatively low concentration (5 ppm) also caused clumping of chromosomes and inhibited mitotic activity in lymphocytes of human blood cultures. Ma and Khan (1972) also reported chromosome clumping and mitotic inhibition in *Tradescantia* pollen tube cultures when concentrations of SO_2 higher than 0.1 ppm were used.

The damaging effects of SO_2 noted in these studies were coupled either with a high-humidity atmosphere or with SO_2 passing through a water-containing medium before reacting with cultured cells. Since SO_2 is readily converted to SO_3 when combined with water, the delterious action of SO_2 is most likely to occur by the SO_3 pathway. As demonstrated by Shapiro et al. (1970), sulfonation of cytosine of DNA molecules may result from SO_3 action followed by deamination of cytosine, causing a C-U transition. It is still not known whether this transition could lead to the breakage of hydrogen bonds or produce pyrimidine dimers in DNA molecules.

Regression techniques applied to chemical data for 38 metropolitan regions in the United States have indicated that concentrations of SO_2 as well as NO_2 were statistically significant predictors of mortality for several categories of diseases of aging including total cancer, cancer of the respiratory organs, and arteriosclerotic heart disease (Hickey et al., 1974). More than half the variance in the criterion was explained by atmospheric concentrations of chemical pollutants, and similar results were obtained by using age-sex-"race" specific subjects of these same populations.

Hickey et al. (1974) proposed a theory to account for these results in which they assumed that the fundamental mechanisms involved are principally genetic, both somatic and intergenerational. It was pointed out that in aqueous solution SO_2 and NO_2 yield the weak acids H_2SO_3 and HNO_2, both of which can function as mutagens. Bisulfite adds reversibly to the 5,6 double bonds of cytosine and uracil, and such adducts of cytosine moieties may alter DNA function, while adducts of cytosine and uracil may alter RNA functions (Ma et al., 1973).

Depression of DNA synthesis and induction of chromosome abnormalities in human lymphocytes by SO_2 (Schneider and Calkins, 1971) and growth inhibition of established cell lines, including HeLa (Thompson and Pace, 1962), by SO_2 and its sodium salts have also been cited.

Jagiello et al. (1975) recently described the effects of SO_2 and its metabolite (Na_2SO_3) *in vitro* and *in vivo* on mouse, ewe, and cow oocytes. Fragmentation with rearrangement at M^1 and M^2 was observed *in vitro* in each species, and it was suggested that this could contribute to a variety of transmissible chromosomal disorders in progeny from germ cells carrying the resultant balanced or unbalanced genomes (Hamerton, 1971). In addition, the anaphase lagging also observed in each species has predictable consequences, with resultant aneuploidies in progeny produced by fertilization of such ova, and these have been shown to be the basis for fetal loss and/or congenital abnormalities in several species (Hamerton, 1971). Jagiello et al. (1975) cautioned that despite the absence of any of these genetically significant abnormalities in the ova in the *in vivo* studies with mouse, the responses of ewe and cow oocytes, which showed both meiotic inhibition and structural damage, suggest that SO_2 and its metabolite should be considered for possible etiologies in contaminated areas with foci of fetal loss or congenital abnormality in these bovids.

Nitrogen Oxides

The major nitrogen-containing compounds in the atmosphere are N_2O, NO, NO_2, NH_3, NH_4^+ as an aerosol, and NO_3^- as an aerosol. The gaseous compounds arise from biological action and organic decomposition in the soil and ocean. Pollutant emissions of NO and NO_2 are major nonnatural combustion sources. On a global scale, biological production of nitrogen oxides (NO_x) of 768×10^6 tons/yr exceeds industrial emission (53×10^5 tons/yr) by a factor of 15 (Robinson and Robbins, 1970a, 1970b). [The total emission of nitrogen oxides was estimated by Robinson and Robbins (1967) as roughly 36% of that of sulfur dioxide.] In the United States, the estimated NO_x emissions (in millions of tons) from anthropogenic sources were: traffic, 8.1; fuel consumption, 10.0; industry, 0.2; and miscellaneous, 2.3 (U.S. DHEW, 1968). Rossano (1969) has calculated the emissions of nitrogen oxides from electrical power plants, industrial power plants, and residential heating to be $\sim$ 10, 10, and 4 kg/ton of burned coal, respectively.

The major biotic source of NO_x is anaerobic bacterial reduction of NO_3 to NO_2 in soil. The resulting NO_2^- in soil is converted to nitrous acid (HNO_2), which decomposes to yield NO and NO_2 (Nelson and Bremmer, 1970).

Nitrous oxide, the most abundant atmospheric nitrogen compound, has a mean concentration of about 0.25 ppm in clean air and 1,000 ppb in polluted air (Fischer, 1972). The major source of N_2O is soil (Adel, 1946, 1951), and an estimated 5.92×10^8 tons/yr is emitted from soil as a result of anaerobic bacterial denitrification (Robinson and Robbins, 1970a, 1970b; Arnold, 1954)–NH_4^+ and NO_3^- into N_2O and N_2. Nitrous oxide is considered to be a very stable and chemically inert gas, undergoing essentially no *chemical* conversions in the atmosphere. Its mean residence time in the atmosphere has been estimated as 4 yr, with its destruction occurring by photodissociation at wavelengths shorter than 2,100 Å (e.g., expected only at altitudes above the ozone layer).

The nitric oxide concentration is much lower than the N_2O concentration, exhibiting a background level of about 0.5 ppb. In areas of high air pollution (e.g., Los Angeles) concentrations of up to 3 ppm ($NO + NO_2$) have been detected (Stern, 1968).

Nitrogen dioxide concentrations range from undetectable to about 1.3 ppb in unpolluted atmospheres and up to 2,000 ppb in polluted ones (Robinson and Robbins, 1970a). Even though the concentration of NO_x in rural areas is $\sim$ 0.2-4 ppb, the concentration is typically 0.1 ppb or more in the morning air of large cities (Berry and Lehman, 1971); thus the local concentrations associated with human activity can be 25-500 times larger than the natural background (Berry and Lehman, 1971).

Of the anthropogenic sources of NO_x, automobiles contribute by far the largest part, about 60% (Agnew, 1968); fixed combustion sources account for most of the remainder. Most of this emission is initially in the form of NO, and a small part, perhaps 1-2%, occurs as NO_2. The NO is the product of high-temperature nitrogen fixation reactions that occur in flames. The directly emitted NO_2 is formed by air oxidation of NO in the exhaust emissions system (Berry and Lehman, 1971).

Once released into the atmosphere, NO is converted to NO_2 by a rapid oxidation process that is not yet completely understood. One of the two major speculative explanations involves the reaction of NO with oxygen atoms. The source of oxygen atoms in the lower atmosphere is the photolysis of NO_2, $NO_2 + h\nu \rightarrow NO + O$, which is also the initiating reaction for almost all photochemical smog reactions (Berry and Lehman, 1971).

The other predominant process is reaction with ozone: $NO + O_3 \rightarrow NO_2 + O_2$. The source of the ozone is supposedly downward diffusion from the stratosphere. According to Robinson and Robbins (1967), in rural areas the balance between NO to NO_2 and the photolytic reduction of NO_2 to NO appears to establish a worldwide ratio of $\sim$ 2-2.5 parts of NO_2 to 1 part of NO. The ozone reaction can apparently account for the oxidation of trace quantities of NO from natural biological sources (Ripperton et al., 1970).

Conversion of NO to NO_2 in urban areas (where it is essentially complete) has been most difficult to explain unequivocally (Berry and Lehman, 1971). The available amount of stratospherically generated ozone is apparently insufficient to account for the predominance of NO_2 in urban air. The initial amount of NO_2 is believed to be formed in exhaust pipes and furnace stacks by thermal oxidation of NO with molecular oxygen in a termolecular process (Berry and Lehman, 1971).

Berry and Lehman (1971) summarized the reaction of NO_2 in a typical *urban* atmosphere as follows:

$$NO_2 + h\nu \rightarrow NO + O$$

$$NO + O + M \rightarrow NO_2 + M$$

$$\text{Secondary reactions} \rightarrow NO_2$$

$$NO_2 + \text{hydrocarbon reactions } (R\cdot) \rightarrow RNO_2$$

The net result is gradual consumption of NO and production of oxygen atoms, which can then initiate the reactions of photochemical smog. The nitrogen is depleted by the reaction of NO_2 with hydrocarbon radicals produced by chain reactions initiated by the oxygen atoms.

Davis et al. (1974) recently examined the extent to which NO_x and SO_2 chemistry occurs as a function of distance following their emission from an isolated 1,000-MW power plant. The power plant plume (examined in the altitude range 200–900 m) carried a significant decrease in ambient O_3 concentrations attributed to reaction of O_3 with NO. The following reaction scheme was proposed:

$$NO + O_3 \rightarrow NO_2 + O_2$$

$$NO_2 + h\nu \rightarrow NO + O$$

$$O + O_2 + M \rightarrow O_3 + M \; (M + N_2)$$

High ambient O_3 concentrations and low UV photon fluxes enhance the rate of NO conversion to NO_2.

Aircraft emissions represent another polluting source of nitrogen oxides. In the United States aircraft emissions (carbon monoxide, hydrocarbons, NO_x and particulate matter) represent 3.3% of all sources, and emission by the air carriers represents only 1.2% (the remainder being caused by military and private aviation) (Hendel, 1973). However, excessive pollution can occur in localized areas around airports. For example, in the vicinity of Los Angeles Airport and Chicago's O'Hare Airport, 32,660 and 29,540 tons/yr of pollutants are released, respectively (Hendel, 1973). It was estimated that 16,000 tons of nitrogen oxides was released by all civil aircraft in the United States in 1967. It should be further noted that the larger engines and higher temperatures in new aircraft are envisioned to make NO_x emissions an even greater problem in the future (Hendel, 1973).

On the basis of the nitrate content of precipitation, which suggests a correlation with electrical processes in the atmosphere, direct production of nitrogen dioxide by electrical discharges also seems possible (Reiter and Reiter, 1958).

Redeposition of NO_2 is assumed to take place by condensation and precipitation processes after it has been converted into nitrate. Its residence time in the atmosphere has been estimated by Junge (1963) to be ~ 2 months.

Ammonia is the remaining principal atmospheric nitrogen gas. As in the case of SO_2 and NO_2, the gaseous form (NH_3) as a rule predominates over the hydrolyzed fraction (NH_4^+). Soil is the major source of atmospheric ammonia (Georgii, 1963), which is produced by microbial deamination of organic matter and reduction of NO_2^- and NO_3^-. The total biological production of NH_3 is estimated to be 1.19×10^9 tons/yr (Robinson and Robbins, 1970).

The concentration of NH_3 averages about 15 ppb in clean air and 2,000 ppb in polluted air (Robinson and Robbins, 1970a, 1970b; Lodge and Pate, 1966), and the concentration of NH_4^+ aerosols averages perhaps 0.1 $\mu g/m^3$, while NO_3^- aerosols may range up to 0.3 $\mu g/m^3$ (the latter appear to be concentrated in the particle size range over 1 μm in radius) (Junge, 1963). The main sink of atmospheric NH_3 is probably transport back to the surface of the earth by precipitation (Israel and Israel, 1974).

Nitrogen dioxide has been shown to induce pulmonary damage in rats and dogs at exposure levels of only a few parts per million (Lodge and Pate, 1966; Stephens et al., 1972) in acute and subacute studies. Exposure to high concentrations of NO_2 is known to produce a potentially lethal reaction in the pulmonary blood vessels, resulting in acute pulmonary edema (Freeman et al., 1969).

The need to examine the long-term effects of exposure to low levels of atmospheric pollution with NO_2 has been stressed (Dowell et al., 1971). Beagles exposed 16 hr daily for 61 months to 1.21 mg/m^3 NO_2 exhibited pulmonary impairment (Lewis et al., 1974). Pathogen-free rats exposed to automotive exhaust containing 23 ppm NO_2 for up to 2 yr exhibited a decrease in body weight and an increased incidence of spontaneous tumors in the aging rats (tentatively attributed to the hydrocarbons in the exhaust gases) (Stupfel et al., 1973). Survival, heart rate, and incidence of renal and aortic lesions were not significantly affected by the exposure.

High levels of NO_2 (50–100 ppm) have been reported to have clearly adverse effects on the human lung, and some have suggested that persistent exposure to very low levels of NO_2 in the atmosphere may eventually have some deleterious effect in humans (*Food and Cosmetics Toxicology*, 1970).

It is important to note other sources of exposure to NO_x as well as the possibility of a "nitrogen oxide-nitrosamine-cancer link" (Fine et al., 1974; *Environmental Health Letters*, 1975). For example, a consistent statistical relation between cancer death rates and ambient NO_2 levels in urban areas has been cited, and the question has been asked whether nitrosamines represent the link between such levels and death rates (*Environmental Health Letters*, 1975). It was also noted in a recent German study that the nitrosamines in air were dependent on the concentration of ambient NO_2 and that "peak NO_2 levels in the German study were 20 times less than what is encountered in peak one to two hour periods in cities such as Chicago, Los Angeles and Denver" (*Environmental Health Letters*, 1975).

From studies on tobacco smoke, NO_x are known to be readily absorbed by the body during inhalation (Bokhoven and Niessen, 1961). Neurath (1972) has suggested that equimolar mixtures of NO_2 and NO, the major oxides of nitrogen present in the environment, are capable of nitrosating secondary and tertiary amines to form the highly carcinogenic and mutagenic *N*-nitrosamines. However, the efficiency of *in vivo* conversion of NO_x to *N*-nitrosamines is unknown.

Atmospheric deposition of large quantities of NO_3^- and NH_4^+ on terrestrial and aquatic environments is also potentially hazardous to the biosphere, because of the subsequent conversion of these substances to NO_2^- and nitrosamines. Nitrosation may result either solely from a chemical process or from microbial metabolic activity (Ayanaba and Alexander, 1973; Ayanaba et al., 1973).

The mutagenic response of N_2O in the *Tradescantia* stamen hair test system as well as the mutagenic potential of aqueous solutions of NO_2 (HNO_2) has been cited by Hickey et al. (1974).

The mutagenic activity of nitrous acid on viral systems has been studied extensively (Freese, 1963; Krieg, 1963; Orgel, 1965), and it has been shown to result from deamination of certain nucleic acid bases and to produce mutations predominantly by base-pair substitutions of the type A-T $\rightarrow$ G-C and G-C $\rightarrow$ A-T. The mutagenicity of nitrous acid toward transforming DNA (Strack et al., 1964; Horn and Herriot, 1962; Bresler et al.; 1968), *E. coli* (Kaudewitz, 1959; Verly et al., 1967), *S. typhimurium* (Reisenstart and Rosner, 1964; Rudner, 1961), *Neurospora* (De Serres et al., 1967; Malling, 1965), *Saccharomyces pombe* (Nashed and Jabbur, 1966; Nasim and Clarke, 1965; Loprieno et al., 1969), *Aspergillus nidulans* (Siddiqi, 1952), phage T_2 (Vielmetter and Wiedner, 1959), T_4 (Tessman, 1959; Benser, 1967), and Φ X174 (Tessman et al., 1964) has been reported.

Tessman (1962) has also shown that nitrous acid can produce mutations that map as extensive deletions and that these account for about 8% of the nitrous acid induced in rII mutants of T_4 bacteriophage.

Studies on the mutagenic effect of nitrous acid on *Neurospora* suggest that this general spectrum of genetic alterations is also found in eukaryotes (as in prokaryotes). Malling (1965) reported that at least 84% of the nitrous acid-induced *ad*-3 mutants of *N. crassa* are base-pair substitutions and that at least 6% of the remaining 16% are unidentified genetic alterations, perhaps due to intralocal deletions.

De Serres et al. (1967) characterized the genetic effects of nitrous acid in *N. crassa* at the molecular level and showed that 72% of nitrous acid-induced *ad*-3B mutants exhibited allelic complementation and had either nonpolarized or polarized complementation patterns, the majority (60.4%) being in the nonpolarized group. The ratio of nonpolarized to polarized complementation patterns is thus about 5 to 1. In addition, a total of 24.3% were leaky, had nonpolarized patterns, and accounted for 40.1% of the mutants in this class. The complementation data of de Serres et al. (1967) in combination with the reversion data of Malling (1965) indicate a direct correlation between the percentage of mutations resulting from base-pair substitutions and the percentage showing allelic complementation.

Nitrous acid has been shown to give rise to a high number of point mutations (Orgel, 1965; Tessman et al., 1964) in bacterial, phage, and plant viral systems and to cause large deletion mutations in T_4 phage of *E. coli* (Tessman, 1962). In the case of *E. coli* phage S13, nitrous acid production of all possible base transitions ($G \rightarrow A$, $A \rightarrow G$, $C \rightarrow T$, $T \rightarrow C$) has been detected genetically (Vanderbilt and Tessman, 1970).

Day (1975) described aspects of the repair of DNA damaged by nitrous acid. Cultured fibroblasts from normal persons or persons afflicted with xeroderma pigmentosum (XP) were used as hosts for adenovirus 2 infection. With xeroderma cells as hosts, nitrous acid-treated virus showed less plaque-forming ability than when normal cells were used, indicating that DNA damaged by nitrous acid is at least partly repaired by normal human cells. The difference in response of XP and normal cells to nitrous acid-damaged virus is rather small (e.g., about twofold) compared with that observed using UV-irradiated virus with the same cells (14–25-fold). This was believed to be because either (1) XP cells are completely deficient in repair of nitrous acid damage, while normal cells are only partly capable of such repair, possibly because of damage in a critical non-DNA component; (2) both normal and XP cells are capable of only half the normal repair.

The recovery of phage T_4 from nitrous acid (pH 4.65) damage was recently described by Harm (1974), who demonstrated that the *px* and *y* gene functions of T_4 were required for repair of lethal effects, suggesting that this system is less specific regarding the type of damage than the V-gene excision repair.

Earlier work of Harm (1962) suggested that about one-sixth of total lethal nitrous acid damage at pH 4.65 is outside the DNA. Vielmetter and Schuster (1960) reported that in the pH range 4.2–4.8 about 15% of the lethal nitrous acid lesions in transducing *Salmonella* phage P22 are in protein.

Harm (1974) suggested that if (under his experimental conditions) only about 85% of all lethal lesions are in DNA, the repairable fraction of DNA lesions would be about 1.18 times as high as the observed fraction of total lesions repaired.

The prevailing DNA alterations by nitrous acid are deaminations of guanine, adenine, and cytosine or hydroxymethylcytosine in the case of T-even phages. They occur in T_2, which has the same nitrous acid sensitivity as T_4 wild type, at a rate of about 3.5 deaminations per lethal nitrous acid lesion at pH 4.20 and about 2.4 at pH 5.0, as calculated by Vielmetter and Schuster (1960). Hence, it was suggested that at pH 4.65 probably not more than 30% of the total deaminations could be lethal.

Harm (1974) suggested that even though T_4 DNA differs to some extent in its G/C ratio from *B. subtilis* DNA, the majority of lethal HNO_2 lesions in T_4 DNA could be either deaminations or cross-linkages, with the latter appearing more likely from the precise one-hit inactivation observed under conditions of no repair.

In addition to the mutagenicity of nitrous acid per se, recognition must also be made of the added mutagenic hazard that might occur through formation of nitrosamines from the reaction of secondary or tertiary amines and nitrite *in vivo*, as demonstrated in the stomachs of humans and laboratory animals and described earlier in this review (see pp. 203–205).

However, the report of the *suppression* of DMN mutagenicity by sodium nitrite (Couch and Friedman, 1974) cited earlier in this review seems to cloud or confuse the assessment of the danger of human exposure to this material since environmental exposure to nitrosamines may occur simultaneously with exposure to agents (nitrite) that may modify its toxicological properties.

Ozone

Ozone is an extremely important trace component found mainly in the stratosphere, which is the region of the atmosphere in the altitude range 10–50 km at high latitudes and 18–50 km at low altitudes (Crutzen, 1972, 1974a, 1974b). The maximum concentrations of O_3 (5×10^{12} molecules/cm³) occur at an altitude of about 25 km (Crutzen, 1974a, 1974b). The mixing ratio of ozone, which is defined as the ratio of the number concentration of ozone to that of all air molecules, is largest at an altitude of about 32 km and is equal to 5–10 ppm (Crutzen, 1974a).

The total amount of global ozone is a function of season and latitude; a very pronounced feature is the occurrence of the largest total amounts of ozone at middle and high latitudes in late winter and spring in the Northern Hemisphere (Crutzen, 1974a, 1974b). This provides strong evidence of the importance of atmospheric wind systems in transporting ozone. Ozone averages ~ 3 ppm of the stratosphere (which has only about 12% of the mass of the atmosphere) (Johnson, 1974). Ozone concentrations increase toward the poles, ranging from 25 ppb in the tropics to 40 ppb in polar regions (Junge, 1963).

Junge (1963) has estimated the lifetime of O_3 in the lower stratosphere to be up to ~ 2 yr and in the troposphere to be 1–1.5 months.

Ozone is a product of photochemical processes in the upper atmosphere, where it is formed by the following reactions:

$$O_2 + h\nu \rightarrow 2\,O\ (\lambda < 240\ \text{nm})$$

$$O + O_2 + M \rightarrow O_3 + M\ (2X)$$
$$\overline{3\,O_2 \rightarrow 2\,O_3}$$

Ozone is both produced and destroyed by photochemical reactions. The photochemical reactions involving ozone are the primary source of local heating in the stratosphere, which sets up the temperature inversion (Johnson, 1974). These reactions determine the distribution of the solar radiation that enters the troposphere. Ozone is essential for the protection of life on the earth from lethal UV radiation of wavelengths shorter than 300 nm. The catalytic destruction of the earth's ozone shield by ozone-attacking catalysts produced by supersonic air transport operations (Crutzen, 1972, 1974a; Johnson, 1971, 1974; Hammond, 1975; Hammond and Maugh, 1974; Grobecker, 1974; Donahue, 1975) and chlorine compounds (Crutzen, 1974, Cicerone et al. 1975; Hammond, 1975; Hammond and Maugh, 1974; Molina and Rowland, 1974; McElroy et al., 1974) (generating nitrogen oxides and free chlorine atoms, respectively) has been the subject of recent controversy in terms of both the vulnerability of O_3 to destruction and the postulated resultant biological effects. If stratospheric O_3 should be reduced, additional UV radiation (290–310 nm) would reach the surface of the earth, and it is postulated that this radiation would not form tropospheric ozone from oxygen (it requires 240-nm radiation to accomplish this), but it could have deleterious biological effects (Johnson, 1971). The most alarming effect might be an increase in the incidence of skin cancer. The National Academy of Sciences in 1973 suggested that a 5% depletion of ozone might produce an additional 8,000 skin cancer cases per year among the white population of the United States (McElroy et al., 1974). A more recent assessment suggests that the percentage increase in the incidence of skin cancers would parallel the increase in the intensity of radiation. A 5% ozone depletion (10% increase in radiation) might cause anywhere from 20,000 to 60,000 additional skin cancer cases per year in the United States alone (Hammond and Maugh, 1974).

The primary mechanisms for the natural destruction of ozone are combinations of free oxygen and ozone to form two oxygen molecules (Hammond and Maugh, 1974). The reconversion of ozone to molecular oxygen is believed by Crutzen (1974a, 1974b) to be catalyzed by cycles that can be written as

$$X + O_3 \rightarrow XO + O_2$$
$$XO + O \rightarrow X + O_2$$
$$\overline{O + O_3 \rightarrow 2\,O_2}$$

     L. Fishbein

where X is H, OH (Bates and Nicolet, 1950), NO (Johnson, 1971; Crutzen, 1971), Cl (Cicerone et al., 1975; McElroy et al., 1974; Molina and Rowland, 1974; Crutzen, 1971, 1974a; Stolarski and Cicerone, 1974; Wofsy and McElroy, 1974; Wofsy et al., 1974), or Br (Crutzen, 1974a).

It is now widely believed that the oxides of nitrogen (NO and NO_2) are the most important natural ozone-attacking catalysts in the environment (Crutzen, 1974a, 1974b; Donahue, 1975; Hammond and Maugh, 1974). For example, NO can destroy ozone through the catalytic cycle (Hammond, 1975): (1) $NO + O_3 \rightarrow NO_2 + O_2$; (2) $O_3 + h\nu \rightarrow O_2 + O$; and (3) $NO_2 + O \rightarrow NO + O_2$. The net result is $2O_3 + h\nu \rightarrow 3O_2$.

While most of this discussion has centered about aspects of stratospheric formation and destruction of ozone and the postulated biological consequences of the latter it is equally important to consider the biological effects of ozone per se, as well as other sources of ozone introduction into the atmosphere and aspects of ozone concentration into urban and nonurban atmospheres.

In regard to other sources of ozone, recent studies of exhaust gases from electric utilities suggest that they participate in free radical reactions to give high ozone levels (*Chemical & Engineering News, 1964*; Davis et al., 1974).

Ozone in ground-level air may be natural ozone of stratospheric origin, which has diffused down through the troposphere, or it may be formed photochemically at low levels (Atkins et al., 1972). Levels of oxidant (chiefly ozone) in excess of 10 parts per hundred million are considered to be evidence of photochemical smog formation (U.S. DHEW, 1973).

Evidence of atmospheric transport of ozone from rural to urban metropolitan areas (Coffey and Stasiuk, 1975), as well as transport of polluted air from U.S. urban areas to yield high nonurban ozone concentrations exceeding the national ambient air quality standards, has been described (*Chemical & Engineering News*, 1974b). In the latter case, it was suggested that once olefins and nitrogen oxides are depleted from polluted air, O_3 in the air may no longer be broken down and generated during transport of polluted air from urban areas to the detection sites. Concentrations of ozone of up to 1,000 ppb have been recorded in polluted areas (Junge, 1963). It should also be noted that ozone has been detected in airplane cabins at altitudes above 30,000 ft; other sources of exposure can include: (1) high-voltage electric equipment, (2) ozonizing equipment for water and food purification, (3) inert-gas shielded arc welding devices, and (4) ozonizing devices for air purification.

The biological effects of ozone on humans and animals have been extensively studied (Freebairn, 1959; Jaffee, 1967a, 1967b; Scheel et al., 1959; Klenfield and Giel, 1956; Stokinger, 1954, 1965; Stokinger and Coffin, 1968). As inhalation of O_3 is the usual mode of exposure, study of O_3 toxicology has been primarily restricted to the respiratory tract. Drastic disturbances in the respiratory activity of animals and humans have been used as indicators of functional injury by ozone (Jaffee, 1967a, 1967b; Stokinger, 1954, 1965). Three long-term effects of repeated exposures to ozone are recognized: (1) chronic pulmonary effects, (2) aging, and (3) lung tumor acceleration.

Ozone has been implicated in the development of adenomas (Stokinger et al., 1957; Werthamer et al., 1970a, 1970b), squamous metaplasia (Freeman et al., 1973), cellular hyperplasia, and atypism (Werthamer et al., 1970a) in the bronchial tree of animals.

The main effect of ozone intoxication in humans is on the respiratory system. It ranges from irritation of the throat to fatal pulmonary edema and hemmorrhages, depending on concentration and exposure. Nasr (1971) recently reviewed aspects of clinical manifestation and differential diagnosis of O_3 poisoning in humans.

Evidence has been accumulated over the years indicating that the biological effects of ozone are more widely distributed and involve a variety of body functions, such as those of the nervous (Trans et al., 1972), circulatory (Stokinger and Scheel, 1962; Pan et al., 1972), hemopoietic (Brinkman et al., 1964; Zelak et al., 1971b) and immunologic (Fairchild, 1967; Fairchild and Graham, 1969) systems.

Radiomimetic changes (Menzel, 1970) have been described for ozone, as well as the oxidation of unsaturated fatty acids (Roehm et al., 1971) and of biologically active reducing substances such as reduced sulfhydryl groups and the cofactors NADH and NADPH (Menzel, 1971).

A variety of studies have suggested that ozone may be a general mutagenic agent (Scott and Lesher, 1943; Zelac et al., 1971a, 1971b; Fetner, 1958, 1962, 1963; Brinkman and Lamberts, 1958; Sachsenmaier et al., 1965; Davis, 1959, 1961; Feder and Sullivan, 1969; MacLean et al., 1973; McLeish, 1953; Pace et al., 1969; Prat et al., 1968).

Decomposition of ozone in water produces the same positive radicals (OH and HO_2) generally considered to be the biologically active products of irradiation of protoplasm, and the cytological and cytogenic effects of ozone would thus appear to be radiomimetic. Ozone has been reported to cause chromosome breakage in *Vicia faba* (Fetner, 1958) and in mammalian cell cultures (Sachsenmaier et al., 1965; Fetner, 1962). For example, ozone-induced chromosome breakage of human cells (KB cells) in culture was reported by Fetner (1963). Chromatid deletions were produced as an exponential function of exposure to ozone. This is in agreement with the concept that chemically produced active radicals would be dependent for expression on penetration to the chromosomes, and hence would be a function of concentration and would obey the law of mass action. Such an exponential response has also been interpreted as evidence of a direct type of effect (McLeish, 1953). The chromatid breakages in human cell cultures exposed to 8 ppm of ozone for 5 or 10 min in the study of Fetner (1962) were apparently identical to those produced by X-rays (200 R, 250 kV), with the difference in time–concentration response between O_3 exposure and X-rays being explained in terms of penetration.

Zelac et al. (1971b) described exposure-adjusted break frequencies for chromosome aberrations produced in circulating blood lymphocytes following exposure of Chinese hamsters to UV generated ozone for 5 hr at 0.2 ppm. Inhaled ozone produced 1.67×10^{-3} breaks/cell-ppm-min, agreeing well with data from *in vitro* exposure of human cells. There was no apparent decrease in break frequency with time for 2 wk after treatment. It was suggested by Zelac et al. (1971a) that if the results of this animal study are directly extended to the human case, the presently permitted ozone exposures (American Industrial Hygiene Association, 1968) (up to 0.1 ppm, 4 ppm-hr/wk), would be expected to result in break frequencies orders of magnitude greater than those resulting from permitted radiation exposures. MacLean et al. (1973) described chromosome breakage following exposure of ozone-treated seawater on spawned, fertilized, meiotic, and cleaving eggs of the commercial American oyster.

In ascites tumors and human cell cultures (McLeish, 1953) and in the duck weed *Lemna perpusilla* (Feder and Sullivan, 1969), ozone was found to inhibit mitotic activity.

Ozone was also found to induce *in vivo* structural changes in the nuclei of myocardial cells of rabbits (Brinkman et al., 1964) and in the nuclei of embryonic chick fibroblasts *in vitro* (Sachsenmaier et al., 1965).

Davis (1959, 1961) has described the mutagenicity of ozone in *E. coli*. Hamelin and Chung (1974) described optimal conditions for mutagenesis by ozone in *E. coli* K_{12}. High yields of induced mutants with over 90% survival were obtained when washed cells, taken from the logarithmic phase of growth, were aerated by a stream of ozone (0.05–1.0 ppm) in buffer at pH 5.0 for 30–60 min. It was postulated that ozone itself is probably directly exerting both lethal and mutagenic effects on the cells through a primary effect on the permeability of the cellular membrane. Ozone has been previously observed to produce specific mutants of *E. coli* exposed in ozonated water (Scott and Lesher, 1943; Davis, 1959, 1961; Vrochnskii, 1964) and to modify markedly pyrimidine bases in *E. coli* nucleic acids, and the study of Hamelin and Chung (1974) demonstrated that specific modifications in the genetic material of *E. coli* were produced before destruction of the cell membrane. Ozone has been classified as a weak mutagen when examined in the *Tradescantia* stamen hair system (Sparrow and Schairer, 1974).

SUMMARY

Comparative data have been presented (wherever available) on the relative amounts, residues, and transport in the environment of a spectrum of naturally occurring mutagenic and potentially mutagenic agents, including mycotoxins (aflatoxins, ochratoxins, sterigmatocystin, *Penicillium* and

Fusarium toxins), pyrrolizidine alkaloids, cycasin, polynuclear aromatic hydrocarbons (benzo[*a*]pyrene, benz[*a*]anthracene, dibenzanthracene), nitrosamines, and atmospheric mutagens (sulfur oxides, nitrogen oxides, and ozone).

While it has been convenient to consider the various mutagenic and potentially mutagenic agents *individually*, it is well recognized that the nature of the environmental burden to humans is through a multifaceted and, in many cases, a continuous exposure. Information as to whether the described agents exert an additive, potentiating, or synergistic mutagenic effect is almost totally lacking.

Information is admittedly sparse, as well as lacking in many regards, concerning environmental reactions and interactions (e.g., in atmosphere, soil, and water) of many of the above mutagens, as well as aspects of their transport, residence times, and stability. The fate of many of these agents (particularly the many halogenated hydrocarbons) in the atmosphere is both largely speculative and provocative at this time.

It must also be acknowledged that in the vast majority of cases, environmental chemical agents have not been extensively and/or adequately tested to permit an evaluation of their relative mutagenic hazard to humans.

REFERENCES

Abraham, E. P. and Florey, H. W. 1949. *Antibiotics*, ed. N. W. Florey, vol. 1, p. 273. London: Oxford Univ. Press.

Adel, A. 1946. A possible source of stmospheric N_2O. *Science* 103–285.

Adel, A. 1951. Atmospheric nitrous oxide and the nitrogen cycle. *Science* 113:624–627.

Agnew, W. G. 1968. Automotive air pollution research. *Proc. R. Soc. Lond. Ser. A.* 307:153–181.

Alam, B. S., Saporschetz, I. B. and Epstein, S. S. 1971a. Formation of *N*-nitrosopiperidine and sodium nitrate in the stomach and the isolated intestinal loop of the rat. *Nature (Lond.)* 232:116–118.

Alam, B. S., Saporschetz, I. B. and Epstein, S. S. 1971b. Synthesis of nitrosopiperidine from nitrate and piperidine in the gastrointestinal tract of the rat. *Nature (Lond.)* 232:199–200.

Alderson, T. and Clark, A. M. 1966. Interlocus specificity for chemicals in *Aspergillus nidulans*. *Nature (Lond.)* 210:593.

Alpert, M. E., Hutt, M. S. R., Wogan, G. N. and Davidson, C. S. 1971. Association between aflatoxin content of food and hepatoma frequency in Uganda. *Cancer* 28:253–260.

Ambio. 1972. Sulphur pollution across national boundaries. 1:15–20.

Ambrose, A. M. and Deeds, F. 1946. Some toxicological and pharmacological properties of citrinin. *J. Pharmacol. Exp. Ther.* 88:173–186.

Amdur, M. O. 1969. Toxicological appraisal of particulate matter, oxides of sulfur and sulfuric acid. *J. Air Pollut. Control Assoc.* 19:638.

Amdur, M. O. 1974. 1974 Cummings Memorial Lecture—The long road from Donora. *Am. Ind. Hyg. Assoc. J.* 35:589–597.

American Industrial Hygiene Association. 1968. Community air quality guides: Ozone. *Am. Ind. Hyg. Assoc. J.* 29:299–303.

Ames, B. N., Sims, P. and Grover, P. L. 1972. Epoxides of carcinogenic polycyclic hydrocarbons are frameshift mutagens. *Science* 176:47–49.

Ames, B. N., Durston, W. E., Yamasaki, E. and Lee, F. D. 1973. Carcinogens are mutagens: A simple test system combining liver homogenates for activation and bacteria for detection. *Proc. Natl. Acad. Sci. U.S.A.* 70: 2281.

Amla, I., Kamala, C. S., Gopalakrishna, G. S., Jayaraj, A. B., Screenivasa-murthy, V. and Parpia, H. A. B. 1971. Cirrhosis in children from peanut meal contaminated by aflatoxin. *Am. J. Clin. Nutr.* 24:609.

Andelman, J. B. and Suess, N. J. 1970. Polynuclear aromatic hydrocarbons in the water environment. *Bull. WHO* 43:479.

Anderman, J. B. and Snodgrass, J. E. 1974. Incidence and significance of polynuclear aromatic hydrocarbons in the water environment. *Crit. Rev. Environ. Control* 43:69–83.

Arcos, J. C., Argus, M. F. and Wolf, G. 1968. *Chemical induction of cancer*, vol. 2. New York: Academic Press.

Arnold, P. W. 1954. Losses of nitrous oxide from soil. *J. Soil Sci.* 5:116–128.

Arrhenius, E. 1973. Mycotoxicosis–An old health hazard with new dimensions. *Ambio* 2:49–56.

Atkins, D. H. F., Cox, R. A. and Eggleton, E. J. 1972. Photochemical ozone and sulfuric acid aerosol formation in the atmosphere over southern England. *Nature (Lond.)*235:372–374.

Auerbach, C. 1940. Tests of carcinogenic substances in relation to the production of mutations in *Drosophila melanogaster. Proc. R. Soc. Edinburgh* 60:164–173.

Auerbach, C., Robson, J. M. and Carr, J. G. 1946. The chemical production of mutations. *Science* 105:243–247.

Avanzi, S. 1963. Chromosome breakage by pyrrolizidine alkaloids and modification of the effects by cysteine. *Caryologia* 16:493.

Ayanaba, A. and Alexander, M. 1973. Microbial formation of nitrosamines *in vitro. Appl. Microbiol.* 25:862.

Ayanaba, A. and Alexander, M. 1974. Transformations of methylamine and formation of a hazardous product, dimethylnitrosamine, in samples of treated sewage and lake water. *J. Environ. Qual.* 3:83–89.

Ayanaba, A., Verstraete, W. and Alexander, M. 1973. Formation of dimethyl-nitrosamine, a carcinogen and mutagen, in soils treated with nitrogen compounds. *Soc. Soil Sci. Am. Proc.* 37:565–568.

Babich, H. and Stotzky, G. 1973. Air pollution and microbial ecology. *Crit. Rev. Environ. Control* 3:129–152.

Badger, G. M., Kinber, R. W. C. and Spotswood, T. M. 1960. Mode of formation of 3,4-benzopyrene in the human environment. *Nature (Lond.)* 187:663–665.

Badger, G. M., Kinber, R. W. C. and Novotny, J. 1962. The formation of aromatic hydrocarbons at high temperatures. *Aust. J. Chem.* 15: 616–625.

Ballantine, J. A., Hassall, C. H. and Jones, G. 1965. The biosynthesis of phenols. Part IX. Asperugin, a metabolic product of *A. rugulosus. J. Chem. Soc.* 4672–4678.

Bamburg, J. R., Marasas, W. F., Riggs, N. V., Smalley, E. R. and Strong, F. M. 1968. Toxic spiroepoxy compounds from Fusaria and other Hypho-mycetes. *Biol. Technol. Bioeng.* 10:445–455.

Bamburg, J. R., Strong, R. M. and Smalley, E. R. 1969. Toxins from moldy cereals. *J. Agric. Food Chem.* 17:443–450.

Barnes, J. M. 1970. Aflatoxin as a health hazard. *J. Appl. Bacteriol.* 33: 285–298.

Barrett, R. W. and Tatum, E. L. 1951. An evaluation of some carcinogens as mutagens. *Cancer Res.* 11:234.

Barrett, R. W. and Tatum, E. L. 1958. Carcinogenic mutagens. *Ann. N.Y. Acad. Sci.* 71: 1072–1084.

Bates, D. R. and Nicolet, M. 1950. Atmospheric hydrogen. *Publ. Astron. Soc. Pac.* 62:106–110.

Begeman, C. R. and Colucci, J. M. 1968. Benzo[a]pyrene in gasoline partially persists in automobile exhausts. *Science* 161:271.

Benser, S. 1967. On the topography of the genetic fine structure. *Proc. Natl. Acad. Sci. U.S.A.* 47:403–426.

Berry, R. S. and Lehman, P. A. 1971. Aerochemistry of air pollution. *Annu. Rev. Phys. Chem.* 22:47–84.

Blokker, P. C. 1973. Recent air pollution problems. In *Environmental quality and safety*, eds. F. Coulston and F. Korte, vol. 2, pp. 38–46. Stuttgart: Thieme.

Blumer, M. 1961. Benzypyrenes in soil. *Science* 134:474.

Bokhoven C. and Niessen H. J. 1961. Amounts of oxides of nitrogen and carbon monoxide in cigarette smoke with and without inhalation. *Nature (Lond.)* 192:458–459.

Borker, E., Insalata, N. F., Leve, C. P. and Witzeman, J. S. 1966. Mycotoxins in feeds and foods. *Adv. Appl. Microbiol.* 8:315.

Borneff, J. and Kunte, H. 1965. Kanzerogene Substanzen in Wasser und Boden. XVII. *Arch. Hyg.* 149:226.

Bourgeois, C. H., Shank, R. C., Grossman, R. A., Johnsen, D. O., Wooding, W. L. and Chandavimol, P. 1971. Acute aflatoxin B. Toxicity in the macaque and its similarities to Reye's syndrome. *Lab. Invest.* 24:206.

Boyland, E. and Weigert, F. 1947. Metabolism of carcinogenic compounds. *Br. Med. Bull.* 4:354.

Bresler, S. E., Kalinin, V. L. and Perumov, D. A. 1968. Inactivation and mutagenesis of isolated DNA, IV. Possibility of integration of lethal damage into the chromosome of *B. subtilis* during transformation. *Mutat. Res.* 5:329.

Brian, W. P. Elson, E. W. and Lowe, D. 1956. Production of patulin in apple fruits by *Pencillium expansion. Nature (Lond.)* 178:263–264.

Brink, N. G. 1965. The mutagenic activity of heliotrine in *Drosophila*, I. Complete and mosaic sex-linked lethals. *Mutat. Res.* 3:66.

Brink, N. G. 1969. The mutagenic activity of the pyrrolizidine alkaloid heliotrine in *Drosophila melanogaster*, II. Chromosome rearrangements. *Mutat. Res.* 8:139.

Brinkman, R. and Lamberts, H. B. 1958. Ozone as a possible radiomimetric toxicant of ozonized air. *Lancet* 1:133–136.

Brinkman, R., Lamberts, H. B. and Veninga, T. S. 1964. Radiometric toxicity of ozonized air. *Lancet* 1:133–136.

Brinkman, R. and Lamberts, H. B. 1958. Ozone as a possible radiomimetic gas. *Nature* 181:1202–1203.

Brookes, P. and Lawley, P. D. 1964. Reaction of some mutagenic and carcinogenic compounds with nucleic acids. *J. Cell. Comp. Physiol. Suppl.* 64:111–118.

Brooks, J. B., Cherry, W. B., Thacker, L. and Alley, C. C. 1972. Analysis by gas chromatography of amines and nitrosamines produced *in vivo* and *in vitro* by *Proteus vulgaris. J. Infect. Dis.* 126:143–153.

Bull, L. B., Culvenor, C. C. J. and Dick, A. T. 1968. *The pyrrolizidine alkaloids*. New York: Wiley.

Butler, W. H. and Wigglesworth, J. S. 1966. The effects of aflatoxin B on the pregnant rat. *Br. J. Exp. Pathol.* 47:242–247.

Campbell, T. C. and Stoloff, L. 1974. Implications of mycotoxins for human health. *J. Agric. Food Chem.* 22:1006–1015.

Candeli, A., Mastrandrea, V., Morozzi, G. and Toccaceli, S. 1974. Carcinogenic air pollutants in the exhaust from a European car operating on various fuels. *Atmos. Environ.* 8:698–705.

Carr, J. G. 1947. Production of mutations in mice by 1:1:5:6-dibenzanthracene. *Br. J. Cancer* 1:152.

Chemical & Engineering News. 1974a. Power plants may be major ozone source. 52:22–27.

Chemical & Engineering News. 1974b. High nonurban ozone concentrations spotted. 52:25.

Chemical & Engineering News. 1974c. Water chlorination, cancer link found. 52:5.

Cicerone, R. J., Stolarski, R. S. and Walters, S. 1975. Stratospheric ozone destruction by man-made chlorofluoromethanes. *Science* 185:1165–1167.

Clark, A. M. 1959. Mutagenic activity of the alkaloid heliotrine in *Drosophila. Nature (Lond.)* 183:731–732.

Clark, A. M. 1963. The brood pattern of sensitivity of the Drosophila testes to the mutagenic action of heliotrine. *Z. Vererbungsl.* 94:115–120.

Cleary, G. J. 1963. Measurement of polycyclic aromatic hydrocarbons in the air of Sydney using very long alumina columns for separation. *Int. J. Air Water Pollut.* 7:753.

Cleary, G. J. and Sullivan, J. L. 1965. Pollution by polycyclic aromatic hydrocarbons in the city of Sydney. *Med. J. Aust.* 1:758.

Clifford, J. E. and Rees, K. R. 1966. Aflatoxin: A site of action in the rat liver cell. *Nature (Lond.)* 209:312–313.

Coady, A. 1965. The possibility of factors of plant (particularly fungal) origin in Ethiopia liver disease. *Ethiopian Med. J.* 3:173–185.

Coffey, P. E. and Stasiuk, W. N. 1975. Evidence of transport of ozone into urban areas. *Environ. Sci. Technol.* 9:59–62.

Cohen, H. J. and Fridovich, I. 1971. Hepatic sulfite oxidase purification and properties. *J. Biol. Chem.* 246:359–366.

Colucci, J. M. and Begeman, C. R. 1965. The automotive contribution to airborne polynuclear aromatic hydrocarbons in Detroit. *J. Air Pollut. Control Assoc.* 15:113.

Commins, B. T. and Waller, R. E. 1967. Observations from a ten-year study of pollution at a site in the city of London. *Atmos. Environ.* 1:49.

Cook, J. W., Hewett, C. L. and Hieger, I. 1933. The isolation of a cancer-producing hydrocarbon from coal tar. *J. Chem. Soc.* 395.

Corn, M. and DeMaio, L. 1964. Sulfate particulates: Size distribution in Pittsburgh air. *Science* 143:803–804.

Couch, D. B. and Friedman, M. A. 1974. Suppression of dimethylnitrosamine mutagenicity by sodium nitrite. *Mutat. Res.* 26:371–376.

Cox, R. A. and Penkett, S. A. 1971. Photo-oxidation of atmospheric SO_2. *Nature, (Lond.)* 229:487.

Cromwell, B. T. and Richardson, M. 1966. Studies on the biogenesis of some simple amines and quarternary ammonium compounds in higher plants. *Vulvariae* Trimethylamine in *Chenopodium vulvariae*. Phytochemistry 5:735.

Crosby, N. T., Foremen, J. K., Palframan, J. F. and Sawyer, R. 1972. Estimation of steam volatile N-nitrosamines in food at the µg/kg level. *Nature (Lond.)* 238:342–343.

Crutzen, P. J. 1971. Ozone production rates in an oxygen-hydrogen-nitrogen oxide atmosphere. *J. Geophys. Res.* 76:7311–7325.

Crutzen, P. J. 1972. SST's—A threat to the earth's ozone shield. *Ambio* 1:41–51.

Crutzen, P. J. 1974a. Estimates of possible variations in total ozone due to natural causes and human activities. *Ambio* 3:201–210.

Crutzen, P. J. 1974b. A review of upper atmospheric photochemistry. *Can. J. Chem.* 52:1569–1581.

Culvenor, C. C. and Smith, L. W. 1965. Alkaloids of *Crotalaria crispata* F. Muell. Ex. Benth., the structures of crispatine and fucuine. *Aust. J. Chem.* 16:239–245.

Culvenor, C. C., Dann, A. T. and Dick, A. T. 1962. Alkylation as the mechanism by which the hepatotoxic pyrrolizidine alkaloids act on cell nuclei. *Nature (Lond.)* 195:570–573.

Culvenor, C. C., Edgar, J. A., Smith, L. W. and Tweeddale, H. J. 1970. Dihydropyrrolizines, III. Preparation and reaction of derivatives related to pyrrolizidine alkaloids. *Aust. J. Chem.* 23:1853–1867.

Cuthbertson, W. F. J., Lauresen, A. C. and Pratt, D. A. H. 1967. Effect of groundnut meal containing aflatoxin on cynomolgus monkeys. *Br. J. Nutr.* 21:893.

Davis, D. D., Smith, G. and Klauber, G. 1974. Trace gas analysis of power plant plumes via aircraft measurement: O_3, NO_x and SO chemistry. *Science* 186:733–736.

Davis, I., 1959. The survival and mutability of *E. coli* in aqueous solutions of ozone. Ph. D. thesis, University of Pennsylvania, Philadelphia.

Davis, I. 1961. Microbiologic studies with ozone mutagenesis of ozone for *E. coli. USAF School Aerosp. Med. Rep.* 60–61.

Day, R. S. 1975. Human cells repair DNA damaged by nitrous acid. *Mutat. Res.* 27:407–409.

Demerec, M. 1947. Mutations in *Drosophila* induced by a carcinogen. *Nature (Lond.)* 159:604.

Demerec, M. 1948a. Mutations induced by carcinogens. *Br. J. Cancer* 2:114.

Demerec, M. 1948b. Induction of mutations in *Drosophilia* by dibenzanthracene. *Genetics* 33:337.

Deo, M. G., Dayal, Y. and Ramalingaswami, V. 1970. Aflatoxins and liver injury in the rhesus monkey. *J. Pathol.* 101:47.

De Serres, F. J., Brockman, H. E., Barnett, W. E. and Kolmark, H. G. 1967. Allelic complementation among nitrous acid-induced AD-3B mutants of *Neurospora crassa. Mutat. Res.* 4:415–424.

Dickens, F. and Jones, H. E. H. 1961. Carcinogenic activity of a series of reactive lactones and related substances. *Br. J. Cancer* 15:85–100.

Dickens, F. and Jones, H. E. H. 1965. Further studies on the carcinogenic action of certain lactones and related substances in the rat and mouse. *Br. J. Cancer* 19:392–403.

Dickens, F., Jones, H. E. H. and Waynforth, H. B. 1966. Oral, subcutaneous and intratracheal administration of carcinogenic lactones and related substances: The intratracheal administration of cigarette tar in the rat. *Br. J. Cancer* 20:134.

Diehl, E. K., Dubreuil, F. and Glenn, R. A. 1970. Polynuclear hydrocarbon emissions from coal-fired installations. *J. Eng. Power* 89:276.

Dolimpio, D. A., Jacobson, C. and Legator, M. S. 1968. Effect of aflatoxin on human leukocytes. *Proc. Soc. Exp. Biol. Med.* 127:559–562.

Donahue, T. M. 1975. The SST and ozone depletion. *Science* 187:1144–1145.

Doster, R. C., Sinnhuber, R. O., Wales, J. H. and Lee, D. J. 1971. Acute toxicity and carcinogenicity of ochratoxin in rainbow trout (*Salmo gairdnerii*). *Fed. Proc.* 30:578.

Dowell, A. R., Kilburn, K. H. and Pratt, P. C. 1971. Short-term exposure to nitrogen dioxide: Effects on pulmonary ultrastructure, compliance and the surfactant system. *Arch. Intern. Med.* 128:74.

Drawert, F. 1965. Components of musts and wines. V. Proof of biogenic amines in wines and their significance. *Vitis* 5:127–130.

Druckrey, H., Steinhof, D., Beuthner, H., Schneider, H. and Klarner, P. 1963. Prufung von Nitrit auf chronisch toxische Wirkung an Ratten. *Arzneim. Forsch.* 13:320.

Druckrey, H., Preussmann, R., Ivankovic, S. and Sehmahl, D. 1967. Organotrope Carcinogene Wirkungen bei 65 Versahiedenen N-Nitroso-Verbindungen an BD-Ratten. *Z. Krebsforsch.* 69:103.

DuPlessis, L. S., Nunn, J. R. and Roach, W. A. 1969. Carcinogen in a Transkeian Bantu food additive. *Nature* (*Lond.*) 222:1198.

Eisenberg, A., Wisenberg, E. and Shuval, H. I. 1970. *The public health significance of nitrate and nitrite in food products.* Jerusalem: Ministry of Health.

Eisenbrand, G., Ungerer, O. and Preussmann, R. 1974. Rapid formation of carcinogenic N-nitrosamines by interaction of nitrite with fungicides derived from dithiocarbamic acid in vitro under simulated gastric conditions and in vivo in the rat stomach. *Food Cosmet. Toxicol.* 12:229–232.

Elespuru, R. K. and Lijinsky, W. 1973. The formation of carcinogenic nitroso compounds from nitrite and some types of agricultural chemicals. *Food Cosmet. Toxicol.* 11:807–811.

Ellis, D. and DiPaolo, J. A. 1967. Aflatoxin B_1: Induction of malformations. *Arch. Pathol.* 83:53–57.

Elmenhorst, H. and Grimmer, G. 1968. Polycyclische Kohlenwasserstoffe aus Zigaretten Rauchen Kondensat. Eine Methode zur Fraktionierung grosser Mengen fur Tierversuche. *Z. Krebsforsch.* 71:66.

Ender, F. and Ceh, L. 1968. Occurrence of nitrosamines in foodstuffs for human and animal consumption. *Food Cosmet. Toxicol.* 6:569.

Environmental Health Letters. 1975. Nader, Dr. Epstein ask EPA to investigate NO_x in air. July 1:6–7.

Epstein, S. S. and Shafner, H. 1968. Chemical mutagens in the human environment. *Nature* (*Lond.*) 219:385–387.

Fahmy, O. G. and Fahmy, M. J. 1971. Mutability of specific euchromatic and heterochromatic loci with alkylating and nitroso compounds in *D. melanogaster. Mutat. Res.* 13:19–34.

Fahmy, O. G. and Fahmy, M. J. 1973. Mutagenic properties of benzo(a)-pyrene and its methylated derivatives in relation to the molecular mechanisms of hydrocarbon carcinogenesis. *Cancer Res.* 33:302–309.

Fahmy, O. G., Fahmy, M. J., Massasso, J. and Ondrej, M. 1966. Differential mutagenicity of the amine and amide derivatives of nitroso compounds in *Drosophila melanogaster. Mutat. Res.* 3:201–206.

Fahrig, R. 1974. Development of host-mediated mutagenicity tests, I. Differential response of yeast cells injected into testes of rats and peritoneum of mice and rats. *Mutat. Res.* 26:29–36.

Fairchild, E. J. 1967. Tolerance mechanisms: Determinants of lung responses to injurious agents. *Arch. Environ. Health* 14:111–126.

Fairchild, E. J. and Graham, S. L. 1969. Thyroid influence on the toxicity of respiratory irritant gases, ozone and nitrogen dioxide. *J. Pharmacol. Exp. Ther.* 139:177–184.

Falk, H. C., Steiner, P. E., Goldfein, S., Breslow, A. and Hykes, R. 1951. Carcinogenic hydrocarbons and related compounds in processed rubber. *Cancer Res.* 11:318–326.

Fazio, T., Damico, J. N., Howard, S. W., White, R. H. and Watts, J. O. 1971. Gas chromatographic determination and mass spectrographic confirmation of N-nitrosodimethylamine in smoke processed marine fish. *J. Agric. Food Chem.* 19:250–253.

Fazio, T., White, R., Dusold, L. and Howard, J. 1973. Nitrosopyrrolidine in cooked bacon. *J. Assoc. Off. Anal. Chem.* 56:919.

Feder, W. A. and Sullivan, F. 1969. Ozone-depression of frond multiplication and floral production in duckweed. *Science* 65: 1373–1374.

Federal Register. 1968. Title 21, Chapter 1, no. 121 1063 and no. 121 0164.

Fetner, R. H. 1958. Chromosome breakage in *Vicia faba* by ozone. *Nature (Lond.)* 181:504–505.

Fetner, R. H. 1962. Ozone-induced chromosome breakage in human cell cultures. *Nature (Lond.)* 194:793–794.

Fetner, R. H. 1963. Mitotic inhibition induced in grasshopper neuroblasts by exposure to ozone. *USAF School Aerosp. Med. Rep.* 63–69.

Fiddler, W., Piotrowski, E. G., Pensabene, J. W., Doerr, R. C. and Wasserman, A. E. 1972. Effect of sodium nitrite concentration on N-nitrosodimethylamine formation in frankfurters. *J. Food Sci.* 37:668–670.

Fine, D. H., Rufeh, F., Lieb, D. and Epstein, S. S. 1974. A possible nitrogen oxide-nitrosamine-cancer link. *Bull. Environ. Contam. Toxicol.* 11:18–19

Fischer, R. 1970. Spektrophotometrisches Verfahren zur raschen Beurteilung von Russen auf Ihrengehalf an polycyclischen, aromatischen Kohlenwasserstoffen. *Z. Anal. Chem.* 249:110.

Fischer, W. H. 1972. Atmospheric chemistry: Trace gases and particulates. *Sci. Total Environ.* 1:314–319.

Fishbein, L. 1972. Natural non-nutrient substances in the food chain. *Sci. Total Environ.* 1:211–244.

Fishbein, L. 1976. Atmospheric mutagens. In *Chemical mutagens*, ed. A. Hollaender. vol. 4, pp. 219–319. New York: Plenum.

Fishbein, L. and Falk, H. L. 1970. Chromatography of the mycotoxins. *Chromatogr. Rev.* 12:42.

Fishbein, L., Flamm, W. G. and Falk, H. L. 1970. *Chemical mutagens*. New York: Academic Press.

Food and Cosmetics Toxicology. 1968. Nitrosamines: A jig-saw puzzle with missing pieces. 6:647.

Food and Cosmetics Toxicology. 1970. The air we breath. 8:218–222.

Food and Cosmetics Toxicology. 1975. Ochratoxins. 13:275–284.

Fowler, M. M. 1968. Pyrrolizidine alkaloid poisoning in calves. *Am. J. Vet. Med. Assoc.* 152:1131–1137.

Frayssenet, C., Lafarge, C., DeRecondo, A. M. and LeBreton, E. 1964. Inhibition de l'hypertrophie compensatrice du foie chez le rat par les toxines d'*Aspergillus flavus*. *C. R. Acad. Sci.* (*Paris*) 259:2143–2146.

Freebairn, H. T. 1959. The toxicity of ozone, a constituent of smog. *J. Appl. Nutr.* 12:2–13.

Freeman, G., Crane, S. C. and Furios, N. J. 1969. Healing in rat lung after subacute exposure to nitrogen dioxide. *Am. Rev. Resp. Dis.* 100:662–676.

Freeman, G., Stephens, R. J. and Coffin, D. L. 1973. Changes in dog's lungs after long-term exposure to ozone. *Arch. Environ. Health* 26:209–216.

Freese, E. 1959. On the molecular explanation of spontaneous and induced mutations. *Brookhaven Symp. Biol.* 12:63–73.

Freese, E. 1963. Molecular mechanism of mutation. *Molecular genetics,* ed. J. H. Taylor, part 1, pp. 207–270. New York: Academic Press.

Freimuth, U. and Glaser, E. 1970. Occurrence of nitrosamines in foods. *Nahrung* 14:357.

Fritz, W. 1968. Formation of carcinogenic hydrocarbons during thermal treatment of foods, II. Roasting of coffee beans and coffee substitutes. *Nahrung* 12:799–804.

Fritz, W. 1968. Formation of carcinogenic hydrocarbons during thermal treatment of foods, III. Baking of bread and biscuits. *Nahrung* 12:805–808.

Fritz, W. 1968. 3,4-Benzopyrene and other polyaromatics in margarine and mayonnaise. *Nahrung* 12:495–496.

Furichi, Y., Wataya, Y., Hayatsu, H. and Ukita T. 1970. Chemical modification of TRNA with bisulfite. A new method to modify isopentenyl adenosine residues. *Biochem. Biophys. Res. Commun.* 41:1185–1191.

Gabliks, J. W., Schaeffer, W., Friedman, L. and Wogan, G. N. 1965. Effect of aflatoxin B1 on cell cultures. *J. Bacteriol.* 90:720–723.

Gabridge, M. G. and Legator, M. S. 1969. A host-mediated microbioal assay for the detection of mutagenic compounds. *Proc. Soc. Exp. Biol. Med.* 130:831–834.

Gabridge, M. G., Denunzio, A. and Legator, M. S. 1969. Cycasin detection of associated mutagenic activity *in vivo. Science* 163:689–691.

Garner, R. C. 1973. Chemical evidence for the formation of a reactive aflatoxin B1 metabolite by hamster liver microsomes. *FEBS Lett.* 36:261–264.

Garner, R. C. and Wright, C. M. 1973. Induction of mutations in DNA-repair deficient bacteria by a liver microsomal metabolite of aflatoxin B1. *Br. J. Cancer* 28:544–551.

Garner, R. C., Miller, E. C. and Miller, J. A. 1972. Liver microsomal metabolism of aflatoxin B1 to a reactive derivative toxic to *Salmonella typhimurium* TA 1530. *Cancer Res.* 32: 2058–2066.

Geissler, E. 1962. Uber die Wirkung von Nitrosaminen auf Mikroorganismen. *Naturwissenschaften* 49:380–388.

Gelboin, H. V.,1969. A microsome-dependent binding of benzo(*a*)pyrene to DNA. *Cancer Res.* 29:1972–1976.

Gelboin, H. V., Kinoshita, N. and Wiebel, F. J. 1972. Microsomal hydroxylases: Induction and role in polycyclic hydrocarbon carcinogenesis and toxicity. *Fed. Proc.* 31:1298–1309.

Georgii, H. W. 1963. Oxides of nitrogen and ammonia in the atmosphere. *J. Geophys. Res.* 68:396–398.

Goldblatt, L. A. 1969. *Aflatoxin.* New York: Academic Press.

Goldblatt, L. A. 1970. Chemistry and control of aflatoxin. *Pure Appl. Chem.* 21:331–353.

Goodman, G. T. 1974. How do chemical substances affect the environment? *Proc. R. Soc. Lond. [Biol.]* 185:127–148.

Goze, A., Sarasin, A., Moule, Y. and Devoret, R. 1975. Induction and mutagenesis of prophage λ in *Escherichia coli* K-12 by metabolites of aflatoxin B1. *Mutat. Res.* 28:1–7.

Graves, R. R. and Hesseltine, C. W. 1966. Fungi in flour and refrigerated dough products. *Mycopathologia* 29:287.

Green, C. R. and Christie, G. S. 1961. Malformations in foetal rats induced by the pyrrolizidine alkaloid heliotrine. *Br. J. Exp. Pathol.* 42:369.

Green, M. H. L. and Muriel, W. J. 1975a. Use of repair-deficient strains of *Escherichia coli* and liver microsomes to detect and characterize DNA damage caused by the pyrrolizidine alkaloids heliotrine and monocrotaline. *Mutat. Res.* 28:331–336.

Green, M. H. L. and Muriel, W. J. 1975b. Use of repair deficient E. coli strains and liver microsomes to characterize mutagenesis by dimethyl nitrosamine. *Chem. Biol. Interac.* 11:63–65.

Green, S., Legator, M. S. and Jacobson, C. 1967. Utilization of a cell line derived from rat kangaroo for cytogenetic studies. *Mamm. Chromosome Newslett.* 8:36.

Greenblatt, M., Mirvish, S. S. and So, B. T. 1971. Nitrosamine studies: Induction of lung adenomas by concurrent administration of sodium nitrate and secondary amines in Swiss mice. *J. Natl. Cancer Inst.* 46:1029–1034.

Grimmer, G. 1966. Cancerogene Kohlenwasserstoffe in der Umgebung des Menschen. *Erdoel Kohle Erdgas Petrochem.* 19:578.

Grimmer, G. and Hildebrandt, A. 1965. Kohlenwasserstoffe in der Umgebung des Menschen, I. Eine Methode zur simultanen Bestimmung von dreizehn polycylischen Kohlenwasserstoffen. *J. Chromatogr.* 20:89.

Grobecker, A. J. 1974. *The effects of stratospheric pollution by aircraft.* Washington, D.C.: Office of the Secretary of Transportation.

Grove, M. D., Yates, S. G., Tallant, W. H., Ellis, J. J. Wolff, I. A., Kosuri, N. R. and Nichols, R. E. 1970. Mycotoxins produced by *Fusarium tricinctum* as possible causes of cattle disease. *J. Agric. Food Chem.* 18:734–736.

Gunther, F. A. and Buzzetti, F. 1965. Occurrence isolation, and identification of polynuclear hydrocarbons as residues. *Residue Rev.* 9:90.

Gunther, F. A., Buzzetti, F. and Westlake, W. E. 1967. Residue behavior of polynuclear hydrocarbons on and in oranges. *Residue Rev.* 17:8.

Haenni, E. O. 1968. Analytical control of polycyclic aromatic hydrocarbons in food and food additives. *Residue Rev.* 24:42

Haenni, E. O. and Hall, M. A. 1960. Tentative ultraviolet absorption limits for mineral oils. *J. Assoc. Agric. Chem.* 43:92–95.

Hamelin, C. and Chung, Y. S. 1974. Optimal conditions for mutagenesis by ozone in *E. coli* K12. *Mutat. Res.* 24:271–279.

Hamerton, J. L. 1971. *Human cytogenetics*, vol. 2, p. 345. New York: Academic Press.

Hammond, A. L. 1972. Chemical pollution: Polychlorinated biphenyls. *Science* 175:175.

Hammond, A. L. 1975. Ozone destruction: Problem's scope grows, its urgency recedes. *Science* 187:1181–1183.

Hammond, A. L. and Maugh, T. H. 1974. Stratospheric pollution: Multiple threats to earth's ozone. *Science* 186:335–338.

Hangebrauck, R. P., von Lehmden, D. J. and Meeker, J. E. 1964. Emissions of polynuclear hydrocarbons and other pollutants from heat-generation and incineration processes. *J. Air Pollut. Control Assoc.* 14:267.

Harm, W. 1962. Vergleichende Untersuchungen an HNO_2—Inaktivierten und UV inaktivierten Bakteriophagen. *Th. Z. Vererbungsl.* 91:52–62.

Harm, W. 1974. Recovery of phage T4 from nitrous acid damage. *Mutat. Res.* 24:205–209.

Harrington, J. S. 1962. Occurrence of oils containing 3,4-benzpyrene and related substances in asbestos. *Nature (Lond.)* 193:43.

Harris, P. N. and Chen, K. K. 1970. Development of hepatic tumors in rats following ingestion of *Senecio longilobus. Cancer Res.* 30:2881–2886.

Hayatsu, H. 1969. The oxygen-catalysed reaction between 4-thiouridine and sodium sulfite. *J. Am. Chem. Soc.* 91:5693–5694.

Hayatsu, H. and Miura, A., 1970. The mutagenic action of sodium bisulfite. *Biochem. Biophys. Res. Commun.* 39:156–160.

Hayatsu, H., Wataya, Y., Kai, K. and Iida, S. 1970a. Reaction of sodium bisulfite with uracil, cytosine and their derivatives. *Biochemistry* 9:2858–2865.

Hayatsu, H. Wataya, Y. and Kai, K. 1970b. The addition of sodium bisulfite to uracil and to cytosine. *J. Am. Chem. Soc.* 92:724–726.

Hayatsu, H., Wataya, Y., Furuichi, Y. and Kawazoe, Y. 1972. Reaction of bisulfite with N-6-(2-isopentenyl-adenosine. *Chemosphere* 1:75–78.

Hedler, L. and Marquardt, P. 1968. Occurrence of diethylnitrosamine in some samples of food. *Food Cosmet. Toxicol.* 6:341.

Heidelberger, C. 1973. Current trends in chemical carcinogenesis. *Fed. Proc.* 32:2154–2161.

Heidelberger, C. and Jones, H. B. 1948. The distribution of radioactivity in the mouse following administration of dibenzanthracene labeled in the 9 and 10 positions with carbon 14. *Cancer* 1:252–260.

Hendel, F. J. 1973. Aerothermochemistry of the terrestrial atmosphere. *Crit. Rev. Environ. Control* 3:129–152.

Hickey, F. J., Clellend, R. C., Boyce, D. E. and Horner, E. B. 1974. Atmospheric sulfur dioxide, nitrogen dioxide and lead as mutagenic hazards to human health. *Mutat. Res.* 26:445–446.

Hince, T. A. and Neale, S. 1974. Effect of N-nitroso-N-methylurea on viability and mutagenic response of repair-deficient strains of *Escherichia coli. Mutat. Res.* 22:235–242.

Holzapfel, C. W. 1968. Isolation and structure of cyclopiazonic acid, a toxic metabolite of *Penicillium cyclopium. Tetrahedron* 24:2101.

Holzapfel, C. W., Purchase, I. F. H., Steyn, P. S. and Gouns, L. 1966. The toxicity and chemical assay of sterigmatocystin, a carcinogenic mycotoxin, and its isolation from two new fungal sources. *S. Afr. Med. J.* 40:1100.

Horn, E. E. and Herriot, R. M. 1962. The mutagenic action of nitrous acid on "single-stranded" (denatured) Hemophilus-transforming DNA. *Proc. Natl. Acad. Sci. U.S.A.* 48:1409.

Howard, J. W. and Haenni, E. O. 1963. Extraction and determination of polynuclear hydrocarbons in paraffin waxes. *J. Assoc. Off. Agric. Chem.* 46:933.

Howard, J. W., Fazio, T. and Watts, J. O. 1970. Extraction and gas chromatographic determination of nitroso dimethylamine in smoked fish. Application to smoked nitrite treated chub. *J. Assoc. Off. Anal. Chem.* 53:269.

Hsieh, D. P. H., Salhab, A. S., Yang, S. and Wong, J. J. 1974. Toxicity of aflatoxin Q1 as evaluated with the chicken embryo and bacterial auxotrophs. *Toxicol. Appl. Pharmacol.* 30:237–242.

Huberman, E., Aspiras, L., Heidelberger, C., Grover, P. L. and Sims, P. 1971. Mutagenicity to mammalian cells of epoxides and other derivatives of polycyclic hydrocarbons. *Proc. Natl. Acad. Sci. U.S.A.* 68:3195–3199.

Hueper, W. C. and Conway, W. D. 1964. *Chemical carcinogenesis and cancers.* Springfield, Ill.: Thomas.

Iball, J. 1939. The relative potency of carcinogenic compounds. *Am. J. Cancer* 35:185.

Inoue, M., Hayatsu, H. and Tanooka, H. 1972. Concentration effect of bisulfite on the inactivation of transforming activity of DNA. *Chem. Biol. Interac.* 5:85–95.

International Agency for Research on Cancer. 1972. Evaluation of carcinogenic risk of chemicals to man. *IARC Monog.* 1:157–163.

International Agency for Research on Cancer. 1973. Evaluation of the carcinogenic risk of chemicals to man: Certain polycyclic aromatic hydrocarbons and heterocyclic compounds. *IARC Monogr.* 3:91–136.

Israel, H. and Israel, G. W. 1974. *Trace elements in the atmosphere.* Ann Arbor, Mich.: Ann Arbor Science.

Jaffee, L. S. 1967a. The biological effects of photochemical air pollutants on man and animals. *Am. J. Public Health* 57:1269–1277.

Jaffee, L. S. 1967b. The biological effects of ozone on man and animals. *Am. Ind. Hyg. Assoc. J.* 28:267–277.

Jagiello, G. M., Lin, J. S. and Ducayen, M. B. 1975. SO_2 and its metabolite: Effects on mammalian egg chromosomes. *Environ. Res.* 9:84–93.

Johnson, H. S. 1971. Reduction of stratospheric ozone by nitrogen oxide catalysts from supersonic transport exhaust. *Science* 173:517–522.

Johnson, H. S. 1974. Pollution of the stratosphere. *Environ. Conserv.* 1:163–176.

Junge, C. E. 1963. *Air chemistry and radioactivity.* New York: Academic Press.

Kada, T. 1973. Cellular metabolism of mutagens. *Igaku No Ayumi* 84:776–782.

Karow, E. O. and Foster, J. W. 1944. An antibiotic substance from species of *Gymnonscus* and *Penicillium. Science* 99:265–266.

Katz, M. and Monkman, L. 1964. The organic fraction of particulate pollution including polycyclic hydrocarbons. *Occup. Health Rev.* 16:3–16.

Kaudewitz, F. 1959. Production of bacterial mutants with nitrous acid. *Nature (Lond.)* 183:1829.

Keen, P. and Martin, P. 1971. Is aflatoxin carcinogenic in man? *Trop. Geogr. Med.* 23:44.

Khanin, M. W. 1956. The etiology and pathogenesis of toxic hepatitis with ascites. *Arkh. Patol.* 18:35–45.

Kingsbury, J. M. 1964. *Poisonous plants of the United States and Canada,* 3d ed. Englewood Cliffs, N.J.: Prentice-Hall.

Klenfield, M. and Giel, C. P. 1956. Clinical manifestations of ozone poisoning: Report of a new source of exposure. *Am. J. Med. Sci.* 231:638–643.

Knotek, Z. and Schmidt, P. 1964. Pathogenesis, incidence and possibilities of preventing alimentary nitrate methemoglobinemia in infants. *Pediatrics* 34:78.

Kobayashi, Y. 1959. Toxicity studies with methylazoxymethanol. *Proc. Jpn. Acad.* 35:501–507.

Kobayashi, A. and Matsumoto, H. 1965. Studies on methylazoxymethanol, the aglycone of cycasin. *Arch. Biochem.* 110:373.

Korzybski, T., Kowszyk-Gindifer, Z. and Kurylowicz, W. 1967. *Antibiotics, origin, nature and properties,* vol. 2. New York: Pergamon.

Kotin, P. and Falk, H. L. 1963. Atmospheric factors in pathogenesis of lung cancer. *Adv. Cancer Res.* 7:475.

Kotin, P., Falk, H. L. and Thomas, M. 1954. Aromatic hydrocarbons–II. Presence in particulate phase of gasoline-engine exhaust and carcinogenicity of exhaust extracts. *Arch. Ind. Hyg.* 9:164–177.

Kraybill, H. F. 1969. The toxicology and epidemiology of mycotoxins. *Trop. Geogr. Med.* 21:1–18.

Kraybill, H. F. and Shimkin, M. B. 1964. Carcinogenesis related to foods contaminated by processing and fungal metabolites. *Adv. Cancer Res.* 8:191.

Kreyberg, L. 1959. 3,4-Benzpyrene in industrial air pollution. *Br. J. Cancer* 13: 618.

Krieg, D. R. 1963. Specificity of chemical mutagenesis. *Progr. Nucleic Acid Res.* 2:125–168.

Krieger, R. I., Salhab, A. S., Dalezios, J. I. and Hsieh, D. P. H. 1975. Aflatoxin B1 hydroxylation by hepatic microsomal preparations from the rhesus monkey. *Food Cosmet. Toxicol.* 13:211–219.

Kroeller, E. 1967. Detection of nitrosamines in tobacco smoke and food. *Dtsch. Lebensm. Rundsch.* 63:303–308.

Krogh, P., Hasselager, E. and Friis, P. 1970. Fungal nephrotoxicity 2. Isolation of two nephrotic compounds from *Penicillium viridicatum*, citrinin and oxalic acid. *Acta Pathol. Microbiol. Scand.* [*B*] 78:401.

Kruger, F. W. 1972. New aspects in metabolism of carcinogenic nitrosamines. In *Topics in chemical carcinogenesis*, eds. W. Nakahara, S. Takayama, T. Sugimura, and J. Odashima, pp. 213–235. Tokyo: Univ. of Tokyo Press.

Kuehn, H. H. 1958. A preliminary survey of the Gymnoascaceae. *Mycologia* 50:417–439.

Lam, Y. and Nicholas, D. J. D. 1969. Nitrate reductase from *Micrococcus denitrificans*. *Biochim. Biophys. Acta* 178:225–234.

Lamb, M. J. and Lilly, L. J. 1971. Induction of recessive lethals in *Drosophila melanogaster* by aflatoxin B1. *Mutat. Res.* 11:430–433.

Lancet. 1968. Nitrites, nitrosamines, and cancer. 1:1071.

Laquer, G. L. and Matsumoto, H. 1966. Neoplasms in female Fischer rats following intraperitoneal injection of methyl azoxymethanol. *J. Natl. Cancer Inst.* 37:217.

Laquer, G. L. and Spatz, M. 1968. Toxicology of cycasin. *Cancer Res.* 28:2262.

Lawley, P. D. and Thatcher, C. J. 1970. Methylation of deoxyribonucleic acid in cultured mammalian cells by N-methyl-N-nitro-nitrosoguanidine. *Biochem. J.* 116:693–707.

Lawther, P. J., Commings, B. T. and Waller, R. E. 1965. A study of the concentration of polycyclic aromatic hydrocarbons in gas works retort houses. *Br. J. Ind. Med.* 22:13.

LeBreton, E., Frayssinet, C., LaFarge, C. and DeRecondo, A. M. 1964. Aflatoxine: Mechanisme de l'action. *Food Cosmet. Toxicol.* 2:675–680.

Lee, K. Y. and Lijinsky, W. 1966. Alkylation of rat liver RNA by cyclic N-nitrosamines *in vivo*. *J. Natl. Cancer Inst.* 37:40.

Legator, M. S. 1966. Biological effects of aflatoxin in cell culture. *Bacteriol. Rev.* 30:471–477.

Legator, M. S. 1969. Mutagenic effects of aflatoxin. *J. Am. Vet. Med. Assoc.* 155:2080–2083.

Legator, M. S. and Withrow, A. 1964. Aflatoxin: Effect on mitotic division in cultured embryonic lung cells. *J. Assoc. Off. Agric. Chem.* 47:1007–1009.

Legator, M. S., Zuffante, S. M. and Harp, A. R. 1965. Aflatoxin: Effect on heteroploid human embryonic lung cells. *Nature (Lond.)* 208:345–348.

Leonard, D. A., Deknudt, G. H. and Linden, G. 1975. Mutagenicity tests with aflatoxins in the mouse. *Mutat. Res.* 28:137–139.

Lewis, T. R., Moorman, W. J., Yang, Y. Y. and Stara, J. F. 1974. Long-term exposure to auto exhaust and other pollutant mixtures. *Arch. Environ Health* 29:102–106.

Lijinsky, W. 1971. Nitrosation of tertiary amines and some biological implications. Paper presented at the Conference on Nitrosamines, Heidelberg, W. Germany.

Lijinsky, W. and Epstein, S. S. 1970. Nitrosamines as environmental carcinogens. *Nature (Lond.)* 225:21–23.

Lijinsky, W. and Ross, A. E. 1969. Alkylation of rat liver nucleic acids not related to carcinogenesis, N-nitrosamines. *J. Natl. Cancer Inst.* 42:1095.

Lillehoj, E. B. and Ciegler, A. 1970. Aflatoxin B1 induction of lysogenic bacteria. *Appl. Microbiol.* 20:782–785.

Lilly, L. J. 1965. Induction of chromosome aberrations by aflatoxin. *Nature (Lond.)* 207:433–434.

Linsell, C. A. and Peers, F. G. 1972. The aflatoxins and human liver cancer. *Recent Results Cancer Res.* 39:125–129.

Lodge, J. P., Jr. and Pate, J. B. 1966. Atmospheric gases and particulates. *Science* 153:408–410.

Loprieno, N., Guglielminetti, R., Bonatti, S. and Abbondandalo, A. 1969. Evaluation of the genetic alterations induced by chemical mutagens in *Schizosaccharomyces pombe*. *Mutat. Res.* 8:65–71.

Louw, C. W. 1965. The quantitative determination of benzo(a)pyrene in the air of South African cities. *Am. Ind. Hyg. Assoc. J.* 26:520.

Loveless, A. 1969. Possible relevance of O-6 alkylation of deoxyguanosine to the mutagenicity and carcinogenicity of nitrosamines and nitrosamides. *Nature (Lond.)* 223:206–207.

Ma, T. H. and Khan, S. H. 1972. Pollen mitosis and pollen tube growth inhibited by SO_2 in cultured pollen tubes of *Tradescantia*. *Annu. Meet. Am. Soc. Cell Biol.* 320:160A.

Ma, T. H., Isbandi, D., Khan, S. H. and Tseng, Y. S. 1973. Low levels of SO_2 enhanced chromatid aberrations in *Tradescantia* pollen tubes and seasonal variations of the aberration rates. *Mutat. Res.* 21:93–100.

MacLean, S., Longwell, A. C. and Biogoslawski, W. J. 1973. Effects of ozone-treated seawater on the spawned, fertilized, meiotic and cleaving eggs of the commercial American oyster. *Mutat. Res.* 21: 283–285.

Maeda, D. and Tonomura, K. 1971. Microbial degradation of tetramethylthiuram disulfide. *Kogyo Gijutsuin Hakko Kenkyusho Kenkyu Hokoku* 33:1–8; *Chem. Abstr.* 74:10620.

Magee, P. N. 1971. Toxicity of nitrosamines: Their possible human health hazards. *Food Cosmet. Toxicol.* 9:207–218.

Magee, P. N. 1972a. Possibilities of hazards from nitrosamines in industry. *Ann. Occup. Hyg.* 15:19–22.

Magee, P. N. 1972b. Possible mechanisms of carcinogenesis and mutagenesis by nitrosamines. In *Topics in chemical carcinogenesis*, eds. W. Nakahara, S. Takayama, T. Sugimura and S. Odashima, pp. 259–275. Tokyo: Univ. of Tokyo Press.

Magee, P. N. and Barnes, J. M. 1967. Carcinogenic nitroso compounds. *Adv. Cancer Res.* 10:163–246.

Magee, P. N. and Hultin, T. 1962. Toxic liver injury and carcinogenesis. Methylation of proteins of rat liver slices by dimethylnitrosamine *in vitro. Biochem. J.* 83:106.

Magee, P. N. and Lee, K. Y. 1964. Cellular injury and carcinogenesis. Aklylation of ribonucleic acid of rat liver by diethylnitrosamine and N-butyl-methyl-nitrosamine *in vivo. Biochem. J.* 91:35.

Maher, U. M. and Summers, W. L. 1970. Mutagenic action of aflatoxin B_1 on transforming DNA and inhibition of DNA template activity *in vitro. Nature (Lond.)* 225:68–70.

Malling, H. V. 1965. Identification of the genetic alterations in nitrous acid induced AD-3 mutants of *Neurospora crassa. Mutat. Res.* 2:320–327.

Malling, H. V. 1966. Mutagenicity of two potent carcinogens, dimethylnitrosamine and diethylnitrosamine in *Neurospora crassa. Mutat. Res.* 3:537–540.

Malling, H. V. 1971. Dimethylnitrosamine: Formation of mutagenic compounds by interaction with mouse liver microsomes. *Mutat. Res.* 13:425–429.

Marcuse, R., Campbell, A. D., Krogh, P. and Purchase, I. 1972. Control of mycotoxins. *IUPAC Symposium*, London, England.

Mariani, A. and Mannucci, A. 1969. Sensitivity of the mitotic cycle to monocrotaline—Preliminary data on *Vicia faba. Caryologia* 22:113–118.

Marquardt, P. and Hedler, L. 1966. Uber das Vorkommen von Nitrosaminen in Weizenmehl. *Arzneim. Forsch.* 16:778–779.

Marquardt, H., Schwaier, R. and Zimmermann, F. 1963. Nicht-Mutagenitat von Nitrosaminen bei *Neurospora crassa. Naturwissenschaften* 50:135–136.

Marquardt, H., Zimmermann, F. K. and Schwaier, R. 1964. Die Wirkung krebsauslosender Nitrosamine und Nitrosamide auf das Adenin-6-45 Ruck-Mutationssystem von *Saccharomyces cerevisiae. Z. Vererbungsl.* 95:82–96.

Masek, V. 1971. Benzo(a)pyrene in the work place atmosphere of coal and pitch coking plants. *J. Occup. Med.* 13:193.

Masuda, Y. and Kuratsune, M. 1971. Polycyclic aromatic hydrocarbons in smoked fish, "Katsuobuschi." *Gann* 57:549.

Matsumoto, H. and Higa, H. H. 1966. Studies on methylazoxy-methanol, the aglycone of cycasin: Methylation of nucleic acids *in vitro. Biochem. J.* 98:20C.

Matsumoto, H. and Strong, F. M. 1963. The occurrence of methylazoxy-methanol in *Cycas circinalis L. Arch. Biochem.* 101:299.

Mattocks, A. R. 1972a. Toxicity and metabolism of Senecio alkaloids. In *Phytochemical ecology*, ed. J. B. Harborne, pp. 179–200. New York: Academic Press.

Mattocks, A. R. 1972b. Acute hepatotoxicity and pyrrolic metabolites in rats dosed with pyrrolizidine alkaloids. *Chem. Biol. Interact.* 5:227–242.

Mayer, V. W. and Legator, M. S. 1969. Production of petite mutants of *Saccharomyces cerevisiae* by patulin. *J. Agric. Food Chem.* 17:454–456.

McElroy, M. B., Wofsy, S. C., Penner, J. E. and McConnell, J. C. 1974. Atmospheric ozone: Possible impact of stratospheric aviation. *J. Atmos. Sci.* 31:287.

McGlashan, N. D., Walters, C. L. and McLean, A. E. M. 1968. Nitrosamines in African alcoholic spirits and oesophageal cancer. *Lancet* 2: 1017.

McKay, H. A. C. 1971. The atmospheric oxidation of sulfur dioxide in water droplets in presence of ammonia. *Atmos. Environ.* 5:7.

McLean, E. K. 1970. Toxic actions of pyrrolizidine (Senecio) alkaloids. *Pharmacol. Rev.* 22:429.

McLeish, J. 1953. The action of maleic hydrazide in *Vicia. Heredity Suppl.* 125–147.

Menzel, D. B. 1970. Toxicity of ozone, oxygen and radiation. *Annu. Rev. Pharmacol.* 10:379–384.

Menzel, D. B. 1971. Oxidation of biologically active reducing substances by ozone. *Arch. Environ. Health* 23:149–153.

Mickelsen, O., Campbell, E., Yang, M., Mugera, G. and Whitehair, C. K. 1964. Studies with cycad. *Fed. Proc.* 23:1363–1365.

Middleton, J. T., Darley, E. G. and Brewer, R. F. 1958. Damage to vegetation from polluted atmosphere. *J. Air Pollut. Control Assoc.* 8:9–15.

Miller, E. C. and Miller, J. A. 1971. The mutagenicity of chemical carcinogens: Correlations, problems and interpretation. In *Chemical mutagens: Principles and methods for their detection*, ed. A. Hollaender, vol. 1, pp. 83–119. New York: Plenum.

Miller, J. A. 1964. Comments on chemistry of cycads. *Fed. Proc.* 23:1361–1362.

Miller, J. A. 1970. Carcinogenesis by chemicals: An overview. *Cancer Res.* 30:559–576.

Miller, J. A. 1973. Naturally occurring substances that can induce tumors. In *Toxicants naturally occurring in foods*, 2d ed., pp. 508–549. Washington, D.C. National Academy of Sciences.

Miller, J. A. and Miller, E. C. 1971. Chemical carcinogenesis: Mechanisms and approaches to its control. *J. Natl. Cancer Inst.* 47:X–XIV.

Miller, M. W. and Berg, G. G. eds. 1969. *Chemical fallout*. Springfield, Ill.: Thomas.

Mirocha, C. J., Christensen, C. M. and Nelson, G. H. 1968. Physiologic activity of some fungal estrogens produced by *Fusarium. Cancer Res.* 28:2319.

Mirvish, S. S. 1972. Studies on N-nitrosation reactions: Kinetics of nitrosation, correlation with mouse feeding experiments and natural occurrence of nitrosatable compounds (ureides and guanidine). In *Topics in chemical carcinogenesis*, eds. W. Nakahara, S. Takayama, T. Sugimura, and S. Odashima, pp. 219–231. Tokyo: Univ. of Tokyo Press.

Mirvish, S. S. 1973. Kinetics of N-nitrosation reacting in relation to tumorigenesis experiments with nitrite plus amines or ureas. In *Proceedings of the meeting on the analysis and formation of nitrosamines*, ed. P. Bogovski. *IARC Publ.* 3:104–108.

Mirvish, S. S., Sams, J., Fan, T. Y. and Tannenbaum, S. R. 1973. Kinetics of nitrosation of the amino acids proline, hydroxyproline and sarcosine. *J. Natl. Cancer Inst.* 51:1833–1839.

Miyahara, S. 1966. Detection of secondary amines in foodstuffs. *Nippon Kagaku Zasshi* 81:19.

Molina, M. J. and Rowland, F. S. 1974. Stratospheric sink for chlorofluoromethanes: Chlorine atom catalysed destruction of ozone. *Nature (Lond.)* 249:810–812.

Moulé, Y. and Frayssinet, C. 1968. Effect of aflatoxin on transcription in liver cell. *Nature (Lond.)* 218:93–95.

Mudd, S. H., Irreverre, F. and Laster, L. 1967. Sulfite oxidase deficiency in man. Demonstration of the enzymatic defect. *Science* 156:1599–1602.

Muenscher, W. C. 1951. *Poisonous plants of the United States*. New York: Macmillan.

Mukai, F., Hawryluk, I. and Shapiro, R. 1970. The mutagenic specificity of sodium bisulfite. *Biochem. Biophys. Res. Commun.* 39:983–988.

Munro, L., Scott, P. M. and Moodie, C. A. 1973. Ochratoxin A. Occurrence and toxicity. *J. Am. Vet. Med. Assoc.* 163:1269.

Myers, T. L. and Strauss, B. S. 1971. Effect of methylmethane sulphonate on synchronized cultures of Hep-2 cells. *Nature New Biol.* 230:143–144.

Napalkov, N. P. and Alexandrov, V. A. 1968. On the effects of blastomagenic substances on the organism during embryogenesis. *Z. Krebsforsch.* 71:32.

Nashed, N. and Jabbur, G. 1966. A genetic and functional characterization of adenine mutants induced in yeast by 1-nitroso-imidazolidone-2 and nitrous acid. *Z. Vererbungsl.* 98:106–110.

Nasim, A. and Clarke, C. H. 1965. Nitrous acid induced mosaicism in *S. pombe. Mutat. Res.* 2:395–402.

Nason, A. 1962. Symposium on metabolism of inorganic compounds. II. Enzymatic pathways of nitrate, nitrite, and hydroxylamine metabolisms. *Bacteriol. Rev.* 26:16–41.

Nasr, A. N. M. 1971. Ozone poisoning in man: Clinical manifestations and differential diagnosis. A review. *Clin. Toxicol.* 4:461–466.

National Academy of Sciences. 1972. *Report of the committee on biological effects of atmospheric pollutants*, p. 131. Washington, D.C.: National Academy of Sciences.

National Academy of Sciences. 1975. *Assessing potential ocean pollutants.* Washington, D.C.: National Academy of Sciences.

National Air Pollution Control Association. 1968. *Sulfur oxide pollution control, federal research and development planning and programming.* Washington, D.C.: Government Printing Office.

National Air Pollution Control Association. 1970. *Air quality criteria for sulfur oxides.* Washington, D.C.: Government Printing Office.

National Industrial Pollution Control Council. 1971. *Air pollution by sulfur oxides.* Washington, D.C.: Government Printing Office.

Neame, P. B. and Pillay, V. K. G. 1964. Spontaneous hypoglycaemia, hepatic and renal necrosis following the intake of herbal medicines. *S. Afr. Med. J.* 38:729–732.

Nelson, D. W. and Bremmer, J. M. 1970. Gaseous products of nitrite decomposition in soils. *Soil Biol. Biochem.* 2:203–208.

Nesheim, S. 1971. *Abstr. 85th Annu. Meet. Assoc. Off. Anal. Chem., Washington, D.C., October 11–14.*

Neurath, G. 1967. Zur Frage des Vorkommens von N-Nitroso Verbindungen im Tabakrauch. *Experientia* 23:400–404.

Neurath, G. B. 1972. Nitrosamine formation from precursors in tobacco smoke. In *N-Nitroso compound analysis and formation*, eds. P. Bogovski, R. Preussman, and E. A. Walker, pp. 134–136. Lyon: International Agency for Research on Cancer.

Neurath, G., Dunger, M., Gewe, J., Luttich, W. and Wichern, H. 1966a. Volatile bases in tobacco smoke. I. *Beitr. Tabakforsch.* 3:563.

Neurath, G., Krull, A., Pirmann, B. and Wandrey, K. 1966b. Volatile bases in tobacco smoke. I. *Beitr. Tabakforsch.* 3:571.

Newberne, P. M. 1965. *Mycotoxins in foodstuffs*, pp. 187–208. Cambridge, Mass.: MIT Press.

Newberne, P. M. 1974. The new world of mycotoxins—Animal and human health. *Clin. Toxicol.* 7:161–177.

Newberne, P. M. and Butler, W. H. 1969. Acute and chronic effects of aflatoxin on the liver of domestic and laboratory animals: A review. *Cancer Res.* 29: 236–250.

Newberne, P. M. and Rodgers, A. E. 1973. Nutrition, monocrotaline and aflatoxin B1 in liver carcinogenesis. *Plant Foods Ferment.* 1:23.

Newberne, P. M. and Shank, R. C. 1973. Induction of liver and lung tumors in rats by the simultaneous administration of sodium nitrite and morpholine. *Food Cosmet. Toxicol.* 11:819–825.

Newsome, J. R., Norman, V. and Keith, C. H. 1965. Vapor phase analysis of tobacco smoke. *Tob. Sci.* 9:102–110.

Norstadt, F. A. and McCalla, J. M. 1963. Phytotoxic substances from a species of *Penicillium*. *Science* 140:410–411.

Ohtsubo, K., Yamada, M. and Saito, M. 1968. Inhibitory effect of nivalenol, a toxic metabolite of *Fusarium nivale* on the growth cycle and biopolymer synthesis of Hela cells. *Jpn. J. Med. Sci. Biol.* 21:185.

Ong, T. 1970. Mutagenicity of aflatoxins in *Neurospora crassa*. *Mutat. Res.* 9:615–618.

Ong. T. 1971. Mutagenic activities of aflatoxin B1 and G1 in *Neurospora crassa*. *Mol. Gen. Genet.* 111:159–170.

Ong, T. and de Serres, F. J. 1972. Mutagenicity of chemical carcinogens in *Neurospora crassa*. *Cancer Res.* 32:1890–1893.

Orgel, L. E. 1965. The chemical basis of mutation. *Adv. Enzymol.* 27:289–346.

Pace, D. M., Landolt, P. A. and Alftonomos, B. T. 1969. Effects of ozone on cells *in vitro*. *Arch. Environ. Health* 18:165–170.

Pan, A. Y., Beland, J. and Jegier, Z. 1972. Ozone induced arterial lesions. *Arch. Environ. Health* 24:229–232.

Park, C. R., Waynforth, H. B. and Magee, P. N. 1973. The activity of some nitroso compounds in the mouse dominant-lethal mutation assay. I. Activity of N-nitroso-N-methylurea, N-methyl-N-nitroso-N-nitroguanidine and N-nitrosomorpholine. *Mutat. Res.* 21:155–161.

Pasternak, L. 1962. Mutagene Wirkung von dimethylnitrosamin bei *Drosophila melanogaster*. *Naturwissenschaften* 49:381.

Pasternak, L. 1963. Untersuchungen uber die Mutagene Wirkung von Nitrosaminen und Nitrosomethyl Harnstoff. *Acta Biol. Med. Ger.* 10:436–438.

Pasternak, L. 1964. Untersuchungen uber die Mutagene Wirkung verschiedener Nitrosamin und Nitrosamid-Verbindungen. *Arzneim. Forsch.* 14:802–804.

Patterson, D. S. P. 1973. Metabolism as a factor in determining the toxic action of the aflatoxins in different animal species. *Food Cosmet. Toxicol.* 11:287–294.

Patterson, D. S. P. and Allcroft, R. 1970. Metabolism of aflatoxin in susceptible and resistant animal species. *Food Cosmet. Toxicol.* 8:45.

Patterson, D. S. P. and Roberts, B. A. 1970. The formation of aflatoxins B2a and G2a and their degradation products during the *in vitro* detoxification by livers of certain avian and mammalian species. *Food Cosmet. Toxicol.* 8:527.

Patterson, D. S. P. and Roberts, B. A. 1972. Aflatoxin metabolism in duck liver-homogenates: The relative importance of reversible cyclopentenone reduction and hemiacetal formation. *Food Cosmet. Toxicol.* 10:501.

Peckham, J. W., Doupnik, B., Jr. and Jones, O. H., Jr. 1971. Acute Toxicity of ochratoxins A and B in chicks. *Appl. Microbiol.* 21:492–494.

Pensabene, J. W., Fiddler, W., Dooley, C. J., Doerr, R. C. and Wasserman,

E. E. 1972. Spectral and gas chromatographic characteristics of some N-nitrosamines. *J. Agric. Food Chem.* 20:275–277.

Phillips, W. E. J. 1968. Nitrate content of foods, public health implications. *Can. Inst. Food Technol. J.* 1:98–103.

Plant, J. E. and Roberts, J. J. 1971. A novel mechanism for the inhibition of DNA synthesis following methylation: The effect of N-methyl-N-nitrosourea on HeLa cells. *Chem. Biol. Interact.* 3:337–342.

Platt, B. S., Stewart, R. J. G. and Gupta, S. R. 1962. The chick embryo as a test organism for toxic substances in food. *Proc. Nutr. Soc.* 21:XXX–XXXI.

Pogodina, O. N. 1966. O Mutagennoy Aktivonsti Kancerogenov Iz Gruppy Nitrosaminov. *Citologya* 8:503–509.

Prat, R., Nofre, C. and Cier, A. 1968. Effects de l'hypochlorite de sodium, de l'ozone et des radiations ionisantes sur les constituents pyrimidiques de *E. coli. Ann. Inst. Pasteur* 114:595–607.

Preusser, E. 1966. Aliphatic amines in the seeds and fruits and in germinating plants of *Vicia faba* and *Zea mays. Biol. Zentralbl.* 85:19–27.

Preussman, R. 1964. Zum oxydativen Abbau von Nitrosaminen mit Enzyme freien Modell-Systemen. *Arzneim. Forsch.* 14: 769–774.

Promchainant, C., Baimai, V. and Nondasuta, A. 1972. The cytogenetic effects of aflatoxin and gamma-rays on human leucocytes *in vitro. Mutat. Res.* 16:373–380.

Pryor, W. A. 1971. Free radical pathology. *Chem. Eng. News* 49:34–51.

Purchase, I. F. H. and Theron, J. J. 1968. Acute toxicity of ochratoxin A to rats. *Food Cosmet. Toxicol.* 6:479.

Purchase, I. F. H. and Van Der Watt, J. J. 1970. Carcinogenicity of sterigmatocystin. *Food Cosmet. Toxicol.* 8:289.

Rall, D. P. 1974. Review of the health effects of sulfur oxides. *Environ. Health Perspect.* 8:97–121.

Reisenstart, A. and Rosner, J. L. 1964. Chemically induced reversions in the Cys-C region of *Salmonella typhimurium. Genetics* 49:343–355.

Reiss, J. 1971. Chromosomen Aberrationen in den Wurzelspitzen von *Allium cepa* Durch Aflatoxin B1. *Experientia* 27:971–972.

Reiter, R. and Reiter, M. 1958. Relations between the contents of nitrate and nitrate ions in precipitations and simultaneous atmospheric processes. In *Recent advances in atmospheric electricity*, ed. L. G. Smith, pp. 175–194. New York: Pergamon.

Ripperton, L. A., Kornreich, L. and Worth, J. J. B. 1970. Nitrogen dioxide and nitric oxide in non-urban air. *J. Air Pollut. Control. Assoc.* 20:584–588.

Robinson, E. and Robbins, R. C. 1967. *Sources, abundance and fate of gaseous atmospheric pollutants. Final report on SRI project PR-6755.* New York: American Petroleum Institute.

Robinson, E. and Robbins, R. C. 1970a. *Gaseous nitrogen compound pollutants from urban and natural sources. J. Air Pollut. Control. Assoc.* 20:303–313.

Robinson, E. and Robbins, R. C. 1970b. Gaseous atmospheric pollution from urban and natural sources. In *Global effects of environmental pollution*, ed. F. Singer, p. 50. New York: Springer-Verlag.

Roehm, J. M., Hadley, J. G. and Menzel, D. B. 1971. Oxidation of unsaturated fatty acids by ozone and nitrogen dioxide, a common mechanism of action. *Arch. Environ. Health* 23:142–148.

Rolle, I., Payer, R. and Soeder, C. J. 1971. Uber die Amine einzelliger Grünalgen. *Arch. Mikrobiol.* 77:185–195.

Rose, F. L. 1958. Discussion of some experimental studies in toxic liver injury paper by Magee, P. N. In *The evaluation of drug toxicity*, eds. A. C. Walpole and A. Spinks, p. 116. London: Churchill.

Rossano, A. T., Jr. 1969. *Air pollution control—Guidebook for management.* Stanford, Conn.: Environmental Science Division, E.R.A., Inc.

Rudner, R. 1961. Mutation as an error in base pairing. I. The mutagenicity of base analogs and their incorporation into the DNA of *Salmonella typhimurium. Z. Vererbungsl.* 92:336.

Sachsenmaier, W., Siebs, W. and Tan, T. A. 1965. Wirkung von Ozon auf Mauseascitestumor Zellen und auf Huhnerfibroblasten in der Gewebekultur. *Z. Krebsforsch.* 67:113–126.

Sakshaug, J., Sognen, E., Hansen, M. A. and Kippang, N. 1965. Dimethylnitrosamine: Its hepatotoxic effect in sheep and its occurrence in toxic batches of herring meal. *Nature (Lond.)* 206:1261–1262.

Sander, J. 1967. Kann Nitrit in der menschlichen Nahrung Ursache einer Krebsentstehung durch Nitrosaminbildung sein? *Arch. Hyg. Bakteriol.* 151:22.

Sander, J. 1968. Nitrosaminsynthese durch Bakterien. *Z. Physiol. Chem.* 349:429–432.

Sander, J. and Bürkle, G. 1969. Induktion maligner Tumoren bei Ratten durch gleichzeitige Verfutterung von Nitrit und sekundaren Aminen. *Z. Krebsforsch.* 73:54–66.

Sander, J. and Seif, F. 1969. Bakterielle Reduktion von Nitrat im Magen des Menschen als Ursache einer Nitrosamin-Bildung. *Arzneim. Forsch.* 19:1091–1093.

Sander, J., Schweinsber, F. and Menz, H. P. 1968. Untersuchungen uber die Entstehung Cancerogener Nitrosamine im Magen. *Hoppe Seylers Z. Physiol. Chem.* 349:1691–1697.

Sarasin, A. and Moulé, Y. 1973. Inhibition of *in vitro* protein synthesis by aflatoxin B1 derivatives. *FEBS Lett.* 29:329–332.

Sasajima, M. 1968. Studies in psychrotolerant bacteria in fish and shellfish. *Tokaiku Suisan Kenkyusho Kenkyu Hokoku* 55:205–204; 1970. *Chem. Abstr.* 73:32608.

Savvina, K. I. 1952. Pathological anatomy of atrophic liver cirrhosis. *Arkh. Patol.* 14:65–70.

Sawicki, E. 1967. Airborne carcinogens and allied compounds. *Arch. Environ. Health* 14:46.

Sawicki, E., McPherson, S. P., Stanley, T. W., Meeker, J. E. and Elbert, W. C. 1965a. Quantitative composition of the urban atmosphere in terms of polynuclear aza heterocyclic compounds and aliphatic and polynuclear aromatic hydrocarbons. *Int. J. Air Water Pollut.* 9:515.

Sawicki, E., Meeker, J. E. and Morgan, M. J. 1965b. The quantitative composition of air pollution source effluents in terms of aza heterocyclic compounds and polynuclear aromatic hydrocarbons. *Int. J. Air Water Pollut.* 9:291.

Schachtschabel, D. O., Zilliken, F., Saito, M. and Foley, G. E. 1969. Inhibition of DNA synthesis and chromosome aberrations in cultured Ehrlich ascites tumor cells following treatment with luteoskyrin. *Exp. Cell. Res.* 57:19.

Scheel, L. D., Dobrogorski, O. G., Mountain, J. M., Svirbely, J. L. and

Stokinger, H. E. 1959. Physiologic, biochemical, immunological, and pathological changes following ozone exposure. *J. Appl. Physiol.* 14:67–80.

Scherr, G. H., Fishman, M. and Weaver, R. H. 1954. Mutagenicity of some carcinogenic compounds for *E. coli. Genetics* 39:141.

Schimmer, O. and Werner, R. 1974. Mutagenic effect of aflatoxin B1 on nuclear and extranuclear DNA in *Chlamydomonas reinhardii. Mutat. Res.* 26:423–425.

Schneider, L. K. and Calkins, G. A. 1971. Sulfur dioxide-induced lymphocyte defects in human peripheral blood cultures. *Environ. Res.* 3:473–483.

Schoental, R. 1957. Hepatotoxic action of pyrrolizidine (Senecio) alkaloids in relation to their structure. *Nature (Lond.)* 179:361–363.

Schoental, R. 1963. Liver disease and "natural" hepatotoxins. *Bull. WHO* 29:823–833.

Schoental, R. 1968. Toxicology and carcinogenic action of pyrrolizidine alkaloids. *Cancer Res.* 28:2237–2246.

Schoental, R. 1970. Hepatotoxic activity of retrorsine, senkirkine and hydroxysenkirkine in newborn rats and the role of epoxides in carcinogenesis by pyrrolizidine alkaloids and aflatoxins. *Nature (Lond.)* 227:401.

Schoental, R. and Bensted, J. P. M. 1963. Effects of whole body irradiation and of partial hepatectomy on the liver lesions induced in rats by a single dose of retrorsine, a pyrrolizidine (Senecio) alkaloid. *Br. J. Cancer* 17:242–247.

Schoental, R. and Coady, A. 1968. *East Afr. Med. J.* 45:557.

Scott, D. B. M. and Lesher, E. C. 1943. Effect of ozone on survival and permeability of *E. coli. J. Bacteriol.* 85:567–576.

Scott, P. M., Van Walbeek, W., Kennedy, B. and Anyeti, D. 1972. Mycotoxins (ochratoxin A, citrinin, and sterigmatocystin) and toxigenic fungi in grains and other agricultural products. *J. Agric. Food Chem.* 20:1103–1109.

Sen, N. P., Smith, D. C., Schwinghamer, L. and Howsam, B. 1970. Formation of nitrosamines in nitrite treated fish. *Can. Inst. Food Technol. J.* 3:66–69.

Sen, N. P., Donaldson, B., Iyengar, J. R. and Panalaks, T. 1973a. Nitrosopyrrolidine and dimethylnitrosamine in bacon. *Nature (Lond.)* 241:473–474.

Sen, N. P., Miles, W. F., Donaldson, B., Panalaks, T. and Iyengar, S. R. 1973b. Formation of nitrosamines in a meat curing mixture. *Nature (Lond.)* 245:104–105.

Sen, N. P., Donaldson, B., Charbonneau, C. and Miles, W. F. 1974. Effect of additives on the formation of nitrosamines in meat curing mixtures containing spices and nitrite. *J. Agric. Food Chem.* 22:1125–1130.

Sentein, R. 1955. Alterations of the mitotic spindle and fragmentation of the chromosomes by the action of patulin on the segmenting eggs of salamanders. *C. R. Soc. Biol. (Paris)* 149:1621–1622.

Shabad, L. M. 1971. Distribution and the fate of the carcinogenic hydrocarbon benzo(a)pyrene (3,4-benzopyrene) in the soil. *Z. Krebsforsch.* 70:204–210.

Shabad, L. M. and Smirnov, G. A. 1969. 3,4-Benzopyrene levels in the soot and exhaust gases of gas-turbine and piston aviation engines. *Gig. Sanit.* 34:98–99.

Shabad, L. M., Cohan, Y. L., Il'Nitskii, A. P., Khesina, A. Y., Shcherbak, N. P.

and Smirnov, G. A. 1971. The carcinogenic hydrocarbon benzo(a)pyrene in the soil. *J. Natl. Cancer Inst.* 47:1179.

Shank, R. C. and Magee, P. N. 1967. Similarities between the actions of cycasin and dimethylnitrosamine. *Biochem. J.* 105:521–527.

Shank, R. C., Bourgeois, C. H., Keschamras, N. and Chandauimol, P. 1971. Aflatoxins in autopsy specimens from Thai children with an acute disease of unknown etiology. *Food Cosmet. Toxicol.* 9:501.

Shank, R. C., Gordon, J. E., Wogan, G. N., Nondasuta, A. and Subhamani, B. 1972a. Dietary aflatoxins and human liver cancer. III. Field survey of rural Thai families for ingested aflatoxins. *Food Cosmet. Toxicol.* 10:71.

Shank, R. C., Wogan, G. N., Gibson, J. E. and Nondasuta, A. 1972b. Dietary aflatoxins and human liver cancer. II. Aflatoxins in market foods and foodstuffs in Thailand and Hong Kong. *Food Cosmet. Toxicol.* 10:61.

Shank, R. C., Siddhichai, B., Subhamani, B., Bhamarapravati, N., Gordon, J. E. and Wogan, G. N. 1972c. Dietary aflatoxins and human liver cancer III. *Food Cosmet. Toxicol.* 10:18.

Shapiro, R., Servis, R. E. and Welcher, N. 1970. Reaction of uracil and cytosine derivatives with sodium bisulfite, a specific deamination method. *J. Am. Chem. Soc.* 92:422–424.

Shapiro, R., Braverman, B., Louis, J. B. and Serivs, E. 1973. Nucleic acid reactivity and conformation, II. Reaction of cytosine and uracil with sodium bisulfite. *J. Biol. Chem.* 248:4060–4064.

Shimkin, M. B., Wieder, R., McDonough, M., Fishbein, L. and Swern, D. 1969. Lung tumor response in strains in mice as a quantitative bioassay of carcinogenic activity of some carbamates and aziridines. *Cancer Res.* 29:2184–2190.

Shotwell, O. L., Hesseltine, C. W., Vandegraft, E. E. and Goulden, M. L. 1971. Survey of corn for aflatoxin, zearalenone and ochratoxin. *Cereal Sci. Today* 16:266.

Shuval, I. and Gruener, N. 1972. Epidemiological and toxicological aspects of nitrates and nitrites in the environment. *Am. J. Public Health* 62:1045–1052.

Siddiqi, D. H. 1952. Mutagenic action of nitrous acid on *Aspergillus nidulans*. *Genet. Res.* 3:303–304.

Singhal, R. P. 1971. Modification of *E. coli* glutamate transfer ribonucleic acid with bisulfite. *J. Biol. Chem.* 246:5848–5851.

Sinios, A. and Wodsak, W. 1965. Die Spinat Vergiftung des Saüglings. *Dtsch. Med. Wochenschr.* 90:1856–1863.

Sippel, W. L. 1964. Crotalaria poisoning in livestock and poultry. *Ann. N.Y. Acad. Sci.* 111:562–570.

Smith, B. M., Wagman, J. and Fish, B. R. 1969. Interaction of airborne particles with gases. *Environ. Sci. Technol.* 3:558–563.

Smith, C. 1967. Comments on comparative patterns of drug metabolism. *Fed. Proc.* 26:1044.

Smith, D. W. E. 1966. Mutagenicity of cycasin aglycone (methyl-azoxy-methanol), a naturally occurring carcinogen. *Science* 152:1273–1274.

Smith, T. A. 1971. The occurrence, metabolism, and functions of amines in plants. *Biol. Rev.* 46:201–241.

Sparrow, A. H. and Schairer, L. A. 1974. Mutagenic response of *Tradescantia* to treatment with X-rays, EMS, DBE, ozone, SO_2, N_2O and several insecticides. *Mutat. Res.* 26:445.

Spatz, M. 1968. Hydrolysis of cycasin by B-D-glucosidase in skin of newborn rats. *Proc. Soc. Exp. Biol. Med.* 128:1005.

                                    L. Fishbein

Spatz, M., McDaniel, E. G. and Laquer, G. L. 1966. Cycasin excretion in conventional and germ-free rats. *Proc. Soc. Exp. Biol. Med.* 121:417–425.

Spatz, M., Daugherty, W. J. and Smith, D. N. E. 1967. Teratogenic effects of methylazoxymethanol. *Proc. Soc. Exp. Biol. Med.* 124:476–478.

Spatz, M., Laquer, G. L. and Holmes, J. M. 1969. Carcinogenic effects of methylazoxymethanol (MAM) in hamsters. *Proc. Am. Assoc. Cancer Res.* 10:86.

Sporn, M. B., Dingman, C. W., Phelps, H. L. and Wogan, G. N. 1966. Aflatoxin B: Binding to DNA *in vitro* and alteration of RNA metabolism *in vivo*. *Science* 151:1539–1542.

Stasny, J. 1942. Nitrogen bases in fermentation alcohol. *Sb. Cesk. Akad. Zemed.* 17:94–101.

Stefanescu, A. and Stanescu, L. 1968. Der Gefährungsgrad unter Einwirkung der aromatischen polynuklearen Kohlenwasserstoffe beim Fabrikations prozess von Russ. II. Die Gefährung durch einige krebserzeugende Kohlenwasserstoffe und ihre Bestimmung in der luft. *Z. Ges. Hyg.* 14:599.

Stephens, E. R., Freeman, G. and Evans, M. J. 1972. Early response of lungs to low levels of nitrogen oxide. *Arch. Environ. Health* 24:160.

Stern, A. C., ed. 1968. *Air pollution*, vol. 1, *Air pollution and its effects*, 2d ed., p. 694. New York: Academic Press.

Steyn, P. S. and Holzapfel, C. W. 1967. Synthesis of ochratoxins A and B. Metabolites of *Aspergillus ochraceus. J. S. Afr. Chem. Inst.* 20:186.

Steyn, M., Pitout, M. J. and Purchase, I. F. H. 1971. A comparative study on aflatoxin B1 metabolism in mice and rats. *Br. J. Cancer* 25:291–297.

Stokinger, H. E. 1954. Ozone toxicity—A review of the literature through 1953. *Arch. Ind. Health* 9:366–383.

Stokinger, H. E. 1965. Ozone toxicology. *Arch. Environ. Health* 10:719–731.

Stokinger, H. E. and Coffin, D. L. 1968. Biologic effects of air pollutants. In *Air pollution*, ed. A. C. Stern, 2d ed., vol. 2, p. 445. New York: Academic Press.

Stokinger, H. E. and Scheel, L. D. 1962. Ozone toxicity: Immunological and tolerance-producing aspects. *Arch. Environ. Health* 4:327–334.

Stokinger, H. E., Wagner, W. O. and Dobrogorski, O. 1957. Ozone toxicity studies, III. Chronic injury to lungs of animals following exposure at a low level. *Arch. Environ. Health.* 16:514–522.

Stolarski, R. S. and Cicerone, R. J. 1974. Stratospheric chlorine: A possible sink for ozone. *Can. J. Chem.* 52:1610–1615.

Strack, H. B., Freese, E. B. and Freese, E. 1964. Comparison of mutation and inactivation rates induced in bacteriophage and transforming DNA by various mutagens. *Mutat. Res.* 1:10.

Stupfel, H., Magnier, M., Romary, F., Tran, M. H. and Moutet, J. P. 1973. Lifelong exposure of SPF-rats to automotive exhaust gas. *Arch. Environ. Health* 26:264–269.

Sullman, S. F. 1971. Mutagenic effects of some plant and fugal toxins. *Int. J. Environ. Stud.* 1:107.

Summers, G. A. and Drake, J. W. 1971. Bisulfite mutagenesis in bacteriophage T4. *Genetics* 68: 603–607.

Surgeon General's Report. 1964. *Smoking and health, Public Health Serv. Publ. No. 1103.* Washington, D.C.: Government Printing Office.

Swann, P. F. and Magee, P. N. 1968. Nitrosamine-induced carcinogenesis. *Biochem. J.* 10:39–47.

Swedish Secretariat. 1972. Sulphur pollution across national boundaries. *Ambio* 1:15–20.

Swenson, D. H., Miller, J. A. and Miller, E. C. 1973. 2,3-Dihydro-2,3,-dihydroxy aflatoxin B1, an acid hydrolysis product of an RNA-aflatoxin B1 adduct formed by hamster and rat liver microsomes *in vitro*. *Biochem. Biophys. Res. Commun.* 53:1260–1267.

Snyder, E. L. and Hoffmann, D. 1963. Ein experimenteller beitrag zur Tabakrauch Kanzerogenesie. *Dtsch. Med. Wochenschr.* 88:623.

Szczech, G. M., Carlton, W. W. and Tuite, J. Ochratoxiocosis in beagle dogs. I. Clinical and clinico-pathological features. *Vet. Pathol.* 10:135–154.

Tasumo, T. 1968. Toxicologic research on substances from *Fusarium nivale*. *Cancer Res.* 28:2393–2396.

Tazima, Y. 1974. Naturally occurring mutagens of biological origin, a review. *Mutat. Res.* 26:225–234.

Teas, H. J. and Dyson, I. G. 1967. Mutation in *Drosophila* by methylazoxymethanol, the aglycone of cycasin. *Proc. Soc. Exp. Biol. Med.* 125:988–990.

Teas, H. J., Sax, H. J. and Sax, K. 1965. Cycasin: Radiomimetic effect. *Science* 149:541–542.

Teranishi, K., Homada, K. and Watanabe, H. 1975. Quantitative relationship between carcinogenicity and mutagenicity of polyaromatic hydrocarbons in *Salmonella typhimurium* mutants. *Mutat. Res.* 31:97–102.

Tessman, I. 1959. Mutagenesis in phages X174 and T4 and properties of the genetic material. *Virology* 9:375–385.

Tessman, I. 1962. The induction of large deletions by nitrous acid. *J. Mol. Biol.* 5:442–445.

Tessman, I., Poddar, R. K. and Kumar, S. 1964. Identification of the altered bases in mutated single-stranded DNA, *in vitro* mutagenesis by hydroxylamine, ethyl methane sulfonate and nitrous acid. *J. Mol. Biol.* 9:352–363.

Thompson, J. R. and Pace, D.M. 1962. The effect of sulfur dioxide upon established cell lines cultured *in vitro*. *Can. J. Biochem. Physiol.* 40:207–217.

Tilak, T. B. G. 1975. Induction of cholangiocarcinoma following treatment of a rhesus monkey with aflatoxin. *Food Cosmet. Toxicol.* 13:247–249.

Tilgner, D. J. and Daun, H. 1969. Polycyclic aromatic hydrocarbons (polynuclears) in smoked fish. *Residue Rev.* 27:19–41.

Torres, F. O., Purchase, I. F. H. and Van Der Watt, J. J. 1970. The aetiology of primary liver cancer in the Bantu. *J. Pathol.* 102:163.

Trams, A. and Künkel, H. A. 1964. Uber das spektrum einiger biochemischer mutanten bei *E. coli* nach Einwirkung von Roentgenstrahlen und Cancerogenen Substanzen. *Biophysik* 1:422–426.

Trams, A. and Künkel, H. A. 1965. Keine Mutationsauslosung Durch N-Nitrosopiperidin und N,N-Dinitrosopiperazin in *E. coli*. *Naturwissenschaften* 52:650–651.

Trans, E. G., Lauter, C. J., Brown, E. A. B. and Young, O. 1972. Cerebral cortical metabolism after chronic exposure to ozone. *Arch. Environ. Health* 24:229–232.

Tucker, T. L. and Hamilton, P. B. 1971. The effects of ochratoxin in broilers. *Poultry Sci.* 50:1637.

Udenfriend, S., Clark, C. T., Axelrod, J. and Brodie, B. B. 1954. Ascorbic acid in aromatic hydroxylation. I. A model system for aromatic hydroxylation. *J. Biol. Chem.* 208:731–739.

Ueno, Y. and Fukushima, K. 1968. Inhibition of protein and DNA synthesis in Ehrlich ascites tumour by nivalenol, a toxic principle of *Fusarium nivale* in growing rice. *Experientia* 24:1032.

Ukai, T., Yamamoto, Y. and Yamamoto, T. 1954. Poisonous substance from a strain of *Penicillium* (Hori-Yamamoto strains). II. Culture method of Hori-Yamamoto strain and chemical structure of its poisonous substance. *J. Pharm. Soc. Jpn.* 74:450–454.

Umeda, M., Yamamoto, J. and Saito, M. 1972. DNA-strand breakage of HeLa cells induced by several mycotoxins. *Jpn. J. Exp. Med.* 42:527–535.

Uraguchi, K., Sakai, F., Tsukioki, M., Noguchi, Y. and Tatsuno, M. 1961. Acute and chronic toxicity in mice and rats of the fungus matter of *Penicillium islandicum sopp* added to the diet. *Jpn. J. Exp. Med.* 31:435–461.

U.S. Department of Health, Education, and Welfare. 1968. *Nationwide inventory of air pollutant emissions. APCA Publ. No. AP-73.* Washington, D.C.: DHEW.

U.S. Department of Health, Education, and Welfare. 1969. *Air quality criteria for sulfur oxides.* Washington, D.C.: DHEW.

U.S. Department of Health, Education, and Welfare. 1973. *Air quality criteria for photochemical oxidants.* Washington, D.C.: DHEW.

Vandenberg, H. W. and Ball, C. R. 1972. The effect of methylazoxy methanol acetate on DNA synthesis and cell proliferation of synchronous HeLa cells. *Mutat. Res.* 16:381–390.

Vanderbilt, A. S. and Tessman, I. 1970. Identification of the altered bases in mutated single stranded DNA. IV. Nitrous acid induction of the transitions guanine to adenine and thymine to cytosine. *Genetics* 66:1–10.

Van Duuren, B. L. 1958a. Identification of some polynuclear aromatic hydrocarbons in cigarette smoke condensate. *J. Natl. Cancer Inst.* 21:1–16.

Van Duuren, B. L. 1958b. The polynuclear aromatic hydrocarbons in cigarette smoke condensate, II. *J. Natl. Cancer Inst.* 21:623–630.

Van Rheenen, D. C. 1962. Determination of biogenic amines in faeces of normal dairy cattle. *Nature* (*Lond.*) 193:170–171.

Van Walbeek, W., Scott, P. M. and Thatcher, F. S. 1968. Mycotoxins from food-borne fungi. *Can. J. Microbiol.* 14:130.

Veleminsky, J. and Gichner, T. 1968. The mutagenic activity of nitrosamines in *Arabidopsis thaliana. Mutat. Res.* 5:429–431.

Verly, W. G., Barbason, H., Dusart, J. and Petispas-Dewandre, A. 1967. A comparative study on the action of ethyl methane sulfonate and HNO_2 on the mutation to streptomycin resistance of *E. coli* K12. *Biochim. Biophys. Acta* 145:752–762.

Vielmetter, W. and Schuster, H. 1960. Die Basenspezifitat bei der Induktion von Mutationen durch Salpetrige Saure im Phagen T2. *Z. Naturforsch.* [*B*] 15:304–311.

Vielmetter, W. and Wiedner, C. M. 1959. Mutagene und inaktivierende Wirkung Salpetriger Saure auf freie Partikel des Phagen T2. *Z. Naturforsch.* [*B*] 14:312–317.

Vlitios, A. J. 1962. Plant growth regulators. In *Chemical and biological hazards in foods,* eds. J. C. Ayres, A. A. Kraft, H. F. Snyder, H. W. Wacker, pp. 89–126. Ames: Iowa State Univ. Press.

Vrochinskii, K. K. 1964. *E. coli* variability in water under the effect of ozone. *Zh. Mikrobiol. Epidemiol. Immunobiol.* 41:79–84.

Waller, R. E. 1963. Acid droplets in town air. *Water Pollut.* 7:773–778.

Warren, F. O. 1966. The pyrrolizidine alkaloids. In *Progress in the chemistry of organic natural products*, eds. W. Herz et al. New York: Springer-Verlag.

Wasserman, A. E., Fiddler, W., Doerr, R. C., Osman, S. F. and Dooley, C. J. 1972. Dimethyl nitrosamine in frankfurters. *Food Cosmet. Toxicol.* 10:681–684.

Weisburger, J. H. and Williams, G. M. 1975. Metabolism of chemical carcinogens. In *Cancer: Comprehensive treatise*, ed. F. F. Becker, vol. 1, pp. 185–234. New York: Plenum.

Werthamer, S., Schwarz, L. H., Carr, J. J. and Soskind, L. 1970. Ozone induced pulmonary lesions. *Arch. Environ. Health* 20:16–21.

Werthamer, S., Schwarz, L. H. and Sosking, L. 1970b. Abnormal epithelial alterations and pulmonary neoplasia induced by ozone. *Pathos* 35:224–230.

White, I. N. H. and Mattocks, A. R. 1972. Reactions of dihydropyrrolizines with DNA *in vitro*. *Biochem. J.* 128:291–297.

Whiting, M. G. 1963. Toxicity of cycads. *Econ. Bot.* 17:270.

Williams, D. J. and Rabin, B. R. 1971. Disruption by carcinogens of the hormones-dependent association of membranes with polysomes. *Nature (Lond.)* 232:102.

Winton, E. F., Tardiff, R. G. and McCabe, L. J. 1971. Nitrate in drinking water. *J. Am. Water Works Assoc.* 63:95–98.

Withers, R. F. J. 1965. The action of some lactones and related compounds on human chromosomes. In *Proceedings of the Symposium on the Mutational Process* , ed. Z. Landa, pp. 359–364. Prague: Czechoslovakian Academy of Sciences.

Witkin, E. M. Mutation and the repair of radiation damage in bacteria. *Radiat. Res. Suppl.* 6:30–53.

Wofsy, S. C. and McElroy, M. B. 1974. HO_x, NO_x, and ClO_x: Their role in atmospheric photochemistry. *Can. J. Chem.* 52:1582–1591.

Wofsy, S. C., McElroy, M. B. and Sze, N. D. 1974. Freon consumption: Implications for atmospheric ozone. *Science* 187:535–537.

Wogan, G. N. 1966. Chemical nature and biological effects of the aflatoxins. *Bacteriol. Rev.* 30:460–470.

Wogan, G. N. 1968. *Mycotoxins in foodstuffs*. Cambridge, Mass.: MIT Press.

Wogan, G. N. 1969. Naturally occurring carcinogens in foods. *Progr. Exp. Tumor Res.* 11:134.

Wogan, G. N. and Pong, R. S. 1970. Aflatoxins. *Ann. N.Y. Acad. Sci.* 174:623.

Wogan, G. N., Edwards, G. S. and Newberne, P. M. 1971. Structure-activity relationships in toxicity and carcinogenicity of aflatoxins and analogs. *Cancer Res.* 31:1936.

Wolff, I. A. and Wasserman, A. E. 1972. Nitrates, nitrites, and nitrosamines. *Science* 177:15–19.

Wynder, E. L. and Hoffmann, D. 1959. A study of tobacco carcinogenesis, VII. The role of higher polycyclic hydrocarbons. *Cancer* 13:1079.

Yates, S. G., Tookey, H. L., Ellis, J. J. and Burkhardt, H. J. 1967. Toxic butenolide produced by *Fusarium nivale* isolated from tall fescue (*Fusarium arundinacea*). *Tetrahedron Lett.* 25:261.

Zachau, H. G. 1969. Transfer ribonucleic acids. *Angew Chem. [Engl.]* 8:711–727.

Zdrazil, J. and Picha, F. 1966. The occurrence of the carcinogenic compounds 3,4-benzpyrene and arsenic in the soil. *Neoplasma* 13:49.

Zedeck, M. S., Sternberg, S. S., Poynter, R. W. and McGowan, J. 1970. Biochemical and pathological effects of methylazoxy-methanol acetate, a potential carcinogen. *Cancer Res.* 30:801.
Zeiger, E. and Legator, M. S. 1971. Mutagenicity of N-nitrosomorpholine in the host-mediated assay. *Mutat. Res.* 12:469–471.
Zelac, R. E., Chromroy, H. L., Bolch, W. E., Dunavant, B. G. and Blevis, H. A. 1971a. Inhaled ozone as a mutagen, II. Effects on the frequency of chromosome aberrations observed in irradiated Chinese hamsters. *Environ. Res.* 4:325–342.
Zelac, R. E., Chromroy, H. L., Bolch, W. E., Dunavant, O. G. and Bevis, H. A. 1971b. Inhaled ozone as a mutagen, I. Chromosome aberrations induced in golden hamsters lymphocytes. *Environ. Res.* 4:262–282.

Chapter 10

ENVIRONMENTAL SOURCES OF CHEMICAL MUTAGENS II. SYNTHETIC MUTAGENS

Lawrence Fishbein
National Center for Toxicological Research
Jefferson, Arkansas

INTRODUCTION

The spectrum of chemical burdens that humans are subjected to is very broad indeed, and can include use categories such as food and feed additives, drugs, pesticides and industrial chemicals (including their trace synthetic and/or degradation impurities) in various forms including solids, liquids, suspensions, dusts, and aerosols. The potential toxicants can enter the environment through air, water, and soil, as well as entering indirectly or directly into food.

It is estimated that about 500 chemicals are introduced each year [Council on Environmental Quality (CEQ), 1971], adding to the burden of the more than $\frac{1}{2}$ million chemicals *currently* in use, of which about 10,000 or so are produced annually in amounts between 500 and 1 million kg (Goodman, 1974). More than 2 million chemicals have been registered for use, mostly in the last three to four decades (CEQ, 1971). It is generally acknowledged that we know little about the toxicological and environmental aspects of these chemicals.

One striking feature of the chemical industry during the past $2\frac{1}{2}$ decades has been the enormous growth of production of organic chemicals. For example, in 1950 the world production (excluding Eastern bloc countries) totaled only approximately 7 million tons. By 1970 it had grown to 63 million tons, and it is estimated that in 1985 it will total approximately 150 million tons (Iliff, 1972).

Most organic chemicals ($\sim 75\%$) are further processed either in their place of manufacture or elsewhere. Over two-thirds of those in the latter category are used in the preparation of end products such as plastics and resins, synthetic fibers, synthetic rubbers, and surface coatings. (These are no longer chemicals in the usually accepted sense of the term.)

Most of the remaining 25% are further processed within industry itself to produce, either alone or in admixture, materials such as detergents, glycols (e.g., antifreeze, brake fluids), and solvents (e.g., aerosol propellants).

From these types of end products, it has been speculated that at present up to 20 million tons of manufactured organic chemicals may enter the environment annually (Iliff, 1972). It is not known precisely what percentage of these chemicals may be hazardous in terms of potential carcinogenicity, mutagenicity, and teratogenicity.

Although the etiology of human neoplasia, with rare exceptions, is unknown, it has been estimated that 50–90% of cancer in humans is caused by exposure to chemicals (*Chemical & Engineering News*, 1975b; Boyland, 1969). Most of the known chemical carcinogens are considered to be products of increasing agricultural and technological sophistication (*Chemical & Engineering News*, 1975b).

Not all chemical mutagens have been demonstrated to be carcinogenic, although most chemical carcinogens (several of which cause cancer in humans) have been found to be mutagens in one of the mutagenicity test procedures in which microbial, mammalian, or other animal cell systems are combined as genetic targets with an *in vitro* or *in vivo* metabolic activation system (Stoltz et al., 1974; Miller and Miller, 1971; Committee 17, 1974).

The major objective of this chapter is to consider a number of representative important synthetic mutagens and potential mutagens from industrial, pesticidal, and metal use categories just as naturally occurring mutagens were considered in Chapter 9.

INDUSTRIAL MUTAGENS

Halogens and Halogenated Derivatives

In recent years there has been concern over the environmental and toxicological effects of a spectrum of halogenated hydrocarbons, primarily the organochlorine insecticides and related derivatives such as DDT, dieldrin, Mirex, and polychlorinated biphenyls (PCBs). This concern has now been extended to practically all of the major commercial chlorinated hydrocarbons, many which are extensively used as solvents, aerosol propellants, degreasing agents, dry-cleaning fluids, fire extinguishers, and so on, and hence are manufactured on a large scale.

World production capacities for the principal chlorinated hydrocarbons are shown in Table 1. Of the compounds in the first column, the fluoro-chloromethanes are extensively used as aerosol propellants and are almost completely lost after use. The others are employed principally as solvents in industrial or domestic applications.

The products listed in Table 1 are characterized by high volatility and low solubility in water; some of their physical properties are shown in Table

TABLE 1 Estimated World Production Capacities (1973)
of Major Chlorinated Hydrocarbons

Hydrocarbon	Capacity (10^3 tons/yr)	Hydrocarbon	Capacity (10^3 tons/yr)
Trichloroethylene	1,010	Vinyl chloride	10,500
Perchloroethylene	1,050	1,2-Dichloroethane	19,500
1,1,1-Trichloroethane		Carbon tetrachloride	1,000
Methylene chloride	400	Chloroform	245
Trichlorofluoromethane	485	Methyl chloride	350
Dichlorodifluoromethane	570		

2. They enter the environment primarily by evaporation into the atmosphere. Some chlorinated hydrocarbons will, however, be found in aqueous effluents from factories handling them and even in household sewage, and hence will pass into municipal drainage systems and sinks.

The aliphatic chlorinated hydrocarbons listed in Table 1 are rapidly transferred both from air to water and from water to air. Irrespective of whether the initial loss of chorinated hydrocarbon is to the atmosphere or the hydrosphere, the transfer processes will lead to wide distribution of these compounds.

TABLE 2 Physical Properties of Some Aliphatic
Chlorinated Hydrocarbons

Hydrocarbon	Boiling point (°C)	Vapor pressure (mm Hg/20°C)	Solubility in water at 20°C (parts in 10^6 w/w)	Partition coefficient water/air at 20°C (w/v per w/v)
Methyl chloride	−24.2	3,756	7,250[a]	3.3
Methylene chloride	40.1	362.4	13,200 (25°C)	8.1
Chloroform	61.3	150.5	8,200	8.6
Carbon tetrachloride	76.8	90.0	785	1.1
Ethylene dichloride	83.6	63.9	8.800	26.4
1,1,1-Trichloroethane	74.1	96.0	480	0.71
Vinyl chloride	−13.9	2,320	60 (10°C)[a]	0.02 (10°C)
Vinylidene chloride	31.9	496.5	400	0.16
Trichloroethylene	87.0	57.9	1,100	2.74
Perchloroethylene	121.2	14.0	150	1.22
Fluorotrichloromethane	23.8	667.4	1,100	0.03
Difluorodichloromethane	−29.8	4,306	280 (25°C)	0.06
Hexachlorobutadiene	215	0.15	~2	0.97

[a]Under 760-mm pressure of organochlorine compound.

Vinyl chloride. Vinyl chloride [chloroethylene; ethylene monochloride; vinyl chloride monomer (VCM)] has attracted a considerable amount of attention since 1973 because of the discovery of its carcinogenic action in humans (Creech and Johnson, 1974). Thirteen deaths by angiosarcoma of the liver have been linked to occupational exposure to gaseous vinyl chloride during polyvinyl chloride (PVC) production operations in the U.S. plastics industry [Environmental Protection Agency (EPA), 1975; Haley, 1975; Heath et al., 1975]. The length of time between first exposure to VCM and diagnosis of the tumor ranged from 12 to 29 yr (mean, 20.3 yr), and the mean total duration of work involving exposure to VCM was 18 yr (Heath et al., 1975). The total VCM work population in the United States, past and present, has been estimated as about 20,000 (Heath et al., 1975).

The hazard of vinyl chloride was originally believed to concern primarily workers in the plastic industries, who may have a particularly high exposure to VCM in certain operations (e.g., cleaning of polymerization kettles), or a long-term exposure to relatively low concentrations in air of VCM at different factory sites. It is now believed that much larger populations are at risk because of (1) significant losses of VCM to the atmosphere at selected sites with subsequent atmospheric transport, (2) proximity to VCM and PVC production areas, (3) consumption of food products containing leachable amounts of unreacted VCM from PVC-packaged materials, and (4) ingestion of water containing unreacted VCM leached from PVC pipes.

World production of VCM in 1971 in various areas was estimated as follows (in millions of kilograms): United States, 1,969; Western Europe, 2,497; Japan, 1,275; Eastern Europe, 817; and other areas, 499—or a total of 7,057 million kg [International Agency for Research on Cancer (IARC), 1974].

At least 97% of the nearly 1,600 million kg of VCM consumed in the United States in 1971 was used for the production of vinyl chloride homopolymer and copolymer (e.g., in saran and other plastics), while the remainder found diverse applications, including use in the production of methyl chloroform, as an additive to specialty coatings, as a component of certain propellant mixtures, as a chemical intermediate, and as a solvent.

Vinyl chloride production in the United States exceeded 2.9 billion kg in 1973 (about one-third of the Western world's supply), and the annual growth rate in this industry is expected to exceed 10% per year through the 1980s. In the United States, VCM is currently produced at 15 plants and PVC at 37 plants (EPA, 1975). Thousands of companies, both large and small, and hundreds of thousands of workers are engaged in the manufacture and/or use of plastic products made from PVC (EPA, 1975).

The bulk of the VCM is produced by catalytic oxychlorination of ethylene (e.g., yielding ethylene dichloride, which is subsequently cracked to VCM and hydrogen chloride) (Haley, 1975; IARC, 1974). A typical commercial product can contain the following impurities (in milligrams per kilogram) (IARC, 1974): unsaturated hydrocarbons, 10; acetalydehyde, 2; dichloro compounds, 16; water, 15; HCl, 2; nonvolatiles, 200; iron, 0.4; phenol, as a stabilizer, 25–50; and trace amounts of organic impurities including acetylene, 1,3-butadiene, methyl chloride, vinylidene chloride, and vinyl acetate (EPA, 1975). The compositions of 15 by-products of VCM production by the oxychlorination process are shown in Table 3.

PVC is produced in the United States at a yearly rate of 2.4 billion kg (about one-third of the Western world's supply) by four major processes: (1) suspension polymerization (78% of total production), (2) emulsion polymerization (12% of total production), (3) bulk polymerization (6% of total production), and (4) solution (4% of total production).

The U.S. consumption of PVC resins in 1972 was divided among building and construction industries (42%), household uses (15%), consumer goods (12%), electrical applications (11%), packaging (9%), and transportation (6%), with miscellaneous uses accounting for the remainder.

Information concerning VCM emissions from both VCM and PVC resin plants is scant. VCM losses of $\sim$ 6% have been estimated, primarily on the basis of material balance studies (EPA, 1975). VCM is distributed into the atmosphere surrounding the emissions source in patterns that depend on the amount of VCM released, the nature of the plant area from which it is released, and meteorological conditions. Currently, emissions of vinyl chloride from VCM and PVC plants are estimated to exceed 90 million kg annually, with 90% of all vinyl chloride atmospheric emissions believed to emanate from

TABLE 3 Composition of By-products of Vinyl Chloride Production by the Oxychlorination Process[a]

By-product	Formula	Weight %
1,1,2-Trichloroethane	$CH_2Cl-CHCl_2$	67
1,2-Dichloroethane (EDC)	CH_2Cl-CH_2Cl	20
1,3-Dichlorobutane	$CH_3CHClCH_2CH_2Cl$	3
1,2-Dichlorobutane	$CH_3CH_2CHClCH_2Cl$	2
1,4-Dichloro-2-butene	$CH_2ClCH=CHCH_2Cl$	2
1,2,4-Trichloro-2-butene	$CH_2ClCH=CClCH_2Cl$	1.1
Pentachloroethane	$CHCl_2CCl_3$	1
Trichloroethylene	$CHCl=CCl_2$	1
Tetrachloroethane, asymmetric	Cl_3CCH_2Cl	1
1,3-Dichloro-2-butene	$CH_3CCl=CHCH_2Cl$	0.5
1,2,4-Trichlorobutane	$CH_2ClCH_2CHClCH_2Cl$	0.3
Bis(2-chloroethyl)ether	$(CH_2ClCH_2)_2O$	0.3
1,3,4-Trichloro-1-butene	$CH_2ClCHClCH=CHCl$	0.3
1,1,2-Trichlorobutane	$CCl_2CHClCH_2CH_3$	0.3
2,3,4-Trichloro-1-butene	$CH_2ClCHClCCl=CH_2$	0.2
		100.0

[a]Adapted from Jensen et al., 1970.

PVC plants (EPA, 1975). (Monomer plants emit less than 10% of the total.) While monomer plants emit less VCM per kilogram of product than polymer plants, this may be partially offset by the tendency for monomer plants to have larger production capacities than polymer plants. For instance, absolute VCM emission levels from polymer plants are ~ two to five times those from monomer plants (EPA, 1975).

Although emissions of VCM from fabricating plants and from fabricated products may also occur, there are apparently no current data to quantify these emissions.

The concentration of residual VCM monomer in PVC powder that is fabricated into final products is also an important determinant of VCM in the parts-per-million range. The entrapped concentration depends on the production process and can range from 100 to 5,800 ppm, which can be liberated during fabrication, particularly during heating (EPA, 1975).

An additional feature of the VCM and PVC industries (in the United States) that is of significance in terms of potential VCM concentration levels in the atmosphere is the clustering of plants (e.g., on the Gulf Coast in the Pasadena-Deer, Texas, and Baton Rouge, Louisiana, areas) (EPA, 1975).

It has been difficult to estimate the areas and quantities of VCM losses, which come primarily from vent streams, storage and transportation loading systems, and seepages from pumps.

Limited measurements of the atmospheric VCM concentration have been made in the vicinity of VCM/PVC production sources (within 0–8 km). In > 90% of the cases the peak concentrations have been below 1 ppm. A few 24-hr average values have been 1–3 ppm, and at distances of 0.8–8 km values were below 1 ppm (EPA, 1975). However, because of the sampling and analytical procedures used, the accuracy of these measurements may be no better than ± 100% (EPA, 1975).

The principal route of exposure to vinyl chloride is believed to be air inhalation, although exposure could also occur through skin contact or ingestion of food and water. Occupational exposure studies have revealed a wide range of VCM concentrations, depending on the manufacturing processes involved. For example, Cook et al. (1971) reported that the air concentration of VCM in a polymerization reactor before ventilation was on the order of 7,800 mg/m^3 (600–1,000 ppm). Concentrations of 1,560–2,600 mg/m^3 (600–1,000 ppm) in a polymerization reactor after washing have been reported by Lange et al. (1974).

Filatova and Gronsberg (1957) reported a concentration of 50–800 mg/m^3 (20–312 ppm) of VCM in the working atmosphere in a plant producing PVC. Air concentrations of VCM in work places in PVC-producing factories were reported to range from 100 to 800 mg/m^3 (40 to 312 ppm) with peaks up to 87,300 mg/m^3 (34,000 ppm) (Filatova and Gronsberg, 1957).

It has recently been reported (*European Chemical News*, 1974) that

PVC leaving certain manufacturing plants may contain 200–400 ppm VCM; on delivery to the customer, the level of VCM is about 250 ppm; and after processing, levels of 0.5–20 ppm are reached, depending on the method of fabrication.

There are other potential sources of exposure to VCM besides factories. Until recently, vinyl chloride was widely employed as a propellant in aerosols for hair sprays, pesticides, and room deodorants (Kuebler, 1958; Iosaki, 1958). The use of aerosol products in enclosed spaces, even in short bursts (e.g., 30 sec), could result in air concentrations of VCM as high as 1,000 mg/m^3 (400 ppm), and these levels could persist for several hours after spraying (*Federal Register*, 1974).

PVC floor coverings and upholstery represent additional sources of human exposure to VCM (Haley, 1975; Dyachuk, 1970; Sledak and Teplyakova, 1974). In addition to the possible carcinogenic response in humans, vinyl chloride exposure has been associated with the clinical syndrome, acro-osteolysis. The signs, symptoms, and clinical findings of this condition have been previously described (Dinman et al., 1971; Harris and Adams, 1967; Juhe and Lange, 1972, 1974.

Other effects reported in humans include liver dysfunction in individuals occupationally exposed to VCM in air in concentrations varying from 10 to 300 ppm over periods up to 25 yr (Kramer and Mutchler, 1972).

Vinyl chloride administered by inhalation is carcinogenic in rats, mice, hamsters, and rabbits, producing liver angiosarcomas in all three rodent species and a range of induced tumors varying to some extent from species to species (Viola et al., 1971; Maltoni and Lefemine, 1974; Maltoni, 1975; Caputo et al., 1974). For example, in rats vinyl chloride produces Zymbal gland carcinomas, nephroblastomas, angiosarcomas, hepatomas, and brain neuroblastomas; in mice, lung adenomas, mammary carcinomas of a peculiar type, angiomas of the liver and other sites, and skin epithelial tumors; in hamsters, skin trichoepitheliomas, lymphomas, and forestomach papillomas and acanthomas; and in rabbits, skin acanthomas and lung adenocarcinomas.

Other salient factors that should be noted include the following: (1) several of the tumor types produced by vinyl chloride in experimental animals are exceedingly rare or exceptional—for example, liver angiosarcomas, nephroblastomas, and neuroblastomas; (2) the lowest reported effective dose that is carcinogenic in rats and mice is 50 ppm; (3) the type of tumor induced, angiosarcoma of the liver, is the same as that observed in workers exposed to vinyl chloride; (4) studies with Sprague-Dawley and Wistar rats appear to suggest that the strain factor considerably affects the neoplastic response (Maltoni, 1975); (5) onset of subcutaneous angiosarcomas and Zymbal gland carcinoma in the offspring of mice exposed during pregnancy for 7 days to 10,000 and 5,000 ppm of vinyl chloride appears to indicate a transplacental effect (Maltoni, 1975).

The mutagenicity of vinyl chloride and/or its metabolites (e.g., chloroethylene oxide, chloroacetaldehyde, and chloroethanol) has been demonstrated recently *in vitro* by Rannug et al. (1974), Bartsch et al. (1975a), and Malaveille et al. (1975), utilizing the reverse mutation system of *Salmonella typhimurium* of Ames et al. (1973) (e.g., strains TA1530, TA1535, and G46 were specifically reverted to *His*[+] prototrophy by single base-pair substitutions or by base-pair insertions or deletions, "frameshifts" utilizing TA1536, TA1537, and TA1538). Loprieno et al. (1975) demonstrated that vinyl chloride in the presence of purified mouse liver microsomes was converted to an active metabolite(s) producing gene mutation(s) in the yeast *Saccharomyces pombe* and gene conversions(s) in two loci of a diploid strain of *S. cerevisiae*. Vinyl chloride has also been found mutagenic in *Drosophila melanogaster* (Verburgt, 1975). Huberman et al. (1975) reported the mutagenicity in Chinese hamster V79 cells of two vinyl chloride metabolites, chloroethylene oxide and chloroacetaldehyde. Chromosome aberrations in a small number of workers exposed to vinyl chloride have been reported by Ducatman et al. (1975) and Funes-Cravioto et al. (1975).

Major exposures came from leaks of unreacted vinyl chloride gas and fumes from PVC slurry and from polymerization reactor cleaning operations (Ducatman et al., 1975). Reactor cleaning involved skin contact with PVC and inhalation of vinyl chloride gas residues. (The latter accounted for the most intense exposures.) There was no record of ambient gas levels in the factor, but it was assumed that these must have exceeded 500 ppm at times, based on reports of odor detection, dizziness, and headaches (Ducatman et al., 1975). The studies of Ducatman et al. (1975) raise the question of whether chromosome damage studies can be at all predictive of environmentally induced carcinogenesis.

Selikoff (1974) suggested that the wives of workers exposed to vinyl chloride may experience a higher-than-normal incidence of stillbirths and miscarriages. For example, the rate of stillbirths and miscarriages was 142 per 1,000 pregnancies among wives of workers at one plant and 72 per 1,000 at another plant. It should be noted that although the husbands were all exposed to vinyl chloride in their work, they were also exposed to other chemicals, tending to obscure a causal relationship with vinyl chloride.

Gothe et al. (1974) recently described the trapping with 3,4-dichlorobenzenethiol of reactive metabolites formed *in vitro* from vinyl chloride. Cell-free liver microsome preparations were exposed to VCM in the presence of air, and the reactive metabolites were trapped with this nucleophilic thiol, which was added to the liver preparation or exposed in a separate vessel to the gas mixture leaving the liver preparation. One of the products formed from the trapping agent was identified as 2,4-dichlorophenyl thioacetaldehyde. The results are consistent with the formation of chloroethylene oxide as a reactive intermediate of vinyl chloride, but can also be interpreted as indicating the formation of chloroacetaldehyde, which is known to be formed from chloroethylene oxide by a slow intramolecular rearrangement.

Malaveille et al. (1975) also demonstrated the alkylating activity of chloroethylene oxide, but not of chloroacetaldehyde, by its rapid reaction with 4-(*p*-nitrobenzyl)pyridine. The half-life of the epoxide (0.32 mM) in an acetone - 0.1 M Tris buffer at pH 7.5 (30% v/v) was determined as 1.6 min after different times of preincubation at 37°C. These data indicate high electrophilic reactivity of chloroethylene oxide, an example of halogen-substituted aliphatic epoxides. It should be noted that the chemical and biological properties of this class of reactive compounds have not been fully elucidated.

Van Duuren (1974) recently proposed that the activated carcinogenic species of vinyl chloride formed in situ is monochloroethylene oxide, and that noncovalent binding to tissue constituents such as serum albumin, microsomal membranes, and other target sites may precede the activation of vinyl chloride to its epoxide.

Jaeger et al. (1974) also proposed that the metabolism of VCM [like that of trichloroethylene (Daniel, 1963)] proceeds through an epoxide intermediate, which is also responsible for the observed hepatotoxicity of vinyl chloride.

Vinylidene chloride. Vinylidene chloride (1,1-dichloroethylene; $CH_2=CCl_2$) (DCE) is a monomeric intermediate in the production of plastics, particularly the saran type, and has been reported as an impurity in VCM.

Inhalation toxicity studies of DCE indicate that it causes hepatic and renal damage (Irish, 1974; Prendergast et al., 1967; Gage, 1970) and that, in general, its toxicity could be considered both qualitatively and quantitatively comparable to that of carbon tetrachloride. However, measurements of lipoperoxidative stimulatory activity indicated that DCE was dissimilar to CCl_4 in terms of a proposed lipoperoxidative mechanism (Jaeger et al., 1973). Caputo et al. (1974) recently reported the carcinogenicity of DCE in rats.

Kramer and Mutchler (1972) reported that simultaneous exposure to both VCM and DCE in some plant workers led to dose-related changes in liver function. The changes in hepatic function may have resulted from DCE exposure alone.

The mutagenicity of DCE has been reported by Bartsch et al. (1975a) in the *S. typhimurium* strains TA1530 and TA1535. DCE exhibited a higher mutagenic effect than that observed with vinyl chloride, when the compound was metabolically activated by rat or mouse liver microsomal enzymes (Bartsch et al., 1975b).

It is quite possible that, like vinyl chloride (Bartsch et al., 1975a), DCE may be mutagenic after activation to an epoxide intermediate such as

$$CH_2-C-Cl_2$$
$$\diagdown O \diagup$$

Trichloroethylene and tetrachloroethylene. Trichloroethylene (trichloroethene; $ClCH=CCl_2$) and tetrachloroethylene (perchloroethylene, $Cl_2C=$

CCl_2) are both widely employed as solvents, dry-cleaning and degreasing agents, and in the manufacture of a variety of organic chemicals, such as polymerized resins of phenol-formaldehyde, urea-formaldehyde, and epoxides in the production of special fiberglasses. Tetrachloroethylene is also used in small amounts as a commodity fumigant, in the synthesis of fluorocarbons, and as a solvent for silicones. The United States produced 434 million lb of trichloroethylene in 1974 with an estimated 95% used for vapor degreasing of metal parts in industrial fabricating plants.

Both trichloroethylene and tetrachloroethylene have extensive utility as solvents for fats, waxes, resins, oils, rubber, paints and varnishes, cellulose esters, and ethers. For example, in the printing and textile industries they are used as fat solvents for duplicating operations and as resin solvents for fabric impregnation, respectively. In the chemical industry and laboratory, both trichloroethylene and perchloroethylene are used for many extraction processes. They are used for food extractions, including decaffeinating coffee, and removing oleoresins from spices (Seltzer, 1975).

Inhalation of trichloroethylene during production, vapor degreasing, and other industrial uses is an occupational hazard, which in the United States is dealt with by the Occupational Safety and Health Administration (OSHA). The permissible ceiling level of trichloroethylene is now 100 ppm in air (time-weighted average during 8 hr) with a 200-ppm maximum for 15-min exposure and a 300-ppm limit (Seltzer, 1975).

It is generally acknowledged that emissions of commercial organic solvent vapors into the atmosphere have been increasing dramatically in the last decade (McConnell et al., 1975; Brunelle et al., 1966; Hamming, 1967; County of Los Angeles, 1971). McConnell et al. (1975) estimated the loss of trichloroethylene and perchlorethylene to the global environment in 1973 to be over 1 million tons each. The National Academy of Sciences (1975) estimated that 90% of the world's production of perchloroethylene ($\sim 10^6$ tons) is released into the lower atmosphere, almost entirely in the Northern Hemisphere, with the points of injection corresponding closely to the population distribution.

Solvent emissions, for example, are believed to account for $> 20\%$ of the total hydrocarbons emitted into the atmosphere in Los Angeles County (Brunelle et al., 1966; Hamming, 1967; County of Los Angeles, 1971), and these emissions averaged about $\frac{1}{6}$ lb per person annually in this county. The release rate of industrial effluents into the air over Los Angeles County has been estimated as 500 tons/day. These emissions are believed to be mainly solvents, of which 25 tons is dry-cleaning fluids and 95 tons is degreasing solvents; the remaining 380 tons is surface coating and miscellaneous compounds.

Concentrations of trichloroethylene vapor in degreasing units have been reported to range from 20 to 500 ppm (at head height above the bath), the highest levels being over the baths, where it was necessary to manually remove articles (Glass, 1961).

Both tri- and tetrachloroethylene are known to be neurotoxic as well as hepatotoxic (Fabre and Truhaut, 1952; Kimmerlle and Eben, 1973). The predominant action of trichloroethylene in humans is that of a narcotic, hence its earlier use as a surgical anesthetic. Acute intoxication has been reported, principally in industry from degreasing operations involving both tri- and tetrachloroethylene.

The U.S. National Cancer Institute (NCI) recently issued a "state of concern" alert, warning producers, users, and regulatory agencies that preliminary evaluation tests at NCI indicated that trichloroethylene (when fed) induces tumors in mice, predominantly hepatocellular carcinomas (Seltzer, 1975) with some metastases to the lungs. (Levels of 2,400 and 1,200 mg/kg for males and 1,800 and 900 mg/kg for females were administered five times a week.)

It has been shown that induction of liver mixed-function oxidases by treatment with phenobarbital or 3-methylcholanthrene enhances the hepatotoxicity of trichloroethylene (Carlson, 1974), possibly through an increased rate and/or altered route of metabolism (Leibman and McAllister, 1967).

The metabolic pathways of trichloroethylene and tetrachloroethylene in the mouse and the rat are believed to involve the intermediate epoxides

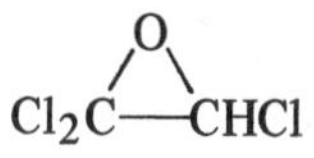

$$Cl_2C \overset{O}{\underset{\diagdown\diagup}{\text{———}}} CHCl \qquad \text{and} \qquad Cl_2C \overset{O}{\underset{\diagdown\diagup}{\text{———}}} CCl$$

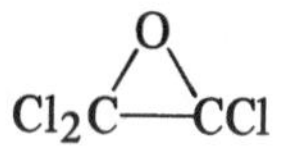

respectively. For example, following exposure of tetrachloroethylene vapor for 2 hr in mice, the urinary metabolites included 52% trichloroacetic acid, 11% oxalic acid, and traces of dichloroacetic acid (Yllner, 1961).

Daniel (1963) and Van Duuren (1974) have also postulated that the metabolism of trichloroethylene proceeds through an epoxide intermediate.

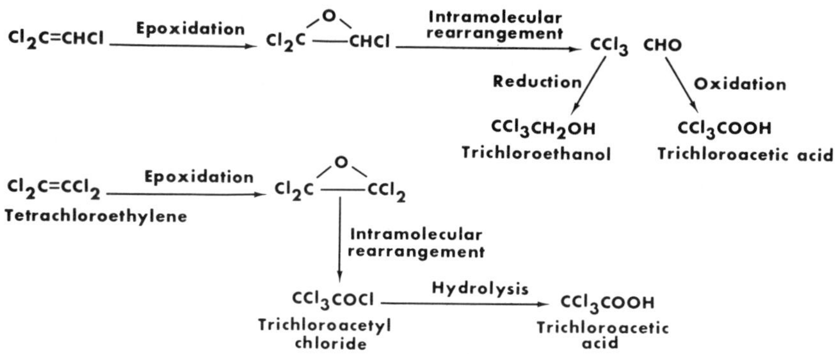

FIGURE 1 Metabolic pathways of trichloroethylene and tetrachloroethylene in the rat.

Figure 1 illustrates metabolic pathways of tri- and tetrachloroethylene in the rat.

It is well known that trichloroethylene is excreted in the urine as trichloroacetic acid and trichloroethanol in all species of animals studied. Bartonicek and Souček (1959) have detected chloroform as a further metabolite in the conversion of trichloroethylene. Its conversion from trichloroacetic acid via decarboxylation is conceivable. Besides these compounds, monochloroacetic acid is also a urinary metabolite of humans.

A point of major importance is the nature of the rearrangement that results in the formation of 2,2,2-trichloroethanol and trichloroacetic acid from 1,1,2-trichloroethylene. This has been shown to be an intramolecular rearrangement of trichloroethylene, with no exchange with the body chloride pool.

It has also been postulated that trichloroethylene oxide is formed when trichloroethylene is oxygenated in the presence of actinic radiation (Powell, 1945). Rearrangement of the oxide yields trichloroacetaldehyde (chloral). Formation of chloral in men exposed to trichloroethylene vapor has been reported (Scansetti et al., 1959). The mutagenicity of chloral hydrate has been described; for example, chloral hydrate has been reported to induce point mutations in *Drosophila* (Barthelmess, 1956) and bacteria (Schull, 1960) and chromosome aberrations in *Vicia faba* (Garrigues, 1940).

It should be noted that trichloroethylene itself and/or its oxide may be mutagenic, according to the considerations discussed above for vinyl chloride (Rannug et al., 1974; Malaveille et al., 1975).

Chloroprene. Chloroprene (1-chloro-2,3-butadiene),

$$CH_2 = \underset{\underset{Cl}{|}}{C} - CH = CH_2$$

is the monomer for neoprene, the specialty rubber. It is prepared by two major routes—addition of hydrogen chloride to vinyl acetylene, or chlorination of butadiene (American Chemical Society, 1973).

Chloroprene has been reported to induce liver injury in several species (Van Oettingen et al., 1936). High rates of skin and lung cancer have been reported among workers in a U.S. plant who have handled chloroprene and its derivatives (*Chemical & Engineering News*, 1975d). Currently about 2,500 workers in the United States are exposed to chloroprene (*Chemical & Engineering News*, 1975d).

The National Institute for Occupational Safety and Health (NIOSH) in the United States has cited (*Chemical & Engineering News*, 1975d) Soviet reports of a large-scale epidemiologic investigation of industrial workers in the Yerevan region of the Soviet Union. During the period 1956–1970, 137 cases of skin cancer were discovered through the examination of 24,989 persons over the age of 25. The study found that 3% of workers exposed to chloroprene and 1.6% of people working in industries using chloroprene derivatives developed skin cancer, compared to only 0.4% of persons working in nonchemical industries. The chloroprene workers who developed skin cancer had an average age of 59.6 yr and an average duration of employment of 9.5 yr.

During the same period, 87 cases of lung cancer were also identified. The group exposed to chloroprene or its derivatives had the highest incidence of lung cancer (1.16%). These workers' average age was 44.5 yr and they had an average duration of employment of 8.7 yr. Of the 34 cases of lung cancer in this group, 18 were among persons having direct and prolonged exposure to chloroprene monomer; the remaining 16 were persons whose exposure was to chloroprene latexes.

Carbon tetrachloride. Carbon tetrachloride is produced in enormous quantities—for example, more than 1.0 billion lb in the United States in 1970 and $\sim$ 140 million lb in Japan in 1974 and in France in 1969 (IARC, 1972). In the United States, the majority of the CCl_4 produced in 1970 was employed in the production of fluorocarbons—700 million lb (69%) for dichlorodifluoromethane (CF_2Cl_2) and about 260 million lb (26%) for trichlorofluoromethane ($CFCl_3$). The remaining 5% of the U.S. production (in 1970) ($\sim$ 50 million lb) was used (1) in grain fumigants (mixed with other chemicals); (2) in fire extinguishers; (3) as a solvent for oils, fats, resins, and rubber cements; (4) as a cleaning agent for machinery and electrical equipment; (5) for degreasing metal fabricated parts; and (6) in organic chlorination processes.

Losses of CCl_4 to the global environment were estimated by McConnell et al. (1975) to be on the order of 1 million tons in 1974.

Carbon tetrachloride has produced liver tumors in the mouse, hamster, and rat following several routes of administration, including inhalation and oral ingestion (IARC, 1972; Warwick, 1971). Prolonged administration of CCl_4 to rats causes centrolobular fatty change and necrosis. Frequent mitotic figures and binucleate cells are evidence of cellular regeneration and hyperplasia (Rubin and Popper, 1967).

A number of cases of hepatomas appearing in men several years after CCl_4 poisoning have also been reported (Rubin and Popper, 1967; Simler et al., 1964; Tracey and Sherlock, 1968). It has been suggested that the selective toxicity of CCl_4 for the livers of animals depends on its metabolism by the liver (Slater, 1966; Rechnagel, 1967) to a reactive chemical species. For example, it was proposed that a free radical, CCl_3, is formed and that this could lead to peroxidation of lipid membranes and produce chemical alterations at other sites (Slater, 1966). Liver tissue reduces CCl_4 to chloroform, and it was also suggested by Butler (1961) that homolytic cleavage of the carbon-chlorine bonds yields free radicals, which could then alkylate the sulfhydryl groups of enzymes. A link between the latter and peroxidative decomposition was established by Rechnagel (1967). Fowler (1968) detected hexachloroethane (CCl_3-CCl_3) in tissues of rabbits following CCl_4 intoxication.

Barthelmess (1970), in his survey of chemical mutagens in the environment, has listed CCl_4 as a chromosome-breaking agent.

Braun and Schoneich (1975) recently reported the synergistic effect of CCl_4 on the mutagenic effectiveness of cyclophosphamide in the host-mediated assay with *S. typhimurium*. CCl_4 did not exhibit any mutagenic effect when assayed in the spot test with *S. typhimurium* strains G46 and TA1950. *In vitro*, CCl_4 did not affect the mutagenicity of cyclophosphamide when tested with these strains of *S. typhimurium*.

Fluorocarbons. Since their introduction 40 yr ago as refrigerants and later as propellants for self-contained aerosol products, the fluorocarbons (fluoroalkanes) have generally been considered to have an extremely low order of biological activity (Clayton, 1967), and as a consequence their use patterns and production have increased enormously. These chemicals, mostly known as Freons, have negligible natural sources and are now used almost exclusively as aerosol propellant gases (65%), as refrigerants (20%), and for a number of other purposes (Crutzen, 1974a), including use as blowing agents for the production of foam. The major fluorocarbons of environmental as well as toxicological concern are trichlorofluoromethane $(CFCl_3; F-11; P-11)$ and dichlorodifluoromethane $(CF_2Cl_2; F-12; P-12)$.

Estimates of both U.S. and worldwide production of these fluorocarbons vary. For example, the total world industrial production of $CFCl_3$ and CF_2Cl_2 in 1973 was reported to amount to 260,000 and 440,000 tons, respectively (Crutzen, 1974b). The 1972 world production rates for $CFCl_3$ and CF_2Cl_2 have been reported as 300,000 and 500,000 tons/yr, respectively (American Chemical Society, 1973; Molina and Rowland, 1974; Rowland and Molina, 1974). Between 1960 and the present, the world production rate was estimated to have grown exponentially, with a doubling time of 3.5 yr (Cicerone et al., 1975; Lovelock et al., 1973).

In the United States, annual production of $CFCl_3$ (F-11) increased from about 300 million lb in 1972 to 325 million lb in 1973 (National Resources Defense Council, 1975), while CF_2Cl_2 (F-12) production increased during this period from 439 million lb to about 487 million lb (U.S. Department of Commerce, 1974; *Chemical & Engineering News*, 1974). It is anticipated that in the foreseeable future, production growth will be about 10% per year. Six U.S. manufacturers currently account for nearly 50% of the world production of $CFCl_3$ and CF_2Cl_2, with about half of this used in aerosol sprays (U.S. Department of Commerce, 1974; *Chemical & Engineering News*, 1974).

Both $CFCl_3$ and CF_2Cl_2 are used as propellants in a broad spectrum of products, as illustrated in the following usage pattern, in *million* units, for 1972 (Sangioyanni, 1974) (a unit is defined as a can or bottle regardless of size): personal products (e.g., cosmetics, perfumes, deodorants), 1,490; household products (e.g., window cleaners, air fresheners, oven cleaners), 699; coating and finishing products (e.g., paint sprays), 270; insect sprays, 135; lubricants and degreasers, 100; and automotive products, 76.

It has been suggested that "hundreds of millions of pounds of P-11, P-12, and similar compounds are used each year in the United States as propellants in pressurized products and thus are released into the atmosphere" (National Resources Defense Council, 1975). Additional quantities of these compounds are released as a consequence of manufacture, transportation, and escape from refrigeration systems, where they are used as refrigerants.

Numerous recent studies have indicated that the fluorocarbons are being added to the environment in steadily increasing amounts (Crutzen, 1974b; Cicerone et al., 1975; McElroy et al., 1974), and since these compounds are chemically inert and relatively insoluble, they are not removed from the lower atmosphere by rainwater. Unlike CCl_4, they seem to have no natural sources or sinks in the troposphere and their lifetimes are apparently controlled by diffusion into the stratosphere, where they can be photodissociated by UV light (Molina and Rowland, 1974).

Calculations by Molina and Rowland (1974) have been substantially confirmed in later studies by Cicerone et al. (1975), who concluded that present usage levels of chlorofluoromethanes (fluorocarbons) could lead to chlorine-catalyzed ozone destruction rates that will exceed natural sinks of ozone by 1985 or 1990.

Wofsy and McElroy (1974) and Wofsy et al. (1974), using several models, speculated that if the use of fluorocarbon propellants continues to increase by about 10% per year, the decrease in atmospheric ozone could be 10% by 1994 and as much as 16% by the year 2000. The atmospheric lifetimes of $CFCl_3$ (F-11) and CF_2Cl_2 (F-12) were estimated as 68 and 45 yr, respectively (Hammond, 1975).

Consequences of ozone depletion, particularly projected increases in the number of deaths due to skin cancer, have been suggested. For example, the National Academy of Sciences (NAS) in 1972 suggested that a 5% depletion of ozone might produce an additional 8,000 skin cancer cases per year among the white population of the United States (McElroy et al., 1974). A more recent assessment suggests that the percentage increase in the incidence of skin cancers would parallel the increase in the intensity of radiation. A 5% ozone depletion (10% increase in radiation) might cause 10,000–60,000 additional skin cancer cases per year in the United States alone (Hammond, 1975).

Although in earlier reports the fluorocarbons were considered to have an extremely low order of biological activity (Clayton, 1967), reports during the 1960s of fatalities attributed to the use and/or abuse of aerosols (Hammond, 1975; Reinhardt et al., 1971), particularly of those used in the treatment of bronchial asthma, have made it necessary to reexamine the toxicity of the propellants.

Belej and Aviado (1975) found that some of the propellants used in aerosols have the potential to produce bronchoconstriction, reduce pulmonary compliance, depress respiratory minute volume, reduce mean blood pressure, and accelerate heart rate in dogs. $CFCl_3$ (F-11), the most widely used low-pressure propellant, was found to be the most toxic one; it exerted all of these undesired effects except bronchoconstriction and a reduction of pulmonary compliance.

Aviado (1975a) summarized the acute inhalation toxicity of $CFCl_3$ for the mouse, rat, dog, and monkey. The most serious sign of toxicity from acute inhalation of F-11 is cardiac arrhythmia, which could be elicited in all four animal species. This may account for the sudden deaths associated with the use and abuse of aerosols (Aviado, 1975b). Blake and Mergner (1974) studied the biotransformation and elimination of $[^{14}C]CFCl_3$ and $[^{14}C]$-CF_2Cl_2 in beagles. Less than 1% of the inhaled fluorocarbon was biodegraded to metabolites in beagles after a short (6–20 min) period of inhalation. Because of limitations posed by the presence of radioactive impurities (e.g., 0.5% $[^{14}C]CCl_4$ and 1.4% $[^{14}C]CHCl_3$ and $[^{14}C]CF_3Cl$ and/or $[^{14}C]CF_4$ in CF_2Cl_2) the possibility that metabolic conversion occurred could not be excluded. However, it was suggested that $CFCl_3$ and CF_2Cl_2, by analogy with fluorocarbon anesthetics, are relatively refractory to biotransformation after inhalation. It was cautioned that extrapolation of these conclusions to data obtained with other routes of administration (e.g., oral) or longer exposure, and/or to other fluorocarbons, should be guarded (Blake and Mergner, 1974).

There is a paucity of data concerning both the carcinogenicity and mutagenicity of the fluorocarbons. Epstein et al. (1967) reported that in mice, combined administration of $CFCl_3$ (F-11) and the insecticidal synergist piperonyl butoxide increased the incidence of malignant hepatoma; they postulated that piperonyl butoxide may so alter the *in vivo* dehalogenation of the propellant that carcinogenic compounds are formed.

Mutation studies with *D. melanogaster* exposed to four fluorinated hydrocarbon gases were described by Foltz and Fuerst (1974). The compounds studied were: Freon C318 (octafluorocyclobutane; $CF_2CF_2CF_2CF_2$), Genetron 23 (fluoroform; CHF_3), Genetron 152A (1,1-difluoroethane; CH_3CHF_2), and perfluorobutene-2 (octafluoro-2-butene; $CF_3CF=CFCF_3$). Two special genetic techniques were employed. The Basc technique, with Muller-5 females and wild-type males (Spencer and Stern, 1948), was used for scoring sex-linked lethal recessive mutations that arise in the germ line of the treated paternal male. All four fluorinated hydrocarbons were found to significantly increase mutation rates in progeny of *Drosophila* over control levels, with Genetron 23 being the most mutagenic of the gases. For each gas studied, pronounced phenotypic effects were observed among progeny of exposed males. While most of the deviant phenotypes found had been previously described in the literature (Lindsley and Grell, 1968), the fused medial "unicorn" antenna phenotype and two tumors had not been previously described. It was not determined whether these phenotypes have a genetic origin. Although varying effects of each gas were noted, it was recognized that an undetermined part of the observed mutagenic effects of the gases may have been due to anoxia and this aspect would warrant further study (Foltz and Fuerst, 1974).

Garrett and Fuerst (1974) described sex-linked mutations in *D. melanogaster* males (Canton-Special strain) after exposure to various mixtures of gas atmospheres. Perfluorobutene-2 was studied in mixtures with compressed air, CO_2, O_2, or N_2 to determine its effects in combination with various components of air. Treatment with 10% perfluorobutene-2 in air produced a recessive mutation rate of 1.78%, compared with 0.25% for compressed air. This was higher than any mutation rate obtained when perfluorobutene-2 was mixed with O_2, N_2, CO_2, or compressed air. Genetron 23, Genetron 152 [as previously described (Foltz and Fuerst, 1974)], nitrous oxide, and sulfur chloride-pentafluoride were all mutagenic to *D. melanogaster* as determined by the Basc technique for the detection of sex-linked lethal recessive mutations.

Polychlorinated biphenyls. Despite the fact that PCBs have been available commercially for 40 yr, it is only within the last 6 yr that they have been recognized to be of significant environmental and potential toxicological concern.

PCBs are manufactured in the United States, Great Britain, France, West Germany, the Soviet Union, Japan, Spain, Italy, and Czechoslovakia and are marketed under a number of commercial trade names such as Aroclor, Clophen, and Phenoclor. The Aroclors (Monsanto Chemical Co., St. Louis, Missouri) are a series marketed under various numbers and consist of mixtures of chlorinated biphenyls and terphenyls. The first 2-digits represent the molecular type; 12 represents chlorinated biphenyls, 25 and 44 refer to blends of chlorinated biphenyls and chlorinated terphenyls (75% and 60% biphenyl, respectively), and 54 represents chlorinated terphenyls. The last 2 digits give the weight percent of chlorine; for example, Aroclor 1242 is a chlorinated biphenyl containing 42% chlorine.

Theoretically, 210 compounds can be prepared in the commercial process for manufacturing PCBs; in the process biphenyls are chlorinated with anhydrous chlorine, with either iron filings or ferric chloride as the catalyst.

The commercial PCBs are very complex mixtures. For example, Aroclor 1260 contains 11 isomers, 5 containing 6 chlorine atoms, 5 containing 7 and 1 containing 8, and Aroclor 1254 was found to contain 18 compounds, 1 containing 3 chlorine atoms, 4 containing 4 chlorines, 4 containing 5 chlorines, 5 containing 6 chlorines, and 4 containing 7 chlorines.

An estimate of the global production (Risebrough and DeLappe, 1972), including PCBs manufactured in the United States, Western Europe, and the Soviet Union, is on the order of 10^{11} g/yr, equivalent to the production of DDT. U.S. production has been the most extensive 1960 through 1971, amounting to ~ 353,000 short tons of PCBs (Monsanto Industrial Chemicals, 1971).

The largest categories of use of PCBs (Fishbein, 1973) have been in capacitors and transformers (as dielectrics) and in certain "plasticizer" applications, including carbonless duplicating paper. The major uses of PCBs before 1970, in order of importance in terms of volume of material used, were in capacitors, plasticizer applications, transformer fluids, hydraulic fluids and lubricants, and heat transfer fluids. They were also used in machine tool cutting oils; high-vacuum oils; specialized lubricants; gasket sealers; epoxy paints; resins; chlorinated rubber; printing inks; waxes; synthetic adhesives; textile dyes; protective coatings for wood, metal, and concretes; sealers in waterproofing compounds; and putty. PCBs have also been incorporated in pesticide formulations, especially in DDVP (dichlorvos), lindane, chlordane, aldrin, dieldrin, and toxaphene, to suppress vaporization and thus extend the "kill-life" of the pesticides, and they have been shown to increase the insecticidal properties of DDT (Lichtenstein et al., 1969).

Risebrough and DeLappe (1972) and Nisbet and Sarafim (1972) recently reviewed the rates and routes of transport of PCBs in the environment (Fig. 2). As with most industrial chemicals, loss figures for PCBs are practically nonexistent. The possible routes into the atmosphere include (1) vaporization from PCB manufacturing and formulation processes and (2) incineration and combustion of PCB-containing products (incineration at 2,000°F or above for 2 sec destroys PCBs, but poorly operated incinerators burning openly may release PCBs into the atmosphere unchanged).

It is estimated that 1,500–2,500 tons/yr of PCBs is emitted into the atmosphere, mainly by vaporization and open burning, resulting in a concentration in urban areas of 50–80 ppm. The rate of terrestrial net input of PCBs through serial fallout in North America will be a little less than the rate of vaporization (about 1,000–2,000 tons/yr). Since the vapor pressure of Aroclor 1254, the dominant airborne PCB commercial mixture, is close to that of DDE, it is estimated, by analogy with DDE, that the half-life of PCBs in soil is on the order of 5 yr (Edwards, 1970).

Aspects of PCB atmospheric concentration and transport over the northeast United States and the North Atlantic and over Iceland were reported by Harvey and Steinhauer (1974) and Bengtson and Sodergren (1974), respectively.

The modes of transport of the PCBs within the environment are complex. For example, vaporized PCBs can be partially absorbed on particulates, transported with the prevailing wind, and deposited on land or in water by particle sedimentation or rain-out; PCBs introduced into water streams can be adsorbed by the waterborne particulates, after which the adsorbed PCBs will diffuse into the bottom sediment, redissolve in the water stream, or be entwined with sediment eroded from the bottom surface. The assimilation, transport, and degradation of PCBs by the biota further complicates the problem.

Hammond (1972) estimated that the escape into the atmosphere and entrance into the waterways of PCBs (with an annual production of roughly 5×10^7 kg/yr) amounted to thousands of tons per year.

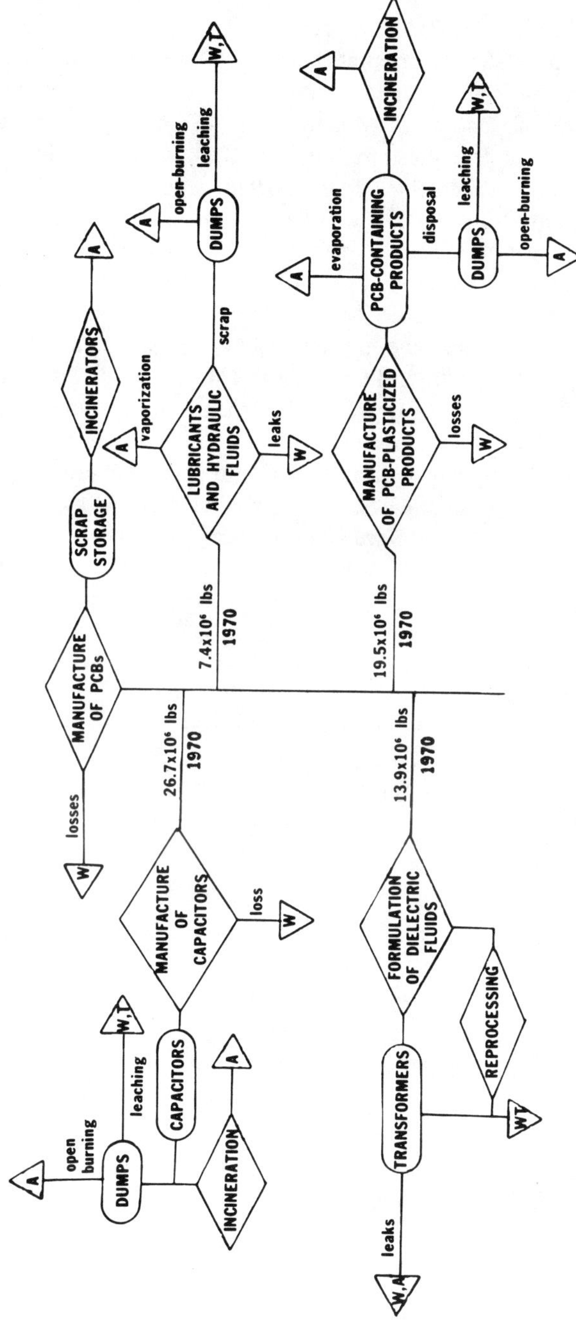

FIGURE 2 Possible routes of loss of PCBs into the environment.

Moilanen and Crosby (1973) recently reported that DDT may be a source of PCBs (Maugh, 1973). For example, it was shown that DDT vapor can be converted to PCBs by irradiation with UV light of the wavelengths present in sunlight in the lower atmosphere (Fig. 3). Extrapolated to the atmosphere, the overall scheme of Moilanen and Crosby (1973) predicts that DDT vapor is converted to small amounts of DDD, which should accumulate in the biosphere, and to a great deal more DDE, which should degrade more slowly than DDT. In turn, DDE vapor is converted at a moderate rate to dichlorobenzophenone [via DDMU: 1-chloro-2, 2-bis(*p*-chlorophenyl)ethylene], and then at a much slower rate to dichlorobiphenyl. Some of the DDE is also converted to 3,6-dichlorofluorenone (whose environmental fate is unknown) and to small amounts of di-, tri-, and tetrachlorobiphenyls. Degradation of DDT vapor as suggested by Moilanen and Crosby (1973) could have profound implications for the fate of pesticides in the environment. For example, atmospheric degradation of DDT by sunlight was considered to be unimportant compared to transport, although the residence time of DDT in the atmosphere is estimated to be approximately 4 yr. It was suggested by Moilanen and Crosby (1973) that much of the DDT and DDE may have been converted to other chemicals, whose presence in the environment would not be attributed to DDT and DDE because of the other sources of these products. It is important to note that although DDE and DDT should be accumulating in the biosphere, since 2.8×10^9 kg of DDT have been dispersed since the early 1940s, global models of pesticide

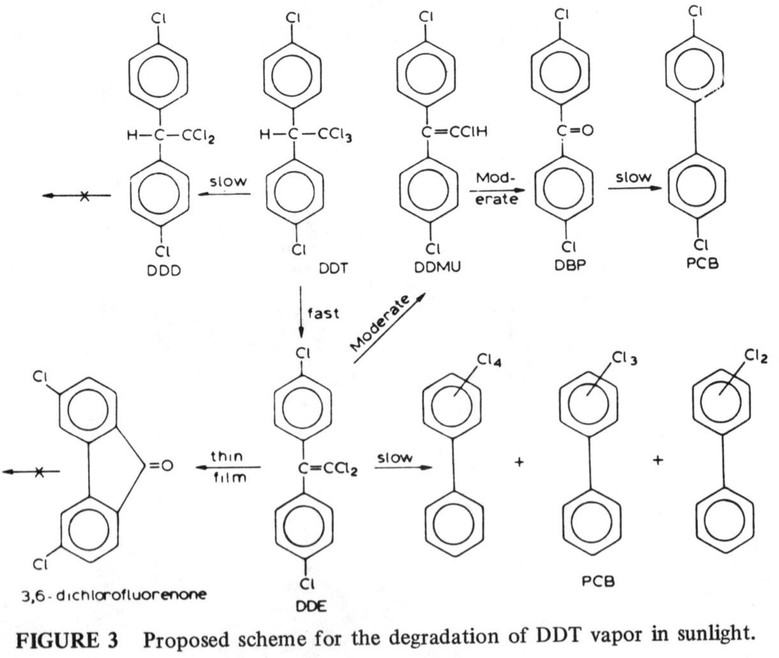

FIGURE 3 Proposed scheme for the degradation of DDT vapor in sunlight.

transport and monitoring of pesticide residues can account for only a small fraction of that amount.

The toxicity of the chlorinated biphenyls has been reviewed by Fishbein (1974a) with particular focus on their carcinogenic, teratogenic, and mutagenic effects. It is important to restress the fact that PCBs are complex mixtures, and there is a paucity of data unequivocally relating a toxic event to a specific chlorinated biphenyl isomer per se.

Peakall et al. (1972) reported that embryos from the second generation of ring doves (*Streptopelia risoria*) fed 10 ppm Aroclor 1254 exhibited a high frequency of chromosomal aberrations and a high incidence of embryonic death.

No chromosomal aberrations were observed in human lymphocyte cultures exposed to Aroclor 1254 at 100 ppm (Hoopingarner et al., 1972), and Keplinger et al. (1971), employing a dominant lethal assay, reported no evidence of mutagenic effects of a number of Aroclors.

Green et al. (1973) described the cytogenetic effects of Aroclor 1242 on rat bone marrow and spermatogonial cells. Aroclor 1242 was administered to albino Osborne-Mendel rats as an acute dosage (po) at 5,000, 2,500, and 1,250 mg/kg or as a subacute regimen at 500 mg/kg and as a solution in corn oil at the other levels.

The results of the bone marrow study showed no significant increases in chromosomal abnormalities or inhibition of cell division. The study of spermatogonial cells showed significant decreases in the number of dividing spermatogonial cells ($p > 0.05$). This effect was noted at 500 X 4 and 500 X 1 dosages. It was concluded that Aroclor 1242 does not produce chromosomal abnormalities in rat bone marrow or spermatogonia, but does cause, at relatively high doses, a decrease in the number of dividing spermatogonial cells.

No discussion of the PCBs in an environmental context would be complete without considering their toxic impurities. For example, Vos et al. (1970) and Vos and Koeman (1970) identified tetra- and pentachlorodibenzofurans and hexa- and heptachloronaphthalenes in commercial lots of PCBs (e.g., Phenoclor DP-6 and Clophen A-60, produced in Germany and France, respectively). Vos and Beems (1971) suggested on toxicological grounds that small quantities of toxic impurities may also be present in Aroclor samples. It is conceivable that chlorinated dibenzofurans are produced from PCBs in the environment. Two possible mechanisms for such transformations involve hydroxy derivatives as intermediates as follows:

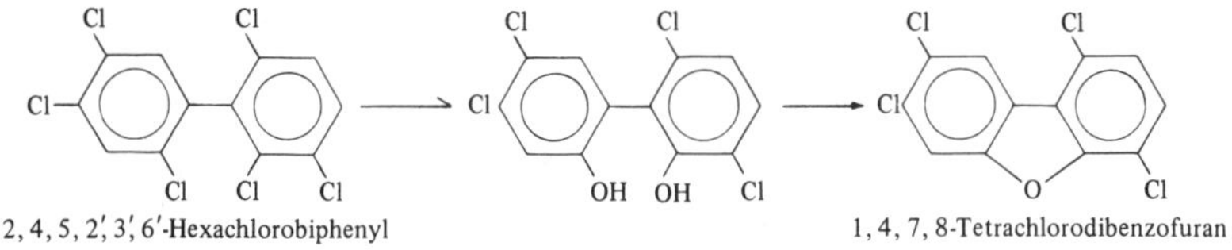

2, 4, 5, 2', 3', 6'-Hexachlorobiphenyl

1, 4, 7, 8-Tetrachlorodibenzofuran

Hydroxylation is a very likely route of metabolism of PCBs. Ring-hydroxylated metabolites of PCBs as well as polar oxygenated compounds have been reported as photolytic products of PCBs. It should be noted that transformation of only 0.002% of a major constituent of an Aroclor mixture to the corresponding chlorinated dibenzofurans would produce concentrations in the mixture corresponding to the values reported by Vos et al. (1970) and Vos and Koeman (1970) as toxicologically significant.

Chlorodioxins. Chlorodioxins (polychlorinated dibenzo-*p*-dioxins) include a large number of compounds (some extremely toxic) that occur primarily as contaminants in technical products such as tri-, tetra-, and pentachlorophenol and a number of other related products. 2,3,7,8-Tetrachlorodibenzo-*p*-*p*-dioxin (TCDD) or other chlorinated dibenzodioxins or chlorinated dibenzofurans may be present in the waste products from chlorination of benzenes, phenols, and polyphenyls since traces have been found in the commercial products (Carter et al., 1975; Kimbrough, 1974; Villaneuva et al., 1974).

TCDD has been the focus of intensive investigations, primarily since its detection in some samples of the herbicide 2,4,5-trichlorophenoxyacetic acid (2,4,5-T) and disclosure of its potent teratogenicity in certain mammals.

As little as 1–10 µg/kg TCDD has been found to be lethal for rabbits (Sparschau et al., 1971). The LD50 of 2,4,5-T containing less than 0.05–0.1 ppm TCDD and administered to mice at 35–130 mg/kg caused both embryotoxic and teratogenic effects (cleft palate) (Roll, 1971), and the LD50 of TCDD in the guinea pig is 0.6 µg/kg (Milnes, 1971).

Jackson (1972) reported that solutions of 0.2 ppb TCDD caused inhibition of mitosis and cytological abnormalities in cells of the African blood lily (*Haemanthus* Kathrinae Baker).

The mutagenic effects of TCDD on bacterial systems have been reported by Hussain et al. (1972). High mutagenic frequencies were observed in *S. typhimurium* strain TA1532, which is known to revert by frameshift mutation. This would indicate that an acridinelike behavior causes the genetic effects of TCDD. It was noted that the strong mutagenic action of TCDD (apparently as a consequence of intercalation) and the efficient induction of microsomal hydroxylases could explain the extraordinarily high toxicity of this compound.

The dioxins found in contaminated samples of 2,4,5-T and in the chlorophenols are formed during the manufacturing process (Fig. 4). During

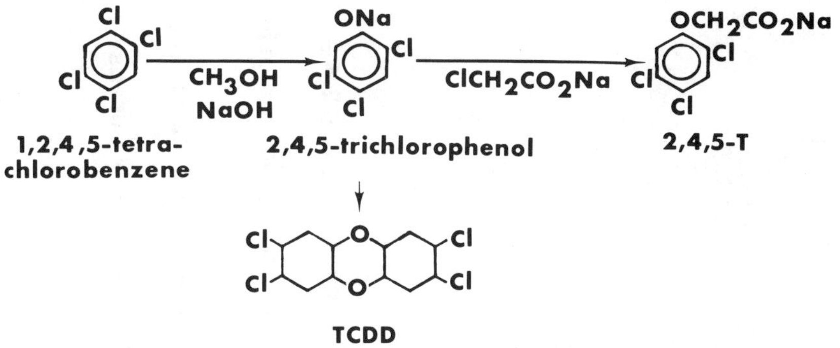

FIGURE 4   Formation of 2,3,7,8-tetrachlorodibenzo-p-dioxin (TCDD) as a by-product in the synthesis of 2,4,5-T.

the process, a reaction between two molecules of 2,4,5-trichlorophenol may occur, resulting in the formation of TCDD. Samples of 2,4,5-T produced by one manufacturer during 1966–1968 often contained $>$ 10 ppm TCDD. More recent samples contain $<$ 0.5 ppm TCDD (Helling et al., 1973). However, TCDD levels as high as 30 ppm in 2,4,5-T have been reported (Jensen and Renberg, 1972). The conditions that enhance TCDD formation are high temperature, high pressure, and alkalinity. The same sort of conditions are necessary for the production of pentachlorophenol (PCP) when hexachlorobenzene is used as the starting material (Fig. 5, reaction 2). Under these conditions, both the dioxins and the chlorinated furans may be formed (Jensen and Renberg, 1972). Alternatively, the chlorophenols can be prepared by direct chlorination of chlorine and phenol (Fig. 5, reaction 3). Application of excessive heat during the manufacture of tetra- and pentachlorophenol can result in the formation of highly chlorinated dioxins.

Accidental production of TCDD as the result of exothermic reaction at a chemical plant in Derbyshire, Great Britain, engaged in the production of 2,4,5-trichlorophenol has been recently reported (May, 1973). Seventy-nine cases of chloracne were recorded following this incident, which were found to be directly related to TCDD produced as a reaction product of the sodium salt of trichlorophenol when the temperature was in excess of $\sim$ 225–250°C.

Kimming and Schulz (1957), Bauer et al. (1940), and Schulz (1968) have described in detail not only chloracne but all the toxic reactions attributed to the chlorinated dioxin, which include liver damage, emphysema, myocardial degeneration, elevated blood pressure, renal damage, reflex irregularities, depression, disturbances of memory sond concentration, and so on. While one human death from pulmonary carcinoma has been rejected as being attributable to chlorinated dioxin exposure, one of intestinal sarcoma has been accepted (May, 1973). It was considered that the dioxin passed into the system by oral inhalation as well as transdermally following exposure during trichlorophenol manufacture.

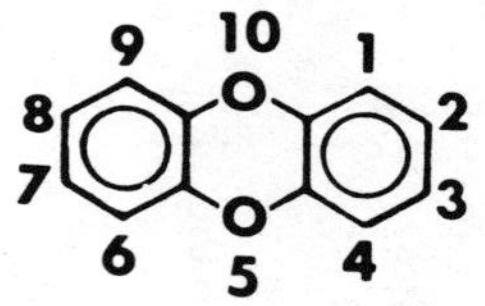

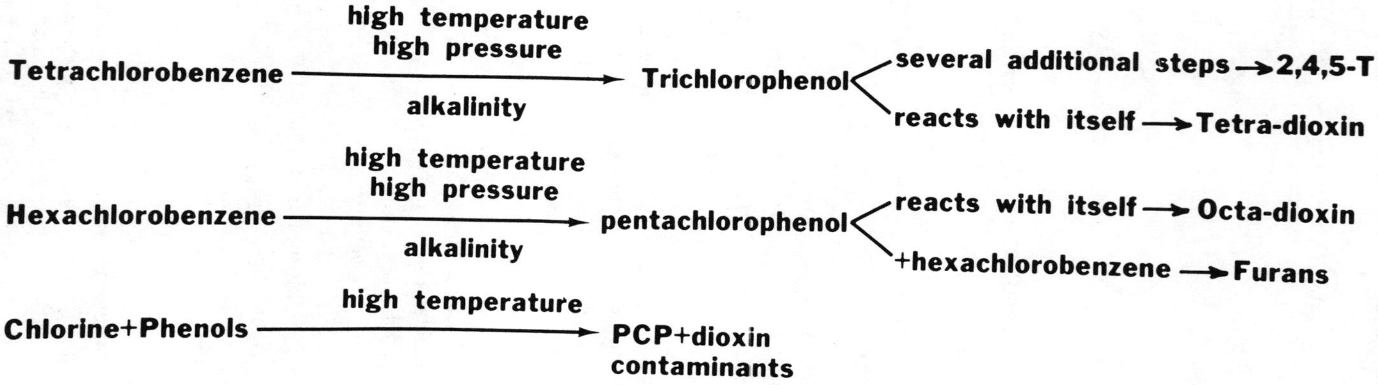

FIGURE 5 Formation of dioxins and furans.

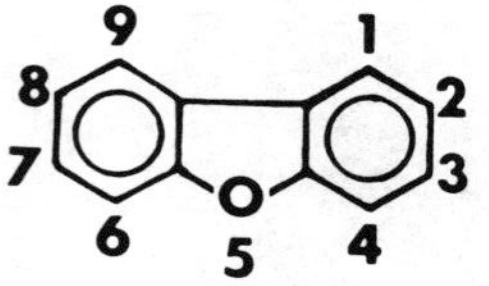

Haloethers. The α-haloethers are highly reactive alkylating agents that have been widely used in industry, primarily as intermediates in organic synthesis (Summers, 1955). They are used in the formulation of water repellents and other textile-treating agents, preparation of ion-exchange resins, and manufacture of polymers and as solvents for polymerization reactions (Summers, 1955; Van Duuren et al., 1968).

The haloethers represent a category of alkylating carcinogens, as well as potential mutagens of increasing interest (Fig. 6). Chloromethyl methyl ether (CMME) has been shown to be a potent tumor initiator (Van Duuren et al., 1968) and induces malignant tumors of the respiratory tract in strain A mice (Leong et al., 1971) and rats and hamsters exposed to 1 ppm for 6 hrs/day, 5 days/wk, throughout their lifetime (Laskin et al., 1975). Comparable studies with bis(chloromethyl) ether (BCME) (Kuschner et al., 1975) have indicated a much higher incidence of tumors induced at one-tenth the concentration of CMME. Since commercial grade CMME may be contaminated with levels of BCME ranging from 1 to 7%, the carcinogenicity demonstrated in rats and hamsters (Laskin et al., 1975) may well reflect the levels of BCME in the CMME preparation used. It should also be noted that hydrolysis of CMME can yield HCl and CH_2O, which can recombine to form BCME. Hence, in operational terms, it was stressed by Laskin et al. (1975) that commercial grade CMME must be considered a carcinogen, albeit of a lower order of activity than BCME.

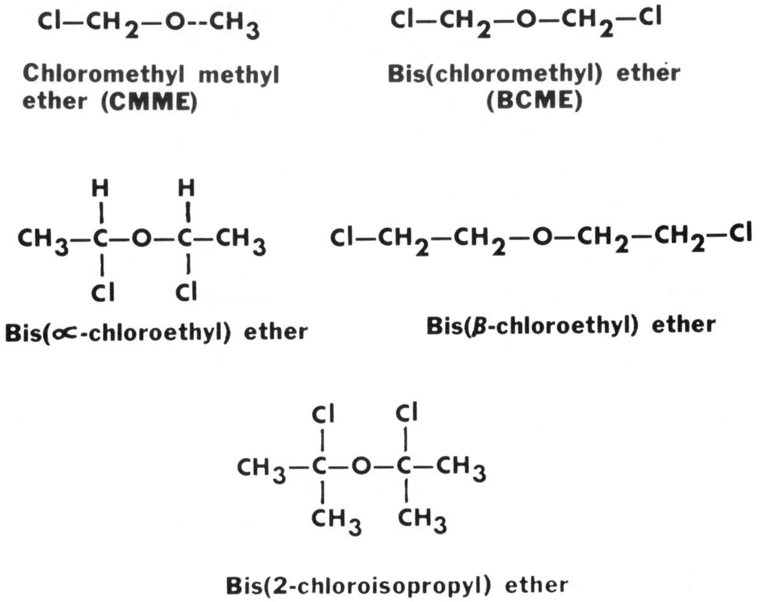

$$Cl-CH_2-O--CH_3 \qquad\qquad Cl-CH_2-O-CH_2-Cl$$

Chloromethyl methyl ether (CMME)   **Bis(chloromethyl) ether (BCME)**

$$CH_3-\underset{\underset{Cl}{|}}{\overset{\overset{H}{|}}{C}}-O-\underset{\underset{Cl}{|}}{\overset{\overset{H}{|}}{C}}-CH_3 \qquad\qquad Cl-CH_2-CH_2-O-CH_2-CH_2-Cl$$

Bis(α-chloroethyl) ether   **Bis(β-chloroethyl) ether**

$$CH_3-\underset{\underset{CH_3}{|}}{\overset{\overset{Cl}{|}}{C}}-O-\underset{\underset{CH_3}{|}}{\overset{\overset{Cl}{|}}{C}}-CH_3$$

Bis(2-chloroisopropyl) ether

FIGURE 6   Structures of haloethers.

BCME has been shown to be a highly potent initiator and complete carcinogen when painted on the skin of mice (Van Duuren et al., 1968) or when administered to mice and rats (Van Duuren et al., 1968, 1969). The induction of lung adenomas by ip injection of BCME in newborn mice (Gargus et al., 1969) and by inhalation (Leong et al., 1971) and the induction of squamous carcinomas of the lung and esthesioneuroepitheliomas in rats by inhalation exposure to BCME (Laskin et al., 1975; Kuschner et al., 1975) have all been reported. In the latter study of Kuschner et al. (1975), tumors of the lung and nasal cavity were produced in male Sprague-Dawley rats at relatively high incidence levels by exposures at the 0.1-ppm level.

The extremely low levels employed and the magnitude of the cancer response with BCME clearly implicate this compound as an extremely potent respiratory carcinogen (Kuschner et al., 1975). A number of recent human epidemiologic studies appear to reinforce this view. Wagoner (1972) found atypical cells in a spectrum of BCME-exposed workers. BCME has been implicated in fatal lung cancers in four employees of an ion-exchange plant in California (Fishbein, 1972). Five cases of lung cancer among 32 workers in Japan exposed to BCME over a 15-yr period have been reported (Sakabe, 1973). Von Thiess et al. (1973) cited an incidence of 6 cases of lung cancer among 18 individuals employed in the laboratory of the research division of a plant in Germany during the period 1954–1967, with 2 additional cases noted among 50 workers in the plant itself.

An increased incidence of lung cancer (about eightfold) has been reported among men exposed to CMME at a chemical manufacturing plant (Figuerova et al., 1973). All had worked as chemical operators in the same building at the chemical plant, where they mixed formalin, methanol, and hydrochloric acid in two 3,800-l kettles to produce CMME. (During the process fumes were often visible, and to check for losses the lids on the kettles were raised several times during each shift.) Both BCME and CMME are now recognized by the U.S. Occupational Safety and Health Administration (1974) as human carcinogens.

There has been conflicting information about the formation of BCME by spontaneous reactions between HCl and formaldehyde in both the gas and the liquid phase. For example, it was reported by the Rohm & Haas Co. in the United States that gaseous formaldehyde and HCl reversibly combine in moist air to form BCME (Rohm & Haas, 1972). For example, it was found that at a room temperature of about 70°F and a relative humidity of 40%, a steady-state level of BCME is reached in less than 1 min. Formaldehyde and HCl can also react rapidly in aqueous and nonaqueous liquid-phase systems to form BCME. In fact, the observation has been made that BCME is formed in Friedel-Crafts reactions of formaldehyde whenever aluminum chloride, zinc chloride, stannous or stannic chloride, or ferric chloride is used as the condensing agent. Other BCME-generating conditions can also arise. For example, BCME has been found above a waste solution from the neutralization of the sodium hydroxide catalyst in phenol-formaldehyde resin manufacture. The base had been neutralized with sulfuric acid and no HCl had been intentionally added anywhere in the process. Its source is believed to be the sodium chloride impurity frequently found in technical grades of caustic acid.

Kallos and Solomon (1973), however, recently reported that mixtures of HCl and formaldehyde in moist air do not form BCME at a detection limit of 0.1 ppb, even with the reactants at their threshold limit values—100 ppm each. However, low parts-per-billion levels of BCME were formed when higher concentrations of these reactants (e.g., 500–300 ppm) were present together in moist air.

Tou and Kallos (1974) recently reported that BCME was not observed in the aqueous or the gas phase (with detection limits of 9 and 1 ppb, respectively) when aqueous HCl and formaldehyde were reacted together at concentrations up to 2,000 ppm at ambient temperature for 18 hr. It was also suggested that BCME could not be present at even a much lower level than 9 ppb in *aqueous solution* (Tou and Kallos, 1974).

However, the formation of BCME should still be considered a possibility whenever formaldehyde is used, since HCl might arise from unexpected sources, as described above, and reaction conditions (both gaseous and aqueous) may prevail to facilitate its formation.

NIOSH has confirmed (*Chemical & Engineering News*, 1975c) the spontaneous formation of BCME from the reaction of formaldehyde and HCl in some textile plants and is now investigating the possible extent of worker exposure to the carcinogen.

The utility of both formaldehyde and HCl is enormous. These compounds can be generated in the processing of other products. Examples other than the extensively used Friedel-Crafts reactions are the treatment of cotton fabrics to improve wash-and-wear properties and wrinkle recovery; the preparation of flameproofing agents such as tetrakis (hydroxymethyl) phosphonium chloride; and the manufacture of agents such as ion-exchange resins, bactericides, dispersing agents, water repellents, and pesticidal synergists such as piperonyl butoxide. BCME is formulated by addition of a chlorine side chain to polystyrene. It is widely used as a chloromethylating agent in organic synthesis.

The α-haloethers are much more reactive than their isomeric β or α isomers in which the halogen atom is situated one or two carbon atoms away from the oxygen-bearing carbon. Because of the high reactivity of these compounds, they have been widely employed in laboratory and industrial syntheses as intermediates in the treatment of textiles, in the manufacture of polymers, as insecticides, as solvents for industrial polymerization reactions, and in the preparation of ion-exchange resins. Kleupfer and Fairless (1972) recently detected a major organic contaminant, bis(2-chloroisopropyl) ether among 40 organic compounds in municipal drinking-water at Evansville, Indiana. The probable source of this haloether was found to be an industrial outfall located about 150 river miles upstream on the Ohio River from the Evansville water intake. The actual concentrations found in the Ohio River at Evansville ranged from 0.5 to 5 µg/l (August and September, 1971). The concentration found in the Ohio River just above the suspected industrial outfall was less than 0.2 µg/l. Bis(2-chloroisopropyl) ether and bis(2-chloroethyl) ether appear to be rather widespread pollutants in the rivers of our nation. In addition to the Ohio River, the compounds have also been found in the Kanawha River at Nitro, West Virginia (Rosen et al., 1963) and in the Mississippi River at New Orleans.

The haloethers are by-products in the manufacture of propylene glycol and ethylene glycol, which are prepared in enormous quantities. Bis(2-chloroethyl) ether is extensively used in the paint and varnish industry as a solvent for many resins, including glyceryl phthalate resins, ester gums, paraffin, gum camphor, castor, linseed and other fatty oils, turpentine, polyvinyl acetate, and ethyl cellulose. It is also used as a solvent for rubber or cellulose esters, but only in the presence of 10–30% alcohol. In the textile industry, it is used for grease-spotting and the removal of paint and tar brand marks from raw wool and is incorporated in scouring and fueling soaps. It is also used as an extractant for lubricating oils in the petroleum industry and as a soil insecticide (fumigant).

Innes et al. (1969) reported the induction of hepatomas in mice fed bis(2-chloroethyl) ether. Bis(2-chloroethyl) ether has been found to be mutagenic in *Drosophila* (Auerbach et al., 1947).

Recent studies (Collier, 1972) indicate that BCME is stable in air at 10 and 100 ppm at 70% relative humidity for at least 18 hr. As a class, α-haloethers are highly reactive; they can react with water, alcohols, amines, proteins, sulfhydryl groups, and so on. This high chemical reactivity is due to the reactivity of the halogen atom in displacement reactions. Van Duuren et al. (1972) have suggested that the α-haloethers be classed with biologically active compounds such as the alkylating agents—for example, nitrogen mustards and epoxide-β-lactones.

Chlorine and chlorinolysis. Approximately 250 million lb of chlorinated hydrocarbon by-products, known as still-bottom material, accumulate each year from organic chemical manufacturing in the United States (Collier, 1972). In addition, the armed forces have accumulated tremendous stockpiles of chlorinated hydrocarbon pesticides [e.g., 24.5 million lb of the defoliant herbicide Orange (a 50-50 mixture of the *n*-butyl esters of 2,4-dichlorophenoxyacetic acid and 2,4,5-trichlorophenoxyacetic acid), 2,4,5-T, DDT, etc.]. Earlier attempts to dispose of these materials by landfill, ocean dispersal, and deep-well injection have proved unsound (*Environmental Science and Technology*, 1974).

A procedure that has been recommended for the decomposition of these materials is chlorinolysis, whereby chlorine is added to the chemical residues, producing high yields of carbon tetrachloride, hydrochloric acid, and carbonyl chloride, as follows:

HCB $\text{C}_6\text{Cl}_6 + \text{Cl}_2 \longrightarrow \text{CCl}_4$

DDT $(\text{ClC}_6\text{H}_4)_2\text{CH-CCl}_3 + \text{Cl}_2 \longrightarrow \text{CCl}_4 + \text{HCl}$

2, 4, 5-T $\text{Cl}_3\text{C}_6\text{H}_2\text{-O-CO-CH}_3 + \text{Cl}_2 \longrightarrow \text{CCl}_4 + \text{HCl} + \text{COCl}_2$

Catalysts are not required for the high-temperature, low-pressure or high-pressure, low-temperature processes, but special reactor materials are necessary to accommodate the highly corrosive reaction products.

More recent concerns have been raised about the use of chlorination as a disinfecting technique (Piecuch, 1974). An estimated 1,000 tons of chlorinated organic compounds, some of them known to induce cancer in laboratory animals (e.g., chloroform and carbon tetrachloride) is discharged annually into U.S. waterways as a result of the chlorination of wastewater. (It should be noted that the wastewater industry relies almost exclusively on chlorine as a disinfectant.) Recent EPA studies have indicated the presence of small quantities of 66 organic chemicals (many of them chlorinated hydrocarbons) in the nation's drinking-water supply (Train, 1974). For example, concentrations of carbon tetrachloride and chloroform in the parts-per-billion range were detected in the municipal drinking water of Cincinnati and New Orleans (*Environmental Science and Technology*, 1974).

Within the typical ranges of pH (5–9) found during the course of most water treatment processes, the active chlorine species could range from entirely hypochlorite ($^-$OCl) to entirely hypochlorous acid (HOCl, $pK_a = 7.5$ at 20°C). It has been noted that chlorine is more readily incorporated into aromatic systems at lower pH values (Liberles, 1968). This parallels the observation of increasing disinfection capability with decreasing pH (White,

1972). Although the active chlorinating species has not yet been unambiguously determined, it is known not to be the Cl^+ ion (Swain and Crist, 1972).

Carlson et al. (1975) described the facile incorporation of chlorine into aromatic systems during aqueous chlorination processes utilized for water renovation. The extent of chlorine incorporation varies with pH and contact time. The extent of chlorine incorporation into monosubstituted aromatics followed well-recognized precepts, whereby aromatics containing "activating" groups such as hydroxyl, ether, amine, or alkyl groups underwent electrophilic aromatic substitution faster than those containing "deactivating" groups such as nitro, chloro, nitrile, and carbonyl groups (DeLaMare and Ridd, 1959; Gaffney, 1974). The biphenyl nucleus was found to incorporate chlorine under a variety of aqueous conditions, with the extent of chlorobiphenyl production depending on pH. Substantial amounts of higher chlorinated isomers were found at increased chlorine concentrations. It is important to stress the fact that under a wide range of aqueous chlorination conditions, the relatively unactivated biphenyl nucleus can be chlorinated, affording the possibility of production of PCBs at waste treatment facilities known to receive biphenyl (Gaffney, 1974). The results of the studies of Carlson et al. (1975) seem particularly significant when it is realized that the chlorinated materials remain after any subsequent standard reductive process, such as treatment with SO_2 for chloramine removal.

Chromosomal effects of chlorine on mammalian cells *in vitro* have been reported by Mickey and Holden (1971). Concentrations of chlorine > 25 ppm produced significantly more chromosome aberrations and endomitotic figures than were observed in controls, and at still higher levels completely inhibited mitosis. The mammalian cells examined were human lymphocytes, Chinese hamster cells, and muntjac cells.

When human lymphocyte cultures were exposed to chlorine at concentrations > 10 ppm, chromatid and chromosome breaks, translocations, dicentric chromosomes, and gaps increased in general with increasing concentrations of chlorine.

The interpretation of these results in terms of an *in vivo* situation is apparently difficult. The concentrations of chlorine utilized in the studies of Mickey and Holden (1971) were higher than those in most drinking water. The efficacy of chlorination depends on the content of free or residual chlorine in the water. Chlorine dosages usually range from 1.2 to 3.6 ppm, but tests of some city water supplies have shown higher concentrations (e.g., 10 ppm) (Mickey and Holden, 1971).

Sodium hypochlorite (NaOCl), which is widely used in industry as an oxidizing agent as well as in households as a bleach and cleanser, has been shown by Wlodkowski and Rosenkranz (1975) to induce base-substitution mutations in *S. typhimurium* TA1530.

Rosenkranz (1973) has also demonstrated that sodium hypochlorite is a preferential inhibitor of DNA polymerase-deficient bacteria (*Escherichia coli, pol* A$_1^-$ strain). The mechanism of action of sodium hypochlorite and the basis of its reaction with DNA remains to be elucidated. Presumably it involves attack of pyrimidine residues across the 5,6 double bond to yield 6-hydroxy-5-chloro-5,6-dihydropyrimidines (Rosenkranz, 1973).

Bromoalkanes. Although the chlorinated hydrocarbons are of primary importance in any environmental health consideration, a number of bromoalkanes are of analogous interest because of their use in antiknock compounds, pesticides, and fumigants. It is especially the latter use area that is of concern because of the possibility of significant losses to the atmosphere and other environmental sinks.

The major bromoalkanes used in fumigants are methyl bromide, ethylene dibromide (EDB; 1,2-dibromoethane; $BrCH_2CH_2Br$), and 1,2-dibromo-3-chloropropane (DBCP; $BrCH_2CHBrCH_2Cl$). At least 8.6 million lb of DBCP and well over 200 million lb of EDB were produced in the United States in 1969 and 1970, respectively (Stanford Research Institute, 1972).

All commercial fumigants are physically or chemically sorbed, the amount depending on the nature and amount of fumigant used, gas-air concentrations, nature of the substrates, moisture content, periods of exposure, and so on (Berck, 1966, 1974; Dumas, 1973; Dumas and Bond, 1975; Brown et al., 1974). Although the major concern has been about fumigant residues per se, as well as degradation products, halohydrins, inorganic bromide, etc., on crops and derived foods (e.g., wheat, flour, bread), it should be noted that the presence of bromine vapors (possibly hydrogen bromide) has been reported in the stratosphere (*Chemical & Engineering News*, 1975). (This may have arisen from the use of bromine compounds in fumigants, gasoline, or the plastics industry.) Information is lacking as to the possible levels of unreacted bromoalkane fumigants in the atmosphere and their transport, although their presence cannot be discounted a priori.

Induction of stomach cancer in rats and mice following chronic oral intubation of EDB and DBCP was reported by Olson et al. (1973). It was suggested that in either EDP or DBCP the bromine atoms are activated so that the compounds probably act as alkylating agents. Current concepts implicate alkylation of DNA, RNA, or other macromolecular cell constituents as one mechanism of carcinogenesis (Miller and Miller, 1971), as well as mutagenesis (Brem et al., 1974).

It has been suggested by Olson et al. (1973) that chronic exposure to either EDB or DBCP could be a health hazard. This would be most pertinent to agricultural and food-storage workers, who disperse these volatile materials through soil or food (the hazard to such workers would probably be largely through inhalation and not through oral exposure).

Ethylene dibromide has been shown to induce *ad-3* mutants in a two-component heterokaryon of *Neurospora crassa* (de Serres and Malling, 1969). Sparrow et al. (1974) described the mutagenicity of EDB in the *Tradescantia* plant test system. EDB gave good dose-response relationships with surface exposures as low as 3.6 ppm [compared to 5 ppm with ethyl methanesulfonate (EMS)]. The genetic basis for the phenotypic changes observed (pink and colorless) is not definitely known, but may be associated with chromosome breakage, gene mutation, chromosome nondisjunction, or somatic crossing-over.

EDB and 1,1-dibromoethane have been shown to be mutagenic for *S. typhimurium* TA1530 and preferentially to inhibit the growth of DNA polymerase-deficient (*pol A$^-_1$*) *E. coli* (Brem et al., 1974). Tessman (1971) reported the induction of transversions and transitions in phage S13 by 1,1-dibromoethane.

Bromoethanol (a potential residue of both ethylene oxide and ethylene dibromide fumigation) has been shown to be mutagenic for *Klebsiella pneumoniae* (Voogd and Vander Vet, 1969) and *S. typhimurium* TA1530 (Rosenkranz et al., 1974) and to inhibit the growth of DNA polymerase-deficient *E. coli* (Rosenkranz et al., 1974).

Fluorine (fluoride). Although fluoride is ubiquitous in the human environment, and its beneficial effects (e.g., reduction of dental cavities) have been known for four decades, airborne fluoride in dusts and gases from both natural and industrial sources can have harmful effects on vegetation, in cattle and other animals, and in humans, primarily by industrial exposure.

Appreciable amounts of gaseous and solid fluorides are discharged into the atmosphere by active volcanoes and fumaroles. In addition to hydrogen fluoride, one of the principal fluoride emissions, many products have been identified, including ammonium fluoride, silicon tetrafluoride, ammonium fluorosilicate [$(NH_4)_2 SiF_6$], and potassium fluoroborate (KBF_4).

Fluoride dusts and gases are emitted to the atmosphere in considerable quantities by a variety of industrial operations, as well as by combustion of coal. The magnitudes of fluoride emissions (in tons per year) in 1968 in the United States (totaling 118,700 tons) from a variety of manufacturing operations were: normal superphosphate fertilizer, 9,700; wet-process phosphoric acid, 3,000; triple superphosphate fertilizer, 300; diammonium phosphate fertilizer, 100; elemental phosphorus, 5,500; phosphate animal feed, 100; aluminum, 16,000; steel (open-hearth furnace), 14,900; brick and tile products, 18,500; glass and frit, 2,700; welding operations, 2,700; nonferrous metal foundries, 18,500; and combustion of coal, 16,000 [National Academy of Sciences (NAS),1971a]. Silicon tetrafluoride (SiF_4) and HF are the chief gas pollutants emitted to the atmosphere in many of these manufacturing processes, such as the production of various phosphate fertilizers.

The manufacture of aluminum [in which alumina is dissolved in molten cryolite ($Na_3 AlF_6$) and reduced electrolytically] contributes significant amounts of gaseous pollutants, including CO, CO_2, SO_2, SiF_4, HF, COS, and CS_2, and hydrocarbons and particulate emissions such as cryolite, alumina, aluminum fluoride, calcium fluoride, chiolite ($Na_5 Al_3 F_{14}$), and $Fe_2 O_3$. Fluorides constitute only a small fraction of all the fumes produced in the manufacture of steel, and are believed to consist chiefly of calcium fluoride and hydrogen fluoride.

Clays used in the manufacture of brick, tile, pottery, and cement generally contain 0.02–0.3% fluorine in the form of hydrated micas such as muscovite and illite. During the firing process (to $\sim 1,100°C$), gaseous HF and SiF_4 are liberated. Estimates of the amounts released in brickmaking, for example, range from ~ 30 to 95% of the fluorine originally present (Semrau, 1957), with gases and dusts from the kilns usually being discharged into the atmosphere without any cleanup.

Samples of coal from various parts of the world have been found to contain 0.001–0.048% fluoride, usually as fluorapatite or fluorspar (Abernethy and Gibson, 1963). An average fluoride content of 0.008% has been found in coal samples from 83 mines in the United States (Abernethy and Gibson, 1967). During combustion, about half the fluoride in the coal is evolved as gaseous HF, SiF_4, and particulate matter. Most of the emissions occur in coal-burning electric power plants.

The manufacture of fluorides constitutes another potential source of loss of fluorides to the atmosphere. In the production of HF by heating fluorspar with sulfuric acid, such gases as SO_2, SiF_4, and CO_2 are produced in addition to HF by decomposition of impurities in the fluorspar. In 1968, about 40% of all HF manufactured in the United States was converted into fluorocarbon compounds and products, including dichlorodifluoromethane (CF_2Cl_2), trichlorofluoromethane ($CFCl_3$), tetrafluoromethane (CF_4), tetrafluoroethylene (C_2F_4), vinyl fluoride (C_2H_3F), and hexafluoropropylene (C_3F_6), and the products include many polymers derived from these and similar compounds (NAS, 1971a).

Hydrogen fluoride is also widely used in the petroleum industry as an alkylation catalyst for producing high-octane gasolines (BF_3 and HF plus BF_3 are also used for this purpose). Volatile fluorides may be released to the atmosphere during loading and unloading operations (e.g., during purging of transfer lines from tank cars) and during disposal of waste products.

Fluoride emissions (e.g., gaseous HF, SiF_4, and particulate fluorides) from welding in shipyards and fabricating plants have been noted when coated electrodes are used (Hanslian and Pleichingerova, 1966).

Gaseous diffusion plants that use uranium hexafluoride (UF_6) to separate uranium isotopes are another potential source of release of fluorine (UF_6, HF, or HF_4) to the atmosphere (NAS, 1971a).

Fluorine-containing pesticides are additional potential sources of fluoride releases to the atmosphere. In this category are products such as sodium fluoride, sodium fluorosilicate, barium fluorosilicate, and cryolite (the latter two used primarily as dusts) (Hanslian and Pleichingerova, 1966), as well as the fumigant sulfuryl fluoride (SO_2F_2) and methyl-containing insecticides including fluoroacetic acid and fluoroacetamide. Trifluralin (α,α,α-trifluoro-2,6-dinitro-N,N-dipropyl-p-toluidine) is a widely used herbicide; for example, 5,184,000 lb was employed in the United States in 1966.

Other sources of fluoride are asbestos and cigarettes; 1,000 g of tobacco contains ~ 25 mg of fluoride; a person smoking 25 cigarettes a day would inhale ~ 0.4 mg fluoride (Waldbott and Oelschlager, 1974).

Although there are no apparent estimates of the amount of fluoride partitioned into the different phases of the environment, its residence times, or its rates of transfer, a gross estimate of two pathways into the environment can be obtained. It has been estimated that 30 million tons of soil is distributed into the atmosphere each year in the United States (Wadleigh, 1968). A mean fluoride concentration of 192 ppm in soil implies an emission of ~ 6,000 tons of fluoride into the atmosphere. Total emissions from industrial processes in the United States for 1968 were estimated at 119,000 tons (NAS, 1971a).

The dispersal of a fluoride in the atmosphere is determined by a variety of factors, including meteorological conditions and the physical state of the fluoride (gas, smoke, aerosol, or dust). A number of inorganic fluorides can be rapidly hydrolyzed by water vapor in the air and converted to less volatile compounds, which are subsequently removed from the atmosphere by condensation or nucleation processes. SiF_4, for example, reacts with water vapor in air to form hydrated silica and fluorosilicic acid: $3SiF_4 + 2H_2O \rightarrow SiO_2 + 2H_2SiF_6$.

Anhydrous HF, another major industrial pollutant, combines with water vapor in the atmosphere to produce an aerosol or fog of aqueous HF. (Both the anhydrous and aqueous forms are easily absorbed by plant and animal tissues.)

Most of the fluorides emitted by industries in the form of particulate matter, such as cryolite, fluorapatite, calcium fluoride, aluminum fluoride, sodium fluoride, and sodium fluorosilicate, are stable compounds that do not hydrolyze readily.

Extremely low levels of fluoride in air have been found in rural areas free of industrial or other types of contamination (usually measured in parts per billion or in micrograms per cubic meter of air; 1 ppb by volume equals ~ 0.8 $\mu g/m^3$). For example, 97% of more than 7,700 air samples from many nonurban areas in the United States in 1966–1967 had no detectable fluoride (when analyzed for total water-soluble fluoride) (Younghans and McMullen, 1970), and the highest concentration found was 0.16 $\mu g/m^3$. In air samples from urban areas, the concentration of fluoride was less than 0.05 $\mu g/m^3$ (the lowest limit of detection) (range, 0.05–1.89 $\mu g/m^3$) in 87% of the samples (NAS, 1971a). It should be noted that higher levels of fluoride contamination than these have occurred in localized areas close to industries. Aluminum factories have been reported as sources of damaging fluoride emissions in the United States, Soviet Union, Great Britain, Italy, France, Germany, and Switzerland (NAS, 1971a).

Fluoride concentrations in air at a number of sites in the industrial areas of Duisburg, Germany, ranged between 0.5 and 3.8 $\mu g/m^3$, with the mean of 1,339 air sample measurements being 1.3 $\mu g/m^3$ (Schneider, 1968).

Average concentrations of airborne gaseous fluoride of 1 and 3.5 ppb (or 0.08 and 2.87 μg/m^3 of fluoride as hydrogen fluoride), corresponding to the 1-month and 24-hr ambient fluoride standards, respectively, of New York State, would contribute about 0.002 mg or < 0.06 mg of fluoride, assuming all of it is absorbed (NAS, 1971a).

Martin (1970) has suggested that fluoride inhaled by the average man in central London is about 0.003 mg in a normal day and may reach 0.03 mg during a day of thick fog with exceptionally heavy pollution. Severe effects of airborne fluoride on humans, such as crippling fluorosis, have been observed, primarily after long-term occupational exposure.

Reports concerning the mutagenic potential of fluorides are relatively few in number. Mohamed et al. (1966a) reported that sodium fluoride had a mutagenic action on the mitotic chromosomes of onion root tips, causing anaphase lags and bridging, tetraploid nuclei, and multipolar anaphases. Such phenomena, when observed in meiotic reduction division, are known to produce monosomies and triploidy or tetraploidy in subsequent progeny. Subsequent studies (Mohamed et al., 1966b; Mohamed, 1968, 1969) revealed the cytological effects of hydrogen fluoride in tomato plants.

Jagiello and Lin (1974) studied the mutagenic potential of sodium fluoride in a variety of female mammalian germ cells. *In vitro* experiments with mouse, sheep, and cow oocytes disclosed a low incidence of anaphase lags, suppression of polar body I, and fragmentation with rearrangement, while only a minor effect on oocyte meiotic maturation was noted *in vivo*. Some of the types of abnormalities seen with all three species exposed to NaF were considered significant to the development of abnormal progeny, seen as abortuses (Carr, 1970) and viable offspring in human populations (Polani, 1961). Of particular note were the cells that were interpreted as containing anaphase lags that could contribute to monosomy (Hamerton, 1971), suppression of PBI in the cause of triploid and tetraploid abortuses (Carr, 1967) and fragmentation with subsequent rearrangement, particularly translocations that have been seen in a variety of mammalian chromosome abnormalities (Cohen, 1972; Lyon and Meredity, 1966).

Mitchell and Gerdes (1973) reported the mutagenicity of sodium fluoride and stannous fluoride (SnF$_2$) to *D. melanogaster*. A direct correlation between the treatment concentration and the frequency of the sex-linked recessive lethal mutation was observed. Significant inductions of these frequencies were found using 5 and 6% NaF and 15–25% SnF$_2$.

Phthalate Esters

The aromatic dicarboxylic esters such as the phthalic, isophthalic, and terephthalic acid esters (PAEs) are the *ortho, meta,* and *para* isomeric esters, respectively, of benzene dicarboxylic acid, and are among the most important industrial chemicals employed. The diesters, of which the most common are shown in Fig. 7, are lipophilic, lyophobic liquids of medium viscosity and high boiling point.

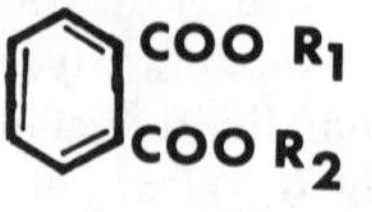

Phthalic acid diester (PAE)

Phthalate esters	*Alcohol radicals*
Dimethyl (DMP)=R_1=R_2=	**$.CH_3$**
Di-*n*-butyl(DnBP)=R_1=R_2=	**$.CH_2.CH_2.CH_2.CH_3$**
Di-*iso*-butyl(DiBP)=R_1=R_2=	**$.CH_2.CH{:}(CH_3)_2$**
Benzyl butyl (BBP)=R_1=	**$.CH_2.CH_2.CH_2.CH_3$**
R_2=	**$.CH_2.C_6H_5$**
Butyl glycolyl butyl (BGBP)=R_1=	**$.CH_2.CH_2.CH_2CH_3$**
R_2=	**$.CH_2.COOCH_2.CH_2.CH_2.CH_3$**
Dimethoxyethyl (DMEP) =R_1R_2=	**$.CH_2.CH_2.OCH_3$**
Dioctyl (DOP)=R_1=R_2=	**$.CH_2.(CH_2)_6.CH_3$**
Di-2-ethylhexyl (DEHP)=R_1=R_2=	**$.CH_2.CH.(CH_2)_4$ / C_2H_5**
Dicyclohexyl (DCHP)=R_1=R_2=	**$.CH$ ($.CH_2.CH_2$ / $CH_2.CH_2$) CH_2**

FIGURE 7 Phthalic acid diester (PAE).

In terms of quantity, use applications, and concomitant environmental considerations, the area of plasticizers (and plastics) is by far the most important aspect of the PAEs. Approximately 10 billion kg of PAEs was produced in 1973 in the United States alone, 50% more than in 1970, with the annual rate expected to increase tenfold in less than 30 yr (*Chemistry and Industry*, 1973). The applications of plastics include home construction, appliances, furnishings, automobiles, apparels, food and medicine containers, and wrappings. The solid waste from such applications amounts to 4.31 billion kg/yr in the United States, a 2.5-fold increase over 1966 (Srinivasan, 1972). Most of the ethylene, propylene, vinyl chloride, and styrene polymers that comprise the bulk of most of the plastics manufactured are generally regarded as biochemically inert. Microbial attack on plastics is farther reduced by the addition of small amounts of biostatics and biocides, such as a variety of heavy-metal organic compounds (Mathur, 1974). Often the most abundant constituents of plastics are members of the PAEs. For example, for PVC plastics, the PAE/resin ratio is usually 1:2. (The PAE plasticizers occur in monomeric forms only loosely linked to the polymers, and hence can be eventually extracted.)

Of the total weight of about 20 different PAEs produced in the United States during 1973 (estimated to be ~450 million kg) (*Chemical & Engineering News*, 1972), about 22.68 million kg will be employed in nonplasticizer applications—for example, as pesticide carriers, insect repellants, in dyes, cosmetics, and fragrances, in munitions, and in lubrications (*Chemical & Engineering News*, 1972).

The production of di(2-ethylhexyl) phthalate (DEHP) in 1970 amounted to ~ 158.8 million kg (or ~ one-fourth of the total phthalate ester plasticizer production), with the closely related diisooctyl phthalate and diisodecyl phthalate accounting for an additional fourth of the market and other phthalates such as *n*-octyl, *n*-decyl, dibutyl, and diethyl phthalates accounting for an additional 20% of the market. DEHP is one of the most widely employed plasticizers for PVC plastics and can constitute up to 40% of the finished product (Autian, 1973).

The expanding usage of PAEs during the last 30 yr and a lack of restrictions on dumping have contributed to the present levels of PAEs in the environment. For example, hundreds of parts per billion of DEHP and BGBP (butylglycolyl butyl phthalate) have been detected in Escambia Bay and the Mississippi River Delta on the Gulf of Mexico (Corcoran, 1973). An empirical calculation by Corcoran (1973) indicated that the total DEHP in the Mississippi River effluent may already be as high as the 1973 total production (158.8 million kg). Samples from a bay of Lake Superior (in an industrial-rural area) were found to contain DEHP at levels of 0.3 ppm, ~ 60 times more than in the water from Lake Huron or the Missouri River (Stalling et al., 1973).

It has been suggested that lyophobic plasticizer pollutants such as the PAEs may interact with lyophilic soil fulvic acids, which may then carry the pollutants into water bodies (Ogner and Schnitzer, 1970).

The observations of Mayer and Sanders (1973), Stalling et al. (1973), and Metcalf et al. (1973) suggest that the level of PAEs present in natural water constitute pollution, since it may be enough to disturb the ecological balance (Mathur, 1974). Accumulation of DEHP in aquatic organisms has been noted, as well as concentration through a food chain (Metcalf et al., 1973).

Approximately 22.68 million kg of PAEs are used as such and constitute a major source of PAE pollution of air since they are added directly into the environment, partly as sprays (Mathur, 1974). The PVC used in packaging is a rich source of PAEs and constitutes more than half of the waste products. Waste plastics comprise only 2–3% of the total urban waste and hence may be incinerated or used in landfills rather than separated for specific treatment or for recycling (Milgrom, 1973). Not all of the PAEs are decomposed during incineration. For example, 300 mg/m^3 of DEHP and 700 ng/m^3 of dibutyl phthalate and BGBP in air samples were detected near a municipal incinerator (Thomas, 1973). Increased surface area and higher temperatures apparently cause losses to air of the normally slightly volatile PAEs (Graham, 1973).

Although DEHP is practically immiscible with water and has a vapor pressure of less than 0.01 mm at room temperature, it (as well as other PAEs) has been found in animal tissues, milk, blood, and other aqueous solutions stored in PVC bags; surface and subsurface soils; river water; and air (Mathur, 1974). In particular, the detection of DEHP residues in human blood stored in PVC bags (Jaeger and Rubin, 1970, 1972, 1973), in milk (Reichle and Tengler, 1968), in various species of fish (Mayer et al., 1972; Stalling et al, 1973), and in bovine tissues (Nazir et al., 1971) has given cause for concern about the potential toxicological hazards associated with the use of PAEs.

DEHP has been found in tissues of 2 patients who had received transfusions of blood stored in plastic bags; the concentrations of DEHP ranged from 2.5 to 27 mg/100 g (dry weight) in the spleen, liver, lungs, and abdominal fat, with the spleen containing the least and abdominal fat the most (Jaeger and Rubin, 1970).

Singh et al. (1972) demonstrated teratogenic effects in rats following ip administration of a number of phthalate esters. Teratogenic effects of phthalate esters have been reported in chicks when the compounds were injected into the yolk sac of developing embryos (Guess et al., 1967; Haberman et al., 1968; Bower et al., 1970).

Mutagenic (dominant lethal) and antifertility sensitivities of mice to DEHP and DMEP (dimethoxy ethyl phthalate) were recently described by Singh et al. (1974). A single ip injection of undiluted DEHP or DMEP (representing one-third, one-half, and two-thirds of the acute LD50) in male ICR mice before mating, was found generally to elicit a dose-related, time-dependent trend of antifertility and mutagenicity, the specific pattern being a function of the compound injected. All three dose levels of DEHP and the high dose of DMEP produced some degree of antifertility (as reflected by reduced incidences of pregnancy) throughout the study. There were fewer implantations per pregnancy and smaller litter sizes, particularly in the first few weeks (postmeiotic stage), with the high dose of the compounds. Mutational effects, expressed by an increase in early fetal deaths and reduced numbers of total implants, were seen at various weeks during the study, but most notably during the first few weeks.

Although DEHP has a low order of acute toxicity (Patty, 1967), subacute studies in the rat have shown that oral administration of DEHP leads to liver enlargement (Nikonorow et al., 1973). A recent study by Lake et al. (1975), in which Wistar rats were treated with DEHP at a dose of 2,000 mg/kg for 21 days, showed a number of biochemical and ultrastructural changes in the liver not generally associated with xenobiotic-induced hepatomegaly. The progressive liver enlargement and the associated proliferation of smooth endoplasmic reticulum were accompanied by an initial increase in the microsomal cytochrome P-450 and protein contents followed by a reversal and depression as the treatment proceeded. A similar biphasic response is produced by dieldrin (Wright et al., 1972).

PESTICIDES

It is generally acknowledged that of the environmental phases, the occurrence and significance of pesticides in air are the least understood. It has been reported that in the United States alone, more than 900 different pesticides (Mrak, 1969) are employed in many thousands of mixtures, as in dusts, wettable powders, emulsifiable concentrates, and so on. Some of the factors affecting the persistence, metabolism, or movement of a particular pesticide can be classified as follows: (1) the chemistry and physical properties of the pesticide per se, its water solubility, vapor pressure, and so on, (2) the purity of the pesticide and the nature of its trace impurities or contaminants, (3) the formulation in which the chemical is applied, (4) its mode of application to plants, soil, or water, and (5) a variety of environmental factors, including soil type, microorganisms, presence of other synthetic chemicals, temperature, moisture, pH, soil cultivation, soil crops, and air movement (Lichtenstein, 1972).

It has become increasingly apparent that the atmosphere is a key transport medium as well as a vast reservoir for pesticides and their residues, metabolites, and degradation products. Although pesticides and their metabolic and/or degradation products may react chemically or photochemically while airborne, the atmosphere is not a medium in which they are biologically active. The biochemical processes occur only after they have become dissolved in liquids or deposited on solid surfaces (Wheatley, 1973).

Adequate mechanisms in the atmosphere permit the redistribution of entrained matter, not necessarily uniformly, on a local, continental, hemispherical, or global scale, provided the material persists and remains airborne for sufficiently long periods (Wheatley, 1973).

Pesticides can enter the atmosphere either intermittently or continuously depending on the source. The former type of release generally occurs (in relatively high concentrations) during their application, at certain stages of batch manufacture, during the handling of concentrates, or when enclosed fumigated spaces are subsequently ventiliated. A more continuous release into the atmosphere occurs as a consequence of the normal weathering processes of pesticide deposits on or in treated substrates (the rates of pesticide loss normally diminishing rapidly as the deposits age). It is important to note that eventually the pesticide lost becomes part of the equilibrium exchange of pesticide molecules between the atmosphere and every substrate-air interface (Wheatley, 1973).

Pesticides may enter the atmosphere either in particulate form (liquids, aerosols, or solids) or as a vapor, either wholly comprised of the pesticide active ingredient or as a carrier matrix in which the pesticide molecules are entrained, absorbed, or adsorbed onto the interstitial surfaces. Normally, both particulate and vapor forms coexist, which compounds the difficulty of determining the quantitative importance of each form in entry or transport mechanisms (Wheatley, 1973).

Carriers for pesticide dusts normally have particle densities of $\sim 2.2\text{–}3$ g/cm^3, so that particles smaller than about 10 μm are particularly drift-prone. Since an appreciable portion of the total weight of dust formulations is usually comprised of 10-μm or smaller particles, they are particularly prone to drift well beyond the application area (Wheatley, 1973; Gerhardt and Witt, 1965).

Vapor-phase losses of pesticides into the atmosphere during application have been scantily studied. However, it is believed that losses of up to half of the amounts of pesticides applied frequently occur during application as a result of direct loss of vapor to the atmosphere. Where comparisons have been made, the greatest losses to the atmosphere have invariably been found for the most volatile compounds. It is significant to note that even DDT, one of the least volatile pesticides, escapes in part by this route, which may well be the most important mechanism whereby pesticides become entrained in vast air-sheds (Wheatley and Hardman, 1965).

Wind erosion of dry soil is considered an important means of intermittent entry of pesticides into the atmosphere (Cohen and Pinkerton, 1966). Pesticide-contaminated soil is constantly being taken up, transported considerable distances at high altitudes by wind, and redeposited, either by sedimentation or by rain, far from its origin. Arable soils in areas of intensive pesticide usage can contain up to a few parts per million of persistent pesticides, the concentrations present being in equilibrium with the frequency and rates of usage (Wheatley et al., 1960).

Intermittent entry of pesticides into the atmosphere can arise from other applications, including those for (1) veterinary purposes, (2) food storage, (3) domestic hygiene, and (4) mothproofing fabrics. For example, fogging techniques used to treat large open areas for public health purposes may be an imporant initial source of pesticides such as DDT and malathion. Additional escapes of pesticides at high concentrations into the atmosphere can occur when food stores, ships, or aircraft are ventilated after fumigation. The dissemination of insecticides such as gamma-benzene hexachloride or DDT by thermal vaporizers can also introduce small amounts of pesticide in the ventilating-air changes. Widespread open burning of straw, stubble, or tree prunings or inefficient incineration of waste citrus peel can result in additional intermittent pesticide releases to the atmosphere (Wheatley and Hardman, 1965; Cook, 1966).

Soils are considered one of the principal sources of *continuous* entry of pesticides into the environment (Edwards, 1966; March, 1965). Residues generally on the order of several parts per million are present in the cultivated layer of arable soils (Wheatley et al., 1960; Decker et al., 1965; Harris et al., 1966). Trace residues are considered to be universally distributed over land masses, the concentrations present representing the net balance between local rates of pesticide input from all sources and rates of decline by all routes, including continual vapor-phase transfer into the atmosphere.

The oceans are considered another ubiquitous, continuous source of pesticide entry into the environment, albeit in trace quantities.

Pesticides occur in air at intermediate concentrations immediately downwind of zones of usage and within the zones during the early phases of residue loss. The insecticides carbaryl, malathion, parathion, and azinphosmethyl have been reported in the air over residential areas in Quebec at concentrations up to 500 $\mu g/m^3$, 300–600 mi from apple orchards, where they were being applied by air-blast equipment (Jegier, 1969).

Tabor (1966) studied atmospheric pesticide concentrations in the air over urban and rural communities in the United States associated with nearby usage. Concentrations of pesticides (primarily DDT and malathion) in associated air samples were mainly in the range of nanograms per cubic meter, although milligram per cubic meter concentrations were sometimes observed during periods of usage.

Evidence of long-distance transport of pesticides (e.g., organochlorines) by air has been obtained by measuring part-per-billion levels in rain (Cohen and Pinkerton, 1966; Tabor, 1966; Tarrant and Tatton, 1968; Risebrough et al., 1968a; Abbott et al., 1966; Wheatley and Hardman, 1965), Antarctic ice (Peterle, 1969), and on remote islands (Risebrough et al., 1968a). For example, the demonstration of pesticides in the air over Barbados in the Caribbean implied transport over 5,000 km of Atlantic Ocean by the northeast trade winds from West Africa (Risebrough et al., 1968a). Evidence of movement on this scale lends credence to the widely held view that contamination of the atmosphere is global. However, it cannot be concluded that the insecticides in the above case originated only in Africa, for they might have come from any part of the world.

Peterle (1969) calculated that up to 2.4×10^6 kg of DDT residues may have accumulated in Antarctic snow, which would indicate that the atmosphere is the only transport system capable of redistributing contaminants extensively over such a remote area.

The *fate* of pesticides in the atmosphere is largely speculative at this time, although a number of important considerations can be identified, including vapor-phase particulate behavior, chemical changes, removal processes, residence times, and extent of redistribution. The capacity of the atmosphere (both within and above the troposphere) to provide a medium within which large quantities of pesticides may be converted or degraded photochemically is for the most part unknown (Crosby, 1973).

DDT and Its Metabolites

The widespread distribution of chlorinated hydrocarbon residues as contaminants in the global ecosystem is an established fact (Wheatley, 1973; Jegier, 1969; Tatton and Ruzicka, 1967; Jensen et al., 1969; Crosby, 1973;

Risebrough et al., 1968a; Sodergren et al., 1972; Woodwell et al., 1956; Miller and Berg, 1969). Their rates of utilization are such that they can contaminate water, soil, and food in concentrations of parts per trillion to parts per million, the extent of pollution depending on the localization and meterological conditions of a given community.

Preeminent in any consideration of the chlorinated hydrocarbon insecticides is DDT [1,1,1-trichloro-2,2-bis(p-chlorophenyl)ethane] and its analogues. More than 4 billion lb of DDT have been used since 1940, about 80% in agriculture and the remainder in the control of insect vectors primarily of malaria, typhus, and the plague. Production of DDT in the United States reached a peak of about 160 million lb in 1961, when DDT was registered for use in the United States in 334 agricultural commodities. The total global production of DDT per year was estimated to be on the order of 10^{11} g, all of which could be released into the environment (NAS, 1971b).

Ironically, the very factors that have made DDT such an effective insecticide—its low vapor pressure (1.5 $\times$ 10^7 mm at 20°C), low water solubility (0.0012 ppm at 25°C), high fat solubility ($\sim$ 100,000 ppm), and *general* stability to photooxidation—have conspired to make it the prototypical environmental pollutant. For example, both DDT and its major metabolite 1,1-dichloro-2,2-bis(p-chlorophenyl)ethylene (DDE) are concentrated in organisms in the trophic webs, increasing roughly tenfold in the concentration stored in lipids and in the percentage of DDE at each trophic level (Woodwell et al., 1956).

Figure 8 illustrates the degradative pathways of DDT in the environment. The residues of DDT and some of its metabolites and degradation products have been shown to be extremely persistent in nature; their half-lives are estimated to be up to 20 yr and perhaps longer under certain conditions (Lichtenstein and Schull, 1959; Woodwell and Martin, 1964; Nash and Woolson, 1967).

The vapor pressure of DDT at 20°C (1.5 $\times$ 10^7 mm Hg) produces an equilibrium concentration of DDT in the atmosphere of about 3 $\times$ 10^6 g/m^3 or about 2 ppb by weight. The dominant mechanism for the removal of DDT from the atmosphere is probably by rainfall. [In the United States and Great Britain concentrations of DDT have been reported to range from 73 to 210 ppm (Tarrant and Tatton, 1968; Wheatley and Hardman, 1965).]

It is not certain how much of the atmospheric transport is actually dust-mediated and how much arises from true pesticide vapors. A detailed analysis of air over 9 U.S. cities in 1967–1968 indicated that the concentration of DDT in air is 1–150 $\times$ 10^{-9} g/m^3 in the winter (Stanley et al., 1971).

The total amount of DDT retained within the biota is considered small compared with the totals that can be retained in other pools within the biosphere and is also small compared with the annual amount of DDT produced. It is estimated that 10^9–10^{10} g of DDT is held within the biota

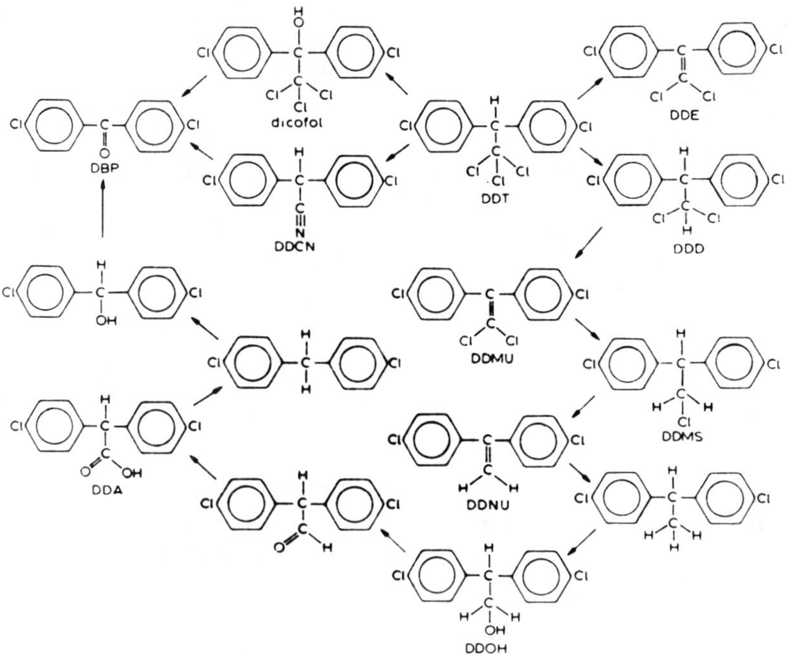

FIGURE 8 Degradative pathways of DDT in the environment.

worldwide (including residues in humans). This is about $\frac{1}{30}$ of the amount produced in 1 yr during the mid-1960s. The worldwide pattern of movement of DDT residues appears to be from the land through the atmosphere into the oceans and into the oceanic abyss.

A number of attempts have been made by modeling to estimate the dynamics of DDT circulation throughout the ecosystem (Woodwell et al, 1971; Harrison et al., 1970; Cramer, 1973). According to Woodwell et al. (1971), if world DDT production ceased after 1974 the concentration of DDT in the lower atmosphere would have reached a peak in 1966 of about 84 ng/m^3, after which concentration of DDT in the atmosphere would decline gradually, reaching 10% of its peak value by 1984. However, if world production and usage of DDT continued and even increased slightly beyond 1974, the average concentration would probably continue to increase slowly until after the year 2000. Accepting the value of Woodwell et al. (1971) of 84 ng/m^3 as the 1966 peak concentration of DDT and the mass of the atmosphere as 5×10^{18} kg, about 4×10^5 tons of DDT is present in the atmosphere. This corresponds to about one-sixth of their estimate for the total production of DDT on a worldwide basis up to 1974 (e.g., 2.8×10^6 tons).

In the case of DDT, the actual mean residence time in the atmosphere seems to be much longer than experimental observations suggest should be the case; this indicates that appreciable recycling of residues may occur between the earth's surface and the atmosphere (Wheatley, 1973).

The evidence for mutagenicity (like that for carcinogenicity) of DDT appears to be equivocal and often conflicting. This may be a consequence of both the different test systems employed and the different purities of test substances, which ranged from purified p,p' isomer of DDT to technical grade material containing a broad spectrum of impurities. The effects of environmental DDT and the genetics of natural populations in the fly *Drosophila pseudoobscura* were studied by Corey et al. (1971) and it was suggested that DDT residues were indirectly responsible for alterations in the genetic content of populations. The conclusions were based on correlations between the chromosomal changes in the fly described over the past 24 yr in the western United States by Dobzhansky (1958) and Dobzhansky et al. (1964, 1966) and the distribution patterns of DDT residues found by Corey et al. (1971) throughout the area.

Vogel (1972) reported that DDT or one of its metabolites, DDA [bis(p-chlorophenyl)acetic acid], induced recessive lethal mutations in *D. melanogaster* and hence could be regarded as weakly mutagenic.

Clark (1974) reported that oral treatment of male Canton-S *D. melanogaster* with technical grade DDT ($\sim$ 80% p,p'-DDT, $\sim$ 19% o,p'-DDT, and 2% p,p'-DDE) caused an increase in dominant lethality in early spermatid and spermatocyte stages. DDT also caused nondisjunction of the X and Y chromosomes at the spermatocyte stage in treated males. Treatment of a population of Canton-S *D. melanogaster* with DDT for 8 months did not cause any increase in frequency of second-chromosome recessive lethal mutations. Luers (1953) could not detect an effect of DDT on the induction of recessive lethals and visible X-chromosome aberrations in treated *D. melanogaster*. DDT has been shown by Vaarama (1947) to induce chromosome breaks in root tips of *Allium cepa*.

A study of a natural population of mice in the foothills of the Andes revealed an unprecedented number of genetic and chromosomal mutants, and DDT was suspected to be the causal agent (Wallace, 1971). Johnson and Jalal (1973) reported DDT-induced chromosomal damage in mice. Treatment of BALB/c mice with 100–400 ppm DDT (mg/kg of body weight) was associated with significantly higher proportions of chromosomal abnormalities in the form of deletions, stickiness, and, rarely, ring and metacentric chromosomes. The study indicated that chromosomal damage to mice occurred frequently at dosages of 150 ppm or higher (the LD50 is 550 ppm). Since the induction of chromosomal damage is closely associated with point mutations in mammals (Epstein and Legator, 1971), DDT would appear to be a potential mutagen. Markaryan (1966) previously reported significantly higher proportions of stickiness and chromosomal damage in mice after treatment with a single dose of DDT at 100 ppm. It was suggested that the effect of 0.06 times the LD50 of DDT in mammalian cells was equivalent to 25 rads of radiation.

Clark (1974), utilizing the dominant lethal assay, found that acute oral doses of technical DDT (2 × 150 mg/kg) in male mice induced dominant lethal mutations in early spermatid and spermatocyte stages. Chronic oral doses of DDT (2 × 100 mg/kg-wk for 10 wk) in male mice caused a persistent increase in the number of dominant lethal mutations. Histological sections showed that chronic treatment of mice with DDT caused changes in seminiferous tubule morphology and degeneration of B-type spermatogonia. Acute treatment of mice with DDT caused an increase in spermatocyte chromosome breakage, stickiness, and precocious separation of the X and Y bivalent.

Clark (1974) pointed out that in both the mouse and *D. melanogaster* no single stage of spermatogenesis is uniquely susceptible to the induction of genetic effects by DDT. This may imply that the mutagenic agent acts by several mechanisms or that its action may be mediated by a mechanism common to different stages of spermatogenesis.

Gray (1970) reported that DDT caused the breakdown of lysosomes, and Allison and Paton (1965) observed that release of hydrolytic enzymes after lysosomal breakdown resulted in chromosome breakage in mammalian cell cultures. Hence, according to Clark (1974), it is possible that the weakly mutagenic effects of DDT treatment observed in the mouse (Swiss albino) and *D. melanogaster* are mediated by lysosomes.

In contrast to these findings, Epstein and Shafner (1971) found that DDT had no effect on CD-1 mice in the dominant lethal assay, while Buselmaier et al. (1973) observed that both DDT and its metabolites gave ambiguous results in this assay.

Palmer et al. (1973) reported that DDT was only marginally positive with respect to the dominant lethal test in rats. A statistically significant effect was found in the proportion of females having one or more dead implants after being mated during week 3 with males given DDT orally in a dose of 100 mg/kg; no significant effects were found in females mated with males treated ip with DDT.

Kelly-Garvert and Legator (1973) described cytogenetic and mutagenic effects of DDT and DDE in a Chinese hamster cell line. In all experiments, DDE consistently produced a significant increase in the mutation frequency over the control level, while DDT proved inactive. The cytogenetic studies also indicated that DDE-treated cells had a significant increase in chromosome aberrations, with exchange figures and chromatid breaks being evident, while DDT produced no significant increase in chromosome abnormalities. The Chinese hamster cell populations exposed to DDE also manifested an increased number of polyploid cells over the control level.

Palmer et al. (1972) reported that chromosome abnormalities were produced by DDT and its metabolites in a cultured mammalian cell line; however, Legator et al. (1973) later reported that no cytogenic abnormalities were found in bone marrow cells of rats treated with DDT.

Fahrig (1974), in surveying the mutagenicity of DDT in various test systems, noted that DDT and its metabolites were genetically inactive in all microorganism test systems.

Clark (1974) noted that DDT was not strongly mutagenic in *N. crassa in vitro*, and *in vivo* the host did not potentiate any mutagenicity. (The fact that the environment of the mouse peritoneal cavity appears mutagenic to conidia of *N. crassa* was suggested as a possible weakness of this assay.

Long-term exposure to *p,p'*-DDT or technical DDT has been reported to induce liver tumors in various mouse strains (Tomatis et al., 1972, 1974a; Terracini et al., 1973; Turusov et al., 1973; Innes et al., 1969; Tarjan and Kemeny, 1969). Lifetime exposure of CF-1 mice to *p,p'*-DDE (the principal metabolite of *p,p'*-DDT) at a dose level of 250 ppm in the diet has recently been reported to result in a high incidence and early appearance of liver tumors (Tomatis et al., 1974b).

Dichlorvos

Dichlorvos [dimethyl 2,2-dichlorovinyl phosphate; Vapona; DDVP; $(CH_3O)_2 PO\cdot OCH=CCl_2$] is prepared by the reaction of trimethyl phosphate and chloral. [It should be noted that both trimethyl phosphate and chloral are mutagenic per se, the former inducing point mutations in *N. crassa* (Epstein, 1969; Epstein and Legator, 1971) as well as being highly active in the dominant lethal test (Epstein et al., 1970), while the latter has been reported to induce point mutations in *Drosophila* (Barthelmess, 1956), bacteria (Schull, 1960), and chromosome aberrations in *V. faba* (Garrigues, 1940).]

DDVP is volatile (145 mg/m^3 at $20°C$) and is slowly released as a vapor from wax resin strands or other suitable materials. It is chiefly in this form that DDVP is used for domestic extermination of insects.

Few pesticides have engendered as much recent concern over the possible health hazards of their widespread use and misuse as DDVP (primarily in the form of resin strips). The resin strips are solid solutions (20%) of Vapona insecticide (93% DDVP) in polyvinyl plastic strips enclosed in foil-covered cardboard holders. The usual constituents of Vapona (Slonka, 1970) are (in percentages): DDVP, 95–97; Dipterex (*O,O*-dimethyl 2,2,2-trichloro-1-hydroxyethylphosphonate), 1.5-3; *O,O*-dimethyl-2-chlorovinyl phosphate, 0.4–0.7; *O,O*-dimethylphosphonate, trace to 0.1; *O,O,O*-trimethylphosphate, 0.3–0.8; and chloral (trichloroacetaldehyde), 0.1–0.5. In addition, the resin releases small quantities of plasticizers and other materials. Vapona has also been used in other formulations as a household aerosol spray (0.5% alone or in combination with either dieldrin or synergized pyrethroids), as an insecticidal fumigant for stored foods and products such as grains and tobacco, for pre- and postharvest crop treatment, and in suitable formulations as an anthelminthic in humans and several other species.

DDVP resin strips function by sustained release of DDVP into a relatively enclosed air space at a *recommended* rate of one strip per 1,000 ft^3, with ventilation limited for at least some period each day, and the strips changed at the end of 3 months. The atmospheric concentration of DDVP from resin strips is apparently limited by vapor-phase adsorption on room surfaces, ventilation, and chemical degradation (Gillett et al., 1972).

DDVP concentrations in air have been determined in a number of studies where Vapona strips were used for the control of cocoa moth (*Ephestia elutella*) and Mediterranean flour moth (*E. kuedniella*) under industrial conditions (Green et al., 1966; Schulten and Kuyken, 1966). The levels of DDVP ranged from < 0.01 to 0.06 µg/l.

Elgar et al. (1972) measured residues of DDVP in the air and in food in shops in Great Britain and France where Vapona strips were used for pest control. The concentrations of DDVP in the air of the shops fell from an average of 0.03 µg/l in the first week to < 0.01 µg/l after 10 wk.

The long-term exposure of factory workers in the production and processing of a DDVP-releasing product to an average concentration of ~ 0.7 mg/m^3 in air has been noted by Menz et al. (1974).

Because of the wide exposure of humans to atmospheres containing DDVP, this pesticide has been the most thoroughly investigated in regard to both its potential alkylating capacity (Löfroth, 1970a; Löfroth et al., 1969; Wennerberg and Löfroth, 1974) and its mutagenicity, with conflicting results.

Dichlorvos has been shown to alkylate DNA (Löfroth et al., 1969), with the types of alkylations produced more closely resembling those of methyl methanesulfonate (MMS) than other common alkylating agents, although DDVP has the additional ability to dimethyl phosphorylate protein (Bedford and Robinson, 1972). On a molar basis, DDVP is about as effective as MMS in alkylating protein but about 15-fold less potent in alkylating DNA (Lawley et al., 1974). A dose on the order of 30 mM of DDVP for 1 hr was computed to produce about 1,400 methylations in the *E. coli* WP2 genome.

DNA strand breakage studies (Bridges et al., 1973; Green et al., 1974) have shown that levels of DDVP (3–13 mM) similar to those of MMS induce breaks in *E. coli* DNA, which can be rapidly repaired by DNA polymerase I. Higher DDVP concentrations (13–26 mM), however, produced nonrandom disintegration of DNA molecules rather than random strand breakage (Green et al., 1974). It was suggested that the ability of DDVP to produce either DNA polymerase I-repairable strand breaks or DNA disintegration did not correlate with the ability to produce gene mutations (Green et al., 1974).

Bridges et al. (1973) compared the lethal and mutagenic effects of DDVP with those of MMS in a series of radiation-sensitive strains of *E. coli*. ExrA, RecA, and PolA strains of *E. coli* exhibited increased sensitivity to both agents. Mutagenesis with both DDVP and MMS was demonstrated to occur by misrepair (e.g., ExrA and RecA strains were not mutated). It was shown that there was much less difference in survival between resistant and sensitive strains with DDVP than with MMS, and DDVP was a much weaker mutagen (Bridges et al., 1973).

Wild (1973) and Mohn (1973) reported definite mutagenicity and clear relationships between DDVP concentration, exposure time, and the mutagenic effect in two other genetic tests in *E. coli*—induction of streptomycin resistance (5.25 m*M* DDVP, 1-10 hr) and induction of 5-methyltryptophan resistance (0.3-3.2 m*M* DDVP, 0.5-6 hr), respectively.

DDVP has been shown to be mutagenic in other bacterial species, for instance, inducing reversions in *Serratia marcescens* with the agar plate test (Dean, 1972a) and in *S. typhimurium* (Dyer and Hanna, 1973). In several bacterial species including *E. coli, S. typhimurium,* and *K. pneumoniae,* the mutation rates to streptomycin resistance were increased (Voogd et al., 1972).

A dose-dependent increase of mitotic gene conversion by 5-40 m*M* DDVP (5 hr) has been demonstrated in the D4 strain of the yeast *Saccharomyces cerevisiae* (Dean et al., 1972; Fahrig, 1973). Although a quantitative relationship between mutagenesis and alkylation of specific sites in DNA has not yet been established, it should be noted that the doses used in the microbial mutation studies above are of the same order as those used in DNA alkylation studies (Lawley et al., 1974; Wennerberg and Lofroth, 1974).

Michalek and Brockman (1969), using the adenine-3 region of *N. crassa,* were unable to demonstrate any mutagenicity of DDVP. However, Dean (1972b) has shown that DDVP (technical, > 97%) at very high concentrations (25-100 mg/ml in dimethyl sulfoxide) is capable of inducing mutations in *S. marcescens* under specific conditions *in vitro.* Dean et al. (1972) emphasize that the conditions in the bacterial test systems, in which DDVP is in intimate contact with the cell and hence more readily available to the bacterial DNA, are vastly different from the situation *in vivo,* where the dichlorvos molecule is confronted by a variety of hydrolytic enzymes (Hutson and Hoadley, 1972). In this regard, a number of recent studies of Dean and his co-workers are of special importance. For example, Dean and Thorpe (1972a) demonstrated the absence of dominant lethal mutations in male CF_1 mice following single and repeated inhalation exposures to DDVP at concentrations of 30 and 55 μg/l of air for 16 hr, or to 2.1 and 5.8 μg/l DDVP for 23 hr daily for 4 wk. These exposures to DDVP produced no mutagenic effects as expressed by increased preimplantation losses or early fetal deaths in subsequent test matings; neither was an impairment of male fertility detected following the exposures to DDVP vapor. It was stressed by Dean and Thorpe (1972a) that the concentration of 5.8 μg/l DDVP used in their repeated exposure study is more than 100 times the average air concentration of 0.04 μg/l found during the domestic use of dichlorvos-impregnated resin strips.

The failure of high doses of DDVP to induce chromosome damage in mice and Chinese hamsters (Dean and Thorpe, 1972b) has also been reported. In this study, mice were exposed to atmospheres containing vapor concentrations of 64-72 μg/l DDVP for 16 hr, or to 5 μg/l for 21 days. Chinese hamsters were exposed by the inhalation and oral routes to high concentrations (32 μg/l and 10-15 mg/kg, respectively). In chromosome preparations made from bone marrow and spermatocytes, the incidence of chromosome abnormalities following exposure did not differ from the control value. Endoxan, used as a positive control, caused chromatic aberrations in bone marrow from both species, but the incidence of meiotic chromosome abnormalities did not differ from the untreated control value.

Genetic studies with DDVP in the host-mediated assay and in liquid medium using *S. cerevisiae* were also described by Dean et al. (1972). Host-mediated assays with *S. cerevisiae* D4 as the test organism were carried out on male CF_1 mice dosed orally with DDVP or EMS (positive control) or exposed to DDVP vapor. After 5 hr, harvested yeast cells were analyzed for mitotic gene conversion at the ade_2 (adenine) and trp_5 (tryptophan) loci. No enhancement of mitotic gene conversion was observed in yeast cells harvested from mice that had been dosed orally with DDVP at 50 or 100 mg/kg, or exposed for 5 hr to atmospheres containing DDVP at 60 or 99 μg/l. However, in mice dosed orally with 400 mg/kg EMS, the rate of mitotic gene conversion was increased at both loci. In *stationary* phase cultures of *S. cerevisiae* treated with DDVP (4 mg/ml), the rate of conversion at both loci was increased. However, no effect was evident with 2 mg/ml DDVP, while 1 mg/ml EMS was positive at both loci. These studies show that high concentrations of DDVP in the culture medium can increase the mitotic gene conversion rate in *S. cerevisiae in vitro*, but the host-mediated assay yields negative results associated with the rapid metabolism of DDVP when given by the oral or inhalation route.

Dean (1972b) studied the effect of various concentrations of DDVP on human lumphocytes (1) when added 24 hr before termination of the cultures, (2) when added before or immediately after mitogenic stimulus with phytohemagglutinin, and (3) when cultures were harvested after 96 hr instead of the customary 72 hr to investigate any delayed effect. DDVP was cytotoxic to cells at concentrations ranging from 5 to 40 μg/ml, and this cytotoxicity was not accompanied by any detectable chromosome aberrations. If the effect of DDVP in cultured cells is direct alkylation of DNA, then according to Dean (1972b) increasing concentrations of the compound should induce chromatid-type aberrations of increasing severity. An increase in single chromatid gaps over the control value was noted in one pair of cultures, although this was not dose-related. Chromatid breakage generally was of low incidence and evenly distributed in control and test cultures. No examples of chromatid interchanges, multiple chromatid aberrations, chromosome pulverization, or any chromosome-type aberrations were seen in any culture.

Formaldehyde and Ethylene Oxide

Formaldehyde is produced in enormous quantities; about 2.2 billion lb is produced in the United States per year, or about half of the world production. Formaldehyde-based resins consume about two-thirds of domestic production and are applied in plastics and to impart permanent-press, wash-

and-wear characteristics to clothing. Other major areas of utility of formaldehyde include use in bactericides and pesticides (fungicides and soil fumigants and for seed treatment) and in the manufacture of textiles, paper, fertilizer, and specialty chemicals (boiling point, 21°C).

The preparation of formaldehyde (by the catalytic oxidation of methanol vapor) as well as a number of its applications—for instance, in fumigant adhesives, coating composition, modification of textiles and paper products, and resin formulations—can be expected to release formaldehyde regionally to the atmosphere in varying concentrations.

Formaldehyde has been found widely in the environment—for instance, in photochemical smog, as described earlier; tobacco smoke (Newsome et al., 1965); incinerator effluents (Stenburg et al., 1961); and automobile (Altshuller et al., 1961) and diesel (Wilson, 1960) exhaust—and in the thermal degradation of epoxy thermoplastic materials (Stuart and Smith, 1965).

The mutagenic properties of formaldehyde have been known for a fairly long period. Formaldehyde reacts specifically with amino groups of proteins or nucleic acids in the cell in different ways (Jensen et al., 1951; Collins and Guild, 1964; Staehelin, 1958). One type of reaction involved in mutagenesis may be the formation of an adenine dimer in which two adjacent adenines in a DNA strand are linked through stable methylene bridges at amino groups (Woodhouse, 1965; Alderson, 1960). It has also been suggested that free radicals produced by autooxidation of the aldehyde could cause certain types of DNA damage (Jensen et al., 1951; Sobels, 1963).

Nishioka (1973) reported that the lethal and mutagenic action of formaldehyde in Hcr^+ and Hcr^- strains of *E. coli* may be subject to the same cellular repair function (excision repair) as damage induced by UV irradiation.

Poverenny et al. (1975) suggested that the action of formaldehyde on bacterial DNA leading to lethality and possibly to mutagenesis is not exerted by formaldehyde per se, but by the products of reaction with amino-containing compounds such as amino acids and proteins. For example, it was shown that treatment of wild strains of *E. coli* and strains deficient in excision repair with a product of the reaction between formaldehyde and amino acids produces inactivation of the cells as well as single-strand breaks in bacterial DNA. The breaks are successfully repaired in wild-type cells but remain unrepaired in bacteria deficient in DNA polymerase I.

Ethylene oxide is a 4-billion-lb/yr (U.S.) chemical made by the action of alkali on ethylene chlorohydrin or by the catalytic oxidation of ethylene in air, which is used in thousands of consumer products. Most germane to considerations of the release of ethylene oxide to the atmosphere are its production per se; its wide employment as a fumigant to sterilize foodstuffs, textiles, medical instruments, and a variety of other objects (Fishbein, 1969); and its applications in agriculture as a pesticide and in the tobacco industry to shorten the aging process and to reduce the nicotine content of tobacco leaves (Fishbein, 1969; Fishbein et al., 1970).

The toxicity and mutagenic potential of ethylene oxide per se are well recognized (Fishbein et al., 1970). For example, ethylene oxide is mutagenic in *Drosophila* (Rapoport, 1948; Bird, 1952), *Neurospora* (Kolmark and Kilbey, 1968; Kolmark and Westergaard, 1953), and barley (Ehrenberg et al., 1956), and induces chromosome aberrations in 1% of maize (Faberge, 1955), barley (Moutschen-Dahmen et al., 1968), and *V. faba* (Loveless, 1953).

Exposure of the mouse to air contaminated with ethylene oxide was used recently by Ehrenberg et al. (1974) to evaluate the potential genetic risk of this alkylating agent. For example, the degree of alkylation of proteins was used to determine the tissue dose D_t (the concentration of free alkylating agent integrated over time) in resting male mice exposed for 1-2 hr to air containing 1-35 ppm of ethylene oxide. The exposure doses were found to be 0.03-2% of the LD50. The results agreed with absorption of all the ethylene oxide in alveolar ventilation, rapid distribution to all organs, and rapid detoxification and excretion (biological half-life, $\sim$ 9 min).

It was suggested on the basis of dose-effect curves for ethylene oxide and X-rays in barley, that a tissue dose of ethylene oxide in humans of 1 mM/hr may be provisionally set equal to 80 rads of LET radiation. Allowing for the difference in alveolar ventilation between mice and humans, this would mean that epoxide operators working in 5 ppm of ethylene oxide for 40 hr/wk would receive a weekly gonad dose of ethylene oxide amounting to about 4 rad-equivalents.

Significant lymphocytosis has been observed in about half the workers employed in the ethylene oxide department of a Swedish factory (Ehrenberg et al., 1974). In a study of effects of ethylene oxide on the blood cell counts in the rat, an $\sim$ 40% decrease of the lymphocyte count was observed in the days following exposure to 1.75 g/m^3 (900 ppm) ethylene oxide. Although the cause of the lymphopenia after treatment with ethylene oxide and the lymphocytosis observed in exposed humans is unknown, the doses involved, according to Ehrenburg et al. (1974), support the idea of a genetic mechanism. A more specifically genetic effect was observed in eight persons overexposed to ethylene oxide. The frequencies of chromosomal aberrations determined in cultured lymphocytes 18 months after the event were believed to be of the magnitude that would have been induced by about 50 rads of sparsely ionizing radiation (e.g., in a reactor accident) (Bender and Gooch, 1966).

In addition to the mutagenic effects of ethylene oxide per se, note must be made of the mutagenicity of its degradation products, primarily ethylene chlorohydrin (2-chloroethanol). This compound is formed by the reaction of ethylene oxide with moisture and chloride ions—for instance, after exposure of foodstuffs to ethylene oxide (Fishbein, 1969; Fishbein et al., 1970; Wesley et al., 1965; Ragelis et al., 1968)—reaching levels of 1,000 ppm.

Rosenkranz and Wlodkowski (1974) reported the induction by ethylene chlorohydrin of mutations of the base substitution type in *S. typhimurium*

T1530 and TA1535. In addition, this compound also preferentially inhibited the growth of DNA polymerase-deficient *E. coli.* Voogdt and Vander Vet (1969) previously described the mutagenicity of ethylene chlorohydrin in *K. pneumoniae.*

METALS

Lead

The pollution of the environment with lead is well documented. With the continuing discharge of lead compounds into the air and water, the rate of increase of lead in the environment has greatly accelerated in the last 50 yr. Today, for example, lead concentrations in urban atmospheres are on the order of 2–8 $\mu g/m^3$, lead in city soils is in the range of several hundred parts per million, while river water in industrialized regions often contains several hundred micrograms of lead per liter. In addition, nearshore seawater contains 0.2 $\mu g/l$ of lead, and plants grown near the roadside are often ten or more times richer in lead than those grown farther away.

The world production of primary ore lead in 1970 was 3.75 million tons, and the consumption of lead in the United States in 1970 amounted to 1,360,000 tons (U.S. Department of Interior, 1971).

Lead is used in industry in (1) the production of weatherproof coverings, pipes, and so on, (2) storage batteries (as accumulator plates), (3) various alloys with tin, copper, and antimony, (4) paints, pigments, and varnishes (as red lead, litharge, white lead, chromates, sulfate, and titanate), (5) flint glass and vitreous enameling, (6) the manufacture of insecticides (lead arsenate), and (7) the manufacture of tetraethyllead. The manufacture of lead-acid storage batteries in 1970 required some 590,000 tons, approximately 44% of the total consumption, but most of the battery lead was recycled and about 350,000 tons was salvaged from old batteries. Tetraethyllead additives for gasoline accounted for about 10% of the world lead consumption in 1970. The largest manufacturer of these additives is the United States, which is currently consuming about 264,000 tons of lead per year, while in Europe the consumption is approximately 200,000 tons/yr. Red lead and litharge pigments, solder, cable covering, ammunition, and caulking lead together made up about 26% of the lead consumption in the United States in 1970.

Lead is disseminated in the environment through mining, smelting, refining, secondary recovery, and use of lead-containing products. Table 4 lists the U.S. lead emissions in 1968. The overwhelming contributor to lead pollutants in the environment is without question the burning of lead alkyl additives in automotive fuels (Chow and Johnstone, 1965; Hicks, 1972; Schubert, 1973; Hall, 1972). For example, lead aerosol emissions in the United States in 1968 were estimated at 184,614 tons, of which some 181,000 tons (98%) was attributed to leaded-gasoline consumption (Hicks,

TABLE 4   Lead Emissions
in the United States
in 1968[a]

Emission source	Lead emitted (tons/year)
Gasoline combustion	181,000
Coal combustion	920
Fuel oil combustion	24
Lead alkyl manufacturing	810
Primary lead smelting	174
Secondary lead smelting	811
Brass manufacturing	521
Lead oxide manufacturing	20
Gasoline transfer	36
Total	184,316

[a]Data from the National Inventory of Air Pollutant Emissions and Controls, on file at the Environmental Protection Agency, Stationary Source Pollution Control Program, Durham, North Carolina.

1972) (in contrast, only 920 tons result from coal burning). Since the advent of leaded gasoline (primarily tetraethyllead) in 1925, more than 6 million tons of lead has been consumed as additives in the United States. Until recently, nearly all the gasoline sold in the United States contained lead alkyl compounds in concentrations ranging from 0.5 to 4.2 g per U.S. gallon. In the internal combustion engine, lead alkyl compounds are burned to form lead halides and oxyhalogenates (with lesser amounts of carbonates and sulfates), and 80% of that lead is emitted from the exhaust pipe as submicrometer aerosols. The manufacture of lead alkyls alone contributes annually in the United States approximately 810 tons of lead alkyls to the atmosphere (Hirschler et al., 1957). According to Jawarowski (1967), the global contribution to atmospheric lead from burning coal is approximately equivalent to that from burning gasoline. However, in the United States, the contribution from gasoline is 20 times that from coal (see above). In Great Britain, approximately 75 times more atmospheric lead originates from gasoline exhausts than from coal, if an estimate of only 120 tons of lead per year from coal burning is correct (Smith, 1972).

The combustion of lead alkyl antiknock compounds since their introduction some 50 yr ago is estimated to have added about 5×10^9 kg of lead to the atmosphere and to have contributed 10 mg/m^2 to the soil (Smith, 1972). It has been suggested that airborne lead forms approximately 0.5–1.5% of the lead content of the U.S. diet (Ter Haar, 1970). Additional sources of lead are the transfer of gasoline, which released 40 tons of lead into the air in 1968; burning waste crankcase oil, which produced 1,000 tons of lead emissions; and incineration of solid wastes, which contributed another 320 tons of lead aerosols. Primary and secondary lead smelting operations in 1968 released 980 tons of lead to the atmosphere. Emission from U.S. industrial sources other than primary and secondary lead smelting accounts for 600 tons of lead annually. The burning of coal (in comparison to leaded gasoline) has not really been a significant contributor to lead aerosols. For example, in recent years, about 500 million tons of coal with an average lead content of 10 ppm were burned annually in the United States; since most of the lead remains in the ash, the atmospheric contribution from coal smoke is approximately 920 tons annually.

Among the factors that may influence the concentration of lead in food are its concentration in the growing environment of plants and food-producing animals, which involves uptake from soil and water and excretion, retention, and distribution of lead by the organism; contamination with lead pollutants through aerial fallout; use of lead compounds in agriculture; and direct contamination during processing, storage, and final preparation. Concentrations in agricultural soils can range from 14 to 96 ppm (Huff, 1952) and in forest areas up to 43 ppm, while the distillation and burning of coal contribute 534–12,340 ppm of lead to the soil (Mahley, 1937). Areas around lead ores have been reported to have concentrations varying from 20 to 10,000 ppm, with similar concentrations near smelters (Huff, 1952).

An important source of lead is water, since this lead is in a soluble and more easily assimilable form for uptake by both plants and animals. The lead levels in seawater (0.08–8 μg/l) (Kehoe, 1960), groundwater (1.5–60 μg/l) (Bagchi et al., 1940), and surface waters (0–55 μg/l) (Durum and Haffty, 1961) can vary enormously. Drinking water can be contaminated with lead as a result of painting of the insides of water storage tanks with lead chromate (Jackson, 1970; Christofferson, 1961).

The pesticide lead arsenate (although greatly restricted in use) is also a source of lead residues in food and tobacco. Other sources include storage batteries, lead-tin solder for sealing cans, and lead pipe for service use. A minor source of lead is glazed pottery used for acid drinks. High contents of extractable lead have been found in stoneware and china (presumably where a lead glaze had been applied), in addition to the expected source, nonvitreous earthenware.

The available evidence indicates that lead is widely distributed in all natural foods. In the United States, lead intake from food and beverages ranges from 100 to 2,000 μg/day for an individual, with long-term averages of 120–350 μg/day (Engel et al., 1971). Lewis (1966) indicated that the lead concentration in milk is slightly higher than it was 20–30 yr ago and suggested that since it is a function of the body burden of the element rather than the concentration in the real diet, the lead concentration in milk might also serve as a useful index of human environmental exposure to lead. [The level of lead in milk in the United States is on the order of 0.05 ± 0.025 ppm (Lewis, 1966).]

Figure 9 is an ecological flow chart for lead showing possible cycling pathways and compartments, and an ecodiagram of lead in the environment and its effects on humans is shown in Fig. 10. This information and the amount and rates of transfer from one compartment of the environment to another permit treatment of the subject in terms of systems analysis.

As far as is known, environmental lead is in the inorganic form and there is no current evidence that a lead alkyl or "methyl"-lead is biosynthesized in the same way as mercury. Geographically, there is a logarithmic increase in the atmospheric lead concentration from midocean to remote high mountains, seashores, and suburban and urban environments. However, in

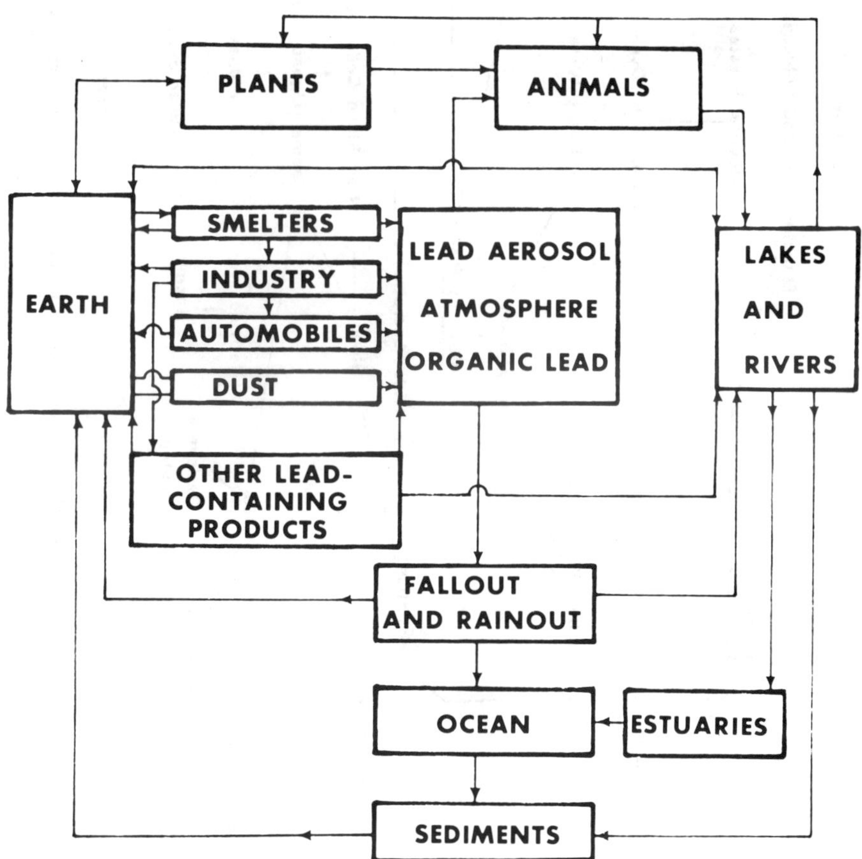

FIGURE 9 Ecological flow chart for lead showing possible cycling pathways and compartments.

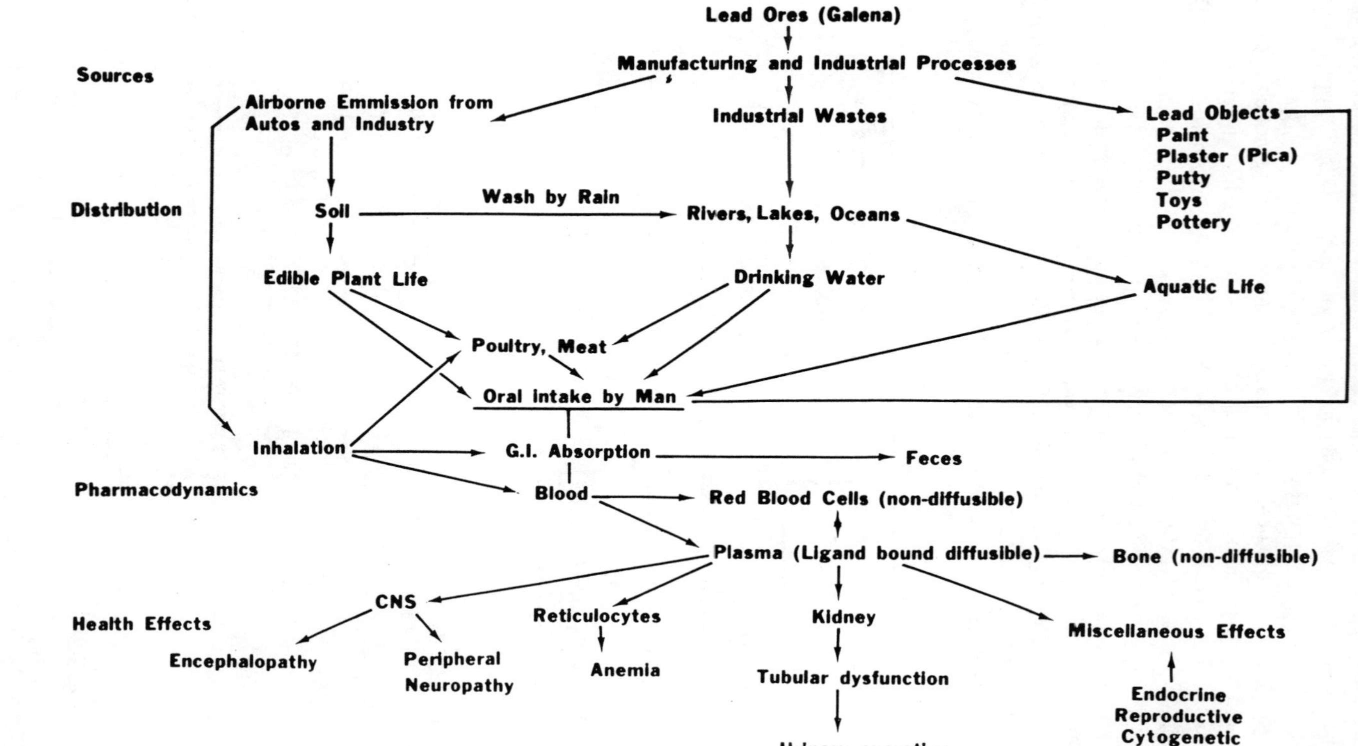

FIGURE 10 Ecodiagram of lead in the environment and its effects on humans.

spite of the rapid increase in the consumption of lead alkyls used in automotive fuels, the concentration of lead in urban air is in general rising only slowly, presumably because of dispersion (NAS, 1972). The disposition of lead emitted to the atmosphere and hence indirectly to other ecological compartments is dependent on both its physicochemical form and the meteorological factors that help dissipate it. Approximately half of the lead-containing particulate matter falls from the air by gravity within a few hundred feet of roadways. The remaining lead consists of aerosols that are largely airborne until removed by precipitation. The mean residence time of lead in the atmosphere is calculated as 7–30 days; much of the lead removed by precipitation and entering aquatic systems is not water-soluble and is removed from water by sedimentation.

Atmospheric lead concentrations at various locations have been reported. These range from 0.0002 $\mu g/m^3$ for Novaya Zemlya in the Soviet Union to 71 $\mu g/m^3$ recorded during a peak traffic period along the Los Angeles, California, freeway. It is interesting to note that before 1960 lead aerosol concentrations of 3 $\mu g/m^3$ would have been found only near highways with very heavy traffic, while today this concentration is commonly found in the urban regions of many large cities (Chow, 1973).

The toxicological effects of inhaled lead have been well documented (Kehoe, 1961; U.S. Department of Health, Education, and Welfare, 1969). It should also be noted that airborne lead forms about 0.5–1.5% of the lead content of the U.S. diet (Ter Haar, 1970), adding to the overall burden of lead.

The role of microorganisms in the biotransfer of lead and almost all aspects of transfer rates between compartments of the ecosystem are areas concerning which there is little or no information. Mosses tend to concentrate airborne lead and can be used as an index of regional lead pollution (Ruhling and Tyler, 1968). The average lead level in sewage effluents is estimated to be 98 $\mu g/l$, with the sludge containing 2,000–8,000 ppm of lead on a dry-weight basis (Ettinger, 1966). Dried municipal sludge is widely used in some areas in Great Britain as a fertilizer, but this usage can lead to virtually permanent contamination of the topsoil by lead, cadmium, and other toxic metals (Chow, 1973).

Huntzicker (1973) has estimated that about 10 tons of lead is deposited each day near the roadways in the Los Angeles metropolitan area. While much of this lead fallout is on the roadways themselves, about 2.1 tons of lead is deposited daily in the coastal waters and about 4.3 tons remains airborne and is blown out of the basin.

The lead discharged through the municipal waste outfalls in Southern California is estimated to be 0.55 ton/day. These values are quite similar to the values obtained for the early atmospheric fallout of lead.

Heavy metals such as lead and mercury are removed from waters quite rapidly after they enter the marine environment from sewer outfalls or rivers, and are associated with the sediments within several kilometers of the input to the marine environment.

Hicks (1972) has reviewed aspects of airborne lead as an environmental toxin. Lead is a highly toxic metal and, unlike other atmospheric pollutants, is a cumulative poison. It is stored primarily in the bones, but also in soft tissues including liver, muscle, kidney, spleen, and aorta (Hardy et al., 1971; Hammond, 1969; Schroeder and Tipton, 1968).

The body stores of lead increase with age, the increase being rapid during the early years and falling off during middle and old age. This stored lead, accumulated in the body tissue over a period of years, is hazardous to health because under a variety of circumstances it can reenter the circulation (Hardy et al., 1971; Hammond, 1969; Chrisholm and Harrison, 1956). Mobilization of stored lead from bone into circulation during pregnancy is of importance since lead can cross the placental barrier and affect the fetus (Barltrop, 1969).

Recent preliminary measurements in the air of central Stockholm have demonstrated that the content of tetraalkyl lead, measured as lead, corresponds to about 10% or more of the content of particulate lead. The observed concentration of alkyl lead (0.1-2 $\mu g/m^3$) is probably far too small to cause *acute* toxic effects in the city population (Ahlberg et al., 1972). However, the recent studies of Ahlberg et al. (1972) demonstrating that organolead compounds are genetically active suggest that health hazards from long-term effects of lead cannot be ruled out. For example, trimethyl, triethyl, and diethyl lead chlorides were found to cause disturbances in the spindle fiber mechanism of *A. cepa* at concentrations of 10^{-6}-10^{-7} M. This is of the same order of magnitude as that of the most active organic mercury compounds and is considerably lower than that of colchicin. Triethyl lead chloride was also observed to cause chromosome loss (presumably due to induced chromosome breakage) in *D. melanogaster* (Ahlberg et al., 1972).

The studies of Ahlberg et al. (1972) indicate that organometal compounds in particular act at very low concentrations and in a similar manner on the spindle fiber mechanism. Presumably, the effects of different metal compounds can be additive, and from the point of view of genetic risk the total load of metals in the environment is therefore of importance.

Contradictory results have been reported with regard to the occurrence of chromosome anomalies in people occupationally exposed to lead. For example, no evidence of increased aberrations was observed in workers in the lead manufacturing industry by Bauchinger and Schmid (1972) and Schmid et al. (1972) or in policemen with increased lead blood levels (Bauchinger and Schmid, 1972). These negative findings have been confirmed in human lymphocytes treated with lead acetate *in vitro* (Schmid et al., 1972) and in mice receiving lead acetate in their drinking water during a 9-month period (Leonard et al., 1972).

However, an increase in chromosome aberrations has been reported by

Forni and Secchi (1972), Schwanitz et al. (1970), and Sperling et al. (1970) in people occupationally exposed to lead, as well as in human lymphocytes treated *in vitro* with lead acetate (Obe and Sperling, 1970). Deknudt et al. (1973) recently described chromosome aberrations in male workers occupationally exposed to lead. In the latter study, peripheral blood lymphocytes of 14 workers from the zinc industry who had presented signs of lead poisoning of different degrees were examined. According to the type and the duration of exposure, the workers examined were classified into three groups: (1) those exposed to a high level of zinc and low levels of lead and cadmium, (2) those exposed to high levels of the three metals, and (3) those exposed to high levels of lead and cadmium in the absence of zinc. It was concluded that exposure to cadmium and zinc did not appear to increase the number of cells with severe chromosome anomalies and that lead intoxication could be considered responsible for the chromosome aberrations observed (dicentrics, rings, chromatid exchanges, and gaps and fragments).

Muro and Goyer (1969) reported that chromosomes of leukocyte cultures from mice fed a diet containing 1% lead acetate showed an increased number of gap and break aberrations. These chromosome abnormalities largely involved only single chromatids, which suggested that the damage occurred after the DNA synthesis phase of the cell cycle. The authors speculated that the chromosome damage inducible by administration of lead salts may contribute to reduction of fertility and to congenital malformations. The significance of these observations for human health is unknown at this time.

Mercury

Reports of the occurrence of mercury in the ecosystem (Fishbein, 1974; Friberg and Vostal, 1972; Johnels and Westermark, 1969; U.S. Department of Interior, 1970; Katz, 1972; International Committee, 1969; Nelson et al., 1971; Goldwater, 1971; Löfroth, 1970b) as well as the toxicological importance of various forms of mercury, primarily methyl mercury, are well documented and are of obvious concern (Friberg and Vostal, 1972; Löfroth, 1970b; Fishbein, 1974b; Bakir et al., 1973; Takeuchi, 1970; Kurland et al., 1960). It is important to note, however, that mercury and methyl mercury are naturally occurring substances to which all living organisms have been exposed (in varying degrees, depending on natural chemical, biological, and physical processes). Any scheme or consideration depicting the distribution and effects of mercury in the environment must certainly attempt to distinguish between the two categories of mercury sources—natural and anthropogenic. The geochemical cycle of mercury is shown in Fig. 11.

Of major environmental significance has been the realization that certain biotransformations involving mercury may occur. The transformation of inorganic mercury to methyl mercury in biological and related systems is well documented (Jensen and Jernelov, 1969; Bertilsson and Neujahr, 1971; Imura et al., 1971; Landner, 1970; Wood et al., 1969). Figure 12 illustrates a cycle of mercury interconversions in nature.

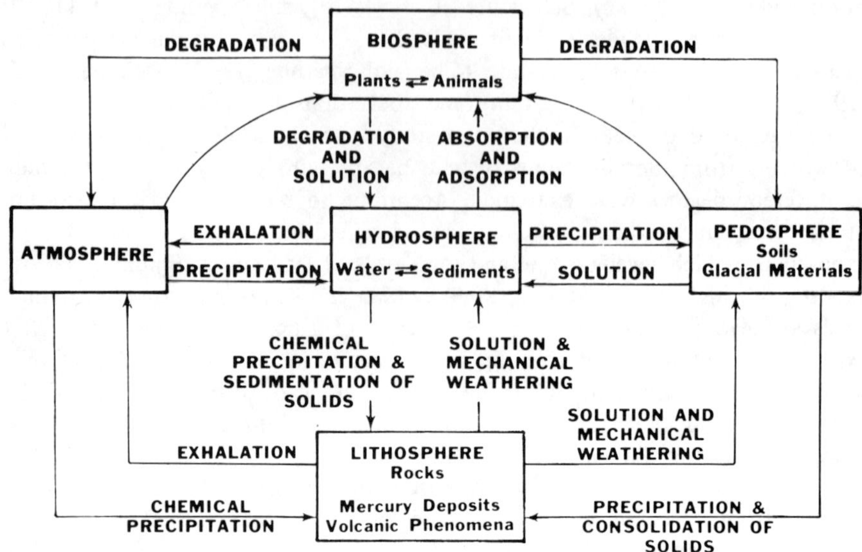

FIGURE 11　Geochemical cycle of mercury.

The world production of mercury amounts to about 10,000 tons/yr, of which about 3,000 tons are used in the United States. The main areas of utility of mercury include the electrolytic preparation of chlorine and caustic soda, agricultural chemicals, pharmaceuticals (diuretics, cathartics, antibacterial agents), hair dressings and preservatives in cosmetics, pulp and paper making (slimicides and algicides), paint (antifouling, pigment), electrical apparatus, catalysts, dental preparations, and amalgams. The production of chlorine and caustic soda is an electrolytic process where large amounts of mercury are used as a flowing cathode (75,000–150,000 lb for a plant with a capacity of 100 tons of chlorine a day) (Fimreite, 1970). It is estimated that the chlor-alkali industry loses to the environment approximately 0.45 lb of mercury per ton of chlorine produced (Murozumi, 1967). This loss, based on projected tonnage figures, may be as much as 3,300 lb/day or 1,200,000 lb/yr. Most of the lost mercury finds its way into streams and lakes and traces of mercury are also carried into the atmosphere with hydrogen gas (20–30 mg/m^3), while usually less than 5 ppm of mercury is retained by the caustic soda.

The manufacturing of electrical apparatus and instruments accounts for a significant portion of the mercury utilized in the United States. The largest specific use is for mercury batteries and alkaline energy cells; the bulk of the remaining mercury is used for manufacturing items such as power tubes, fluorescent lamps, germicidal lamps, mercury-pool rectifiers, and mercury switches, relays, and gauges (D'Itri, 1972). The paint industry accounts for a significant amount of mercury consumption. In 1968 it accounted for 14.4%

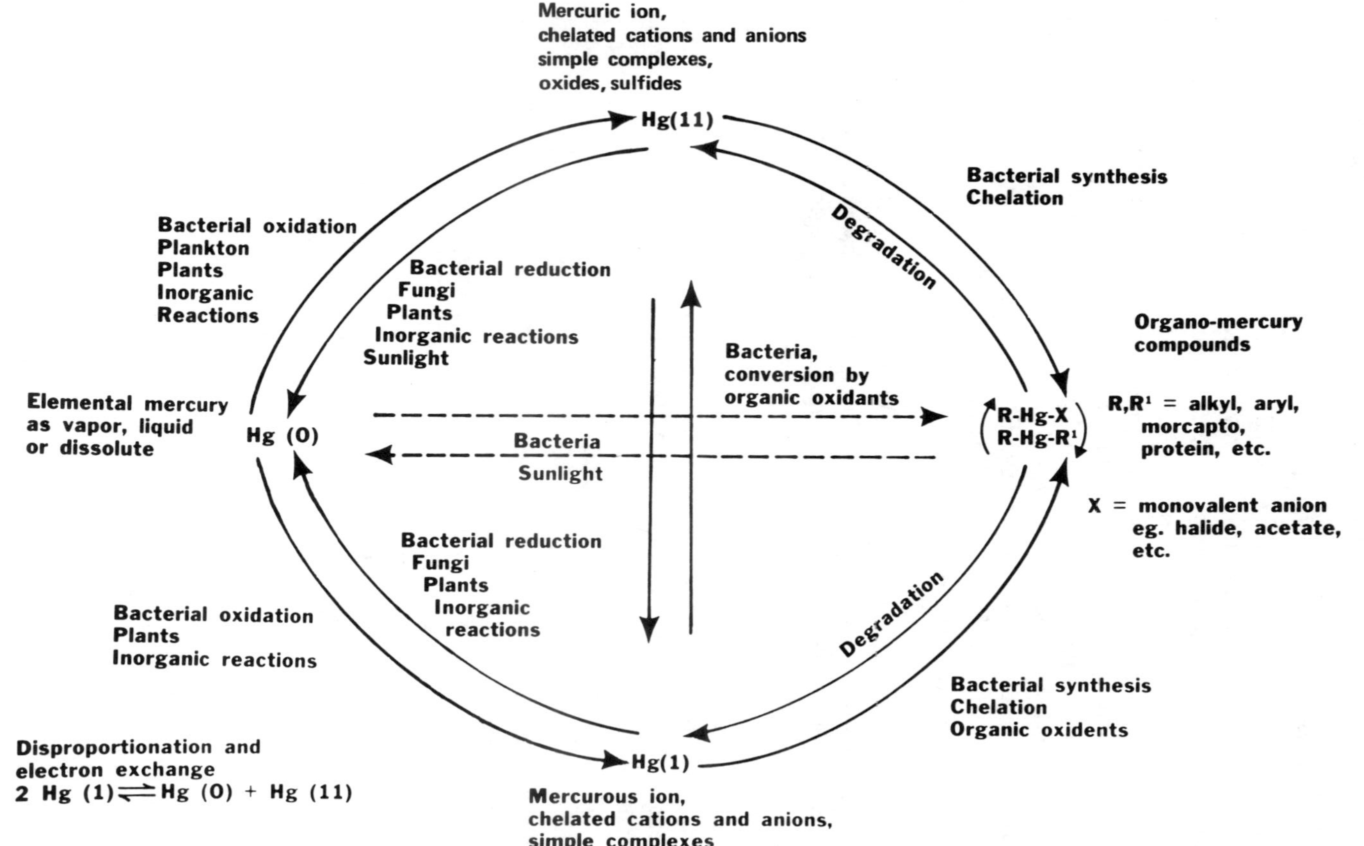

FIGURE 12 Cycle of mercury interconversions in nature.

of the U.S. consumption, which was 803,000 lb (D'Itri, 1972). Organomercurials are used in concentrations between 100 and 15,000 ppm to inhibit bacterial activity prior to paint applications and to retard fungus attacks on painted surfaces under moist or humid conditions. It has been reported (Krenkel, 1973) that a surface freshly painted with latex paint emits significant quantities of mercury to the atmosphere. For example, when 1.2 gal paint containing 0.28 g of a mercurial fungicide was applied in an enclosed room with a volume of 57.8 m^3, the concentration of mercury in the air immediately after painting ranged from 3.8 to 4.0 $\mu g/m^3$, and after 150–200 hr the concentration diminished to 1.3–1.7 $\mu g/m^3$. However, based on a ventilation analysis, it was concluded that mercury-containing vapors would remain in the air almost indefinitely. Foote (1972) recently measured the concentrations of elemental gaseous mercury in homes, offices, and laboratories in the Dallas area and found that they were substantially higher than the ambient natural background concentration (about 3 ng of mercury per cubic meter of air in San Francisco, Washington, and Dallas). Mercury concentrations in homes 3 yr after painting with latex-base interior paint containing diphenylmercury dodecenyl succinate have averaged 0.07 $\mu g/m^3$, an indication that the cleanup of spilled mercury was incomplete.

It is important to note that many basic chemicals contain small amounts of mercury originating from the raw materials. Significant contributions of mercury to the environment can result from large consumption of these materials. For example, utilization of 10,000 tons of sulfuric acid per year (containing 0.5 ppm mercury) would yield 50 kg of mercury.

Mercury has also been detected in chlorinated hydrocarbons, glycols, acetic acid, carbon dioxide, fertilizers, sulfuric acid, sulfide ores, industrial catalyst wastes (e.g., in production of acetaldehyde and vinyl chloride), and bituminous shales and crude oils.

Levels of mercury in the lower part of the atmosphere appear to range between 0 and 10 ng/m^3 (Friberg and Vostal, 1972; Weiss et al., 1971). Because of its high vapor pressure, mercury, primarily as the native metal, enters the atmosphere from rocks, deposits, waters, and volcanic vents. It has been calculated that the atmosphere contains 50 million lb of mercury (U.S. Geological Survey, 1970). Most of the mercury emitted to the atmosphere is washed out by rain, although its atmospheric residence time is not known.

It has been postulated that if all the mercury presently contributed to the environment went into the oceans, it would take 125 yr for the oceans' mercury concentration to double (Krenkel, 1973).

Although little is known about the nature of atmospheric mercury compared to that of other pollutants, it is believed that much of it is in the form of dimethyl mercury $[(CH_3)_2 Hg]$, resulting from volatilization from the hydrosphere and the lithosphere. However, both methyl mercury $[CH_3 Hg^+]$ and elemental mercury also volatilize (Nelson et al., 1971). Natural sources of atmospheric mercury include volcanic action (Eshleman et al., 1971; Saha,

1972) and volatilization from aquatic and terrestial environments (Saha, 1972). Eventually, atmospheric mercury, both organic and inorganic, is deposited by precipitation and fallout on both terrestial and aquatic environments. It is also interesting to note that high atmospheric mercury concentrations in the San Francisco Bay area have been found to coincide with high smog levels (Krenkel, 1973).

Sources of anthropogenic mercury emissions include combustion of fossil fuels (Joensuu, 1971; Billings and Matson, 1972), asphalt plants (Klein, 1972), and chlor-alkali plants (Nelson et al., 1971; Saha, 1972). Fossil fuels in the United States contain mercury in concentrations ranging from a few parts per billion to several parts per million. Annual consumption of 500 million tons of coal (containing an average concentration of at least 1 ppm) would contribute 1 million lb of mercury to the environment, or about 450 metric tons (Nelson et al., 1971). This value does not include the mercury released during refinement or the mercury from crude oil, the products of which may contain higher concentrations of mercury. Altogether, combustion of fossil fuel, roasting of sulfide ores, and cement production are estimated to release up to about 5×10^3 tons of mercury per year (Johnels et al., 1967; Rook et al., 1971).

Mercury released by natural weathering processes has been estimated by Joensuu (1971) to be at most 230 tons/yr. Weiss et al. (1971) suggest that natural degassing of mercury from the earth into the atmosphere yields in the range of 25×10^3 tons/yr and that this process has increased to some extent in recent decades. The fraction of the total flux attributable to industrial activity is small ($\sim 0.03\%$), but, within a confined area, short-term fallout of mercury originally discharged as a result of industrial activity may be significant. Local variations in mercury levels may also occur because of the uneven geochemical distribution of mercury (Eshleman et al., 1971) (Fig. 11).

Figures 13 and 14 illustrate the dissipative and recyclable uses of mercury in the United States for 1968 and the principal pathways of mercury contamination and environmental movement, respectively, while Fig. 15 shows the *estimated* rates of anthropogenic imposition on the ecological cycle of mercury in the United States. The data are little more than estimates, but give some idea of the relative risks. For example, food is shown as supplying only $\frac{1}{15}$ of the total impact of methyl mercury on humans.

Although methyl mercury overshadows the other organomercury compounds in terms of toxicity and environmental considerations, it is important to delineate the potential genetic hazards of the organomercurials as a whole.

Ramel (1967, 1969, 1972) reviewed the genetic effects of methyl mercury and other mercury compounds and cited the prominent effect of methyl mercury—its interference with the mitotic spindle, causing chromosome doubling or defective distribution of individual chromosomes during cell division, which leads to daughter cells with one or more missing or additional chromosomes (c-mitosis). For example, methyl mercury has been shown to

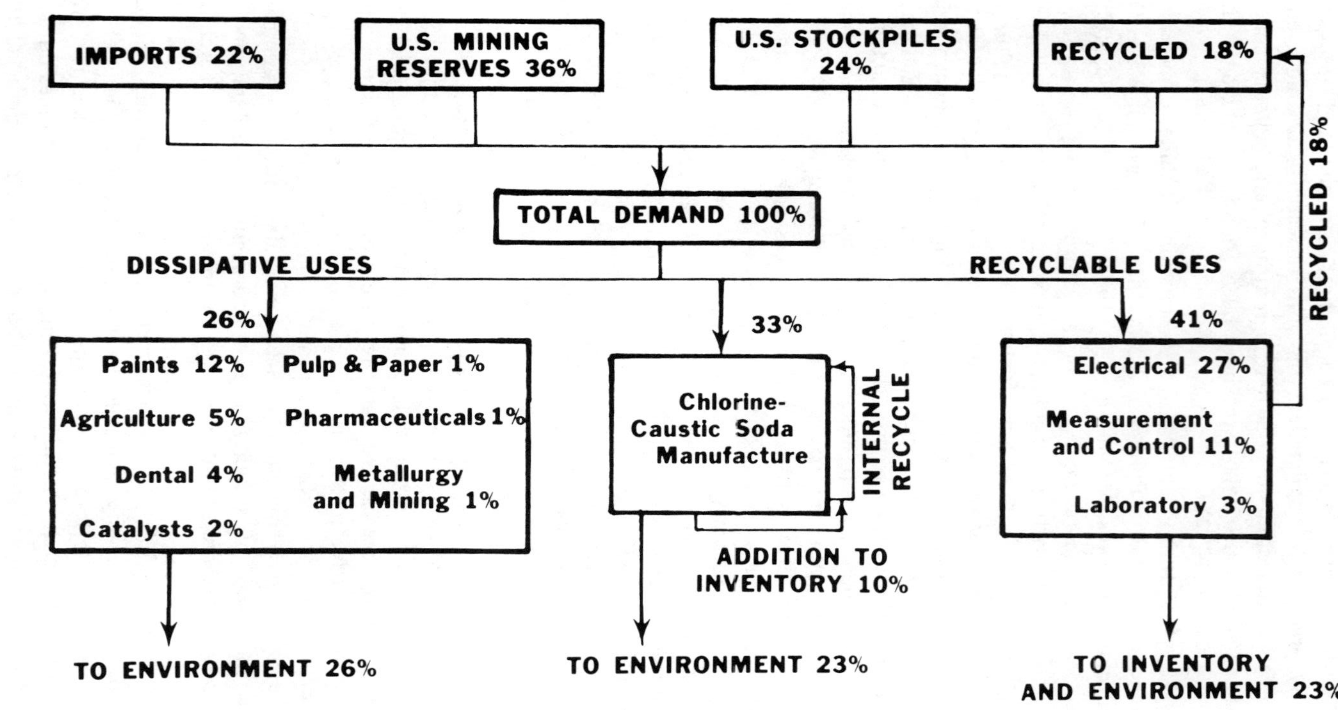

FIGURE 13 Dissipative and recyclable uses of mercury in the United States in 1968.

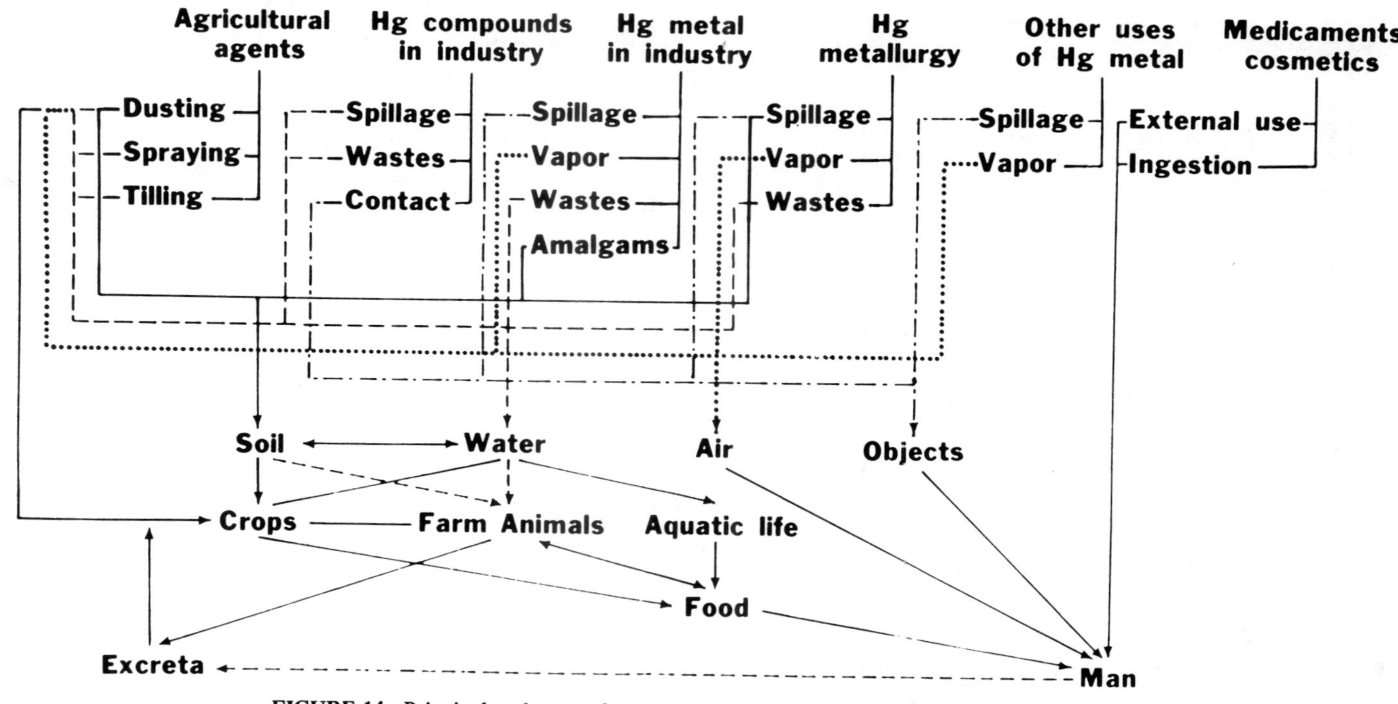

FIGURE 14   Principal pathways of mercury contamination and environmental movement.

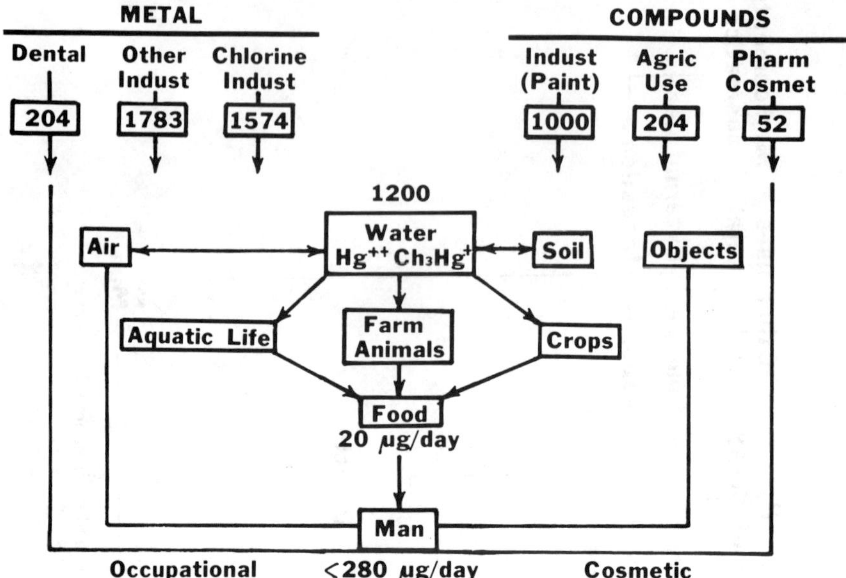

FIGURE 15 Estimated rates of anthropogenic imposition on the ecological cycle of mercury in the United States. Values are in 1,000 lb/yr, unless otherwise indicated.

disturb mitosis in plant cells (Ramel, 1969, 1972; Fiskesjo, 1969), in human leukocytes treated *in vitro* (Fiskesjo, 1970), and in human tissue culture (Umeda et al., 1969), causing polyploidy and aneuploidy. Nondisjunction of meiosis has been observed in *Drosophila* (Ramel and Magnusson, 1969). The chromosome-breaking effect has been attributed to a direct reaction between the mercury compound and the chromosome material, while the effects on cell division have been assumed to be due to interaction with the sulfhydryl groups of the protein units forming the cell spindle (Ramel, 1972).

Methyl mercury-induced chromosome damage in humans has been reported by Skerving et al. (1974). Lymphocytes of blood cultures from 23 subjects exposed to methyl mercury through intake of fish from contaminated waters were compared with those from 16 "nonexposed" subjects. There were statistically significant correlations between frequencies of cells with chromatid-type aberrations, "unstable" chromosome-type aberrations, and aneuploidy on the one hand and blood-cell mercury levels on the other. The significance of these findings for the health of the subjects and their offspring is not known. In 11 of the exposed subjects, no statistically significant correlation between variations in blood-cell mercury and chromosome aberrations could be established during sampling periods of 6 months to 3 yr.

Skerving et al. (1974) also raised the possibility that methyl mercury has cytogenetic effects on the embryo and fetus, since it is known to readily pass the placenta (Harada, 1968). Theoretically, spontaneous abortions, stillbirths, and congenital disorders are possible effects. While similar lesions might be expected from germ cells, it is not known whether germ-cell damage occurs in mammals (Skerving et al., 1974).

Arsenic

Arsenic is widely distributed (generally in small amounts) in the environment, particularly throughout the soils and waters of the world. Traces of arsenic are found in foods, particularly seafood, and in some meats and vegetables (Fishbein, 1972).

Environmental sources of arsenic include arsenic trioxide (the compound used in the preparation of many arsenic compounds), released and obtained primarily as a by-product of the smelting of sulfide ores of copper, zinc, or lead; combustion of coal and petroleum; production of glass, wood preservatives, nonferrous alloys, antifouling paints, and pyrotechnics; and the production and use of arsenic-containing pesticides and herbicides. For example, arsenic acid is used as a defoliant and desiccant (e.g., in the treatment of cotton before machine picking). Three alkylated arsenical herbicides, monosodium methanearsonate, disodium methanearsonate, and hydroxydimethylarsine oxide (cacodylic acid), find wide application in selective and general weed control programs. The estimated U.S. production of the three arsenical compounds in 1971 was 16.8×10^6 kg (Lawless et al., 1972). Cacodylic acid can be degraded oxidatively to CO_2 and AsO_4^{3-} in aerobic soils and reductively to a volatile organoarsenical, probably dimethylarsine (DMA), in aerobic and anerobic soils (Woolson and Kearney, 1973).

The reductive microbial pathway starting with As_2O_3 involves a series of reduction and methylation steps, and includes methanearsonate and cacodylic acid as intermediates in the formation of DMA (McBride and Wolfe, 1971). Figure 16 illustrates the proposed scheme of McBride and Wolfe (1971) for the methylation of arsenic by microorganisms in waterways (methyl

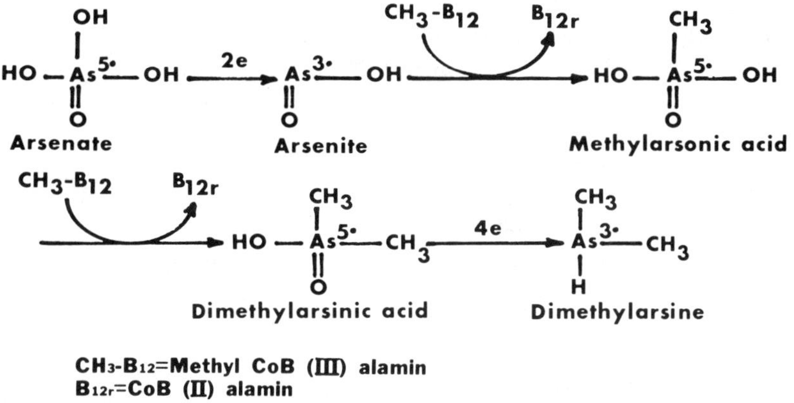

FIGURE 16 Methylation of arsenic by microorganisms in waterways.

cobalamine serving as the methyl donor in the reaction system). The apparent similarity between dimethylmercury and DMA suggests that the latter might undergo bioaccumulation in the aquatic food chains. Isensee et al. (1973) demonstrated that while cacodylic acid and dimethylarsine could be bioaccumulated by algae, *Daphnia magna*, snails, and fish, no biomagnification could be demonstrated in *model* ecosystems.

Arsenic-containing compounds such as arsanilic acid, sodium arsanilate, and 4-hydroxy-3-nitrophenylarsonic acid, are widely used in rations for poultry, cattle, and swine. It is usual to incorporate these arsenic derivatives at a level of approximately 90–250 g/ton of feed.

Arsenical compounds have long been suspected of causing cancer in humans (Buchanan, 1962). Lee and Fraumeni (1969) reported an overall threefold increase in respiratory cancer among 8,000 smelter workers exposed to arsenic trioxide. The increase was as high as eightfold among employees who were heavily exposed to arsenic and worked for more than 15 yr. It should be noted that the influence of sulfur dioxide or unidentified chemicals varying concomittantly with the arsenic exposure could not be discounted.

Ott et al. (1974) recently reported significant increases in respiratory cancer among workers engaged in formulating and packaging insecticides containing arsenic (e.g., lead arsenate, calcium arsenate, copper acetoarsenite, and magnesium arsenate). NIOSH (1973) has estimated that 1.5 million workers in the United States are potentially exposed to inorganic arsenic.

Excess cancer has also been reported to be associated with exposure to arsenicals in a number of British and German studies (Hill and Fanning, 1948; Robson and Jelliffe, 1963; Roth, 1957, 1958). For example, lung cancer and clinical arsenicalism were found in association among German vineyard workers who used insecticides containing arsenic in spraying and dusting operations between 1925 and 1942. In addition, a significant increase in lung cancer was found among inhabitants of the wine-producing areas of the Moselle River (where arsenic-containing insecticides were used) but not among residents of the wine-producing areas of the Ahr River, where pesticides containing arsenic were not used.

Added dimensions to the extent of arsenic exposure can be gleaned from the fact that until the early 1950s arsenical pesticides had been sprayed on tobacco crops in the United States. Use of these products has led to contamination of cigarettes with arsenic (Satterlee, 1956). The arsenic content of cigarettes rose from 12.6 μg per cigarette in 1932 to 42 μg in 1950–1951. These levels could lead to rather high concentrations of arsenic in the lung during smoking. Although in recent years arsenic levels have declined to an average of 7.2 μg/g of tobacco (Lee and Murphy, 1969), Peruvian tobaccos were found to contain arsenic levels of 22 μg per cigarette as recently as 1966 (Arata and Quispe, 1969).

In the epidemiologic studies to date, both the trivalent compounds (e.g., arsenic trioxide) and the pentavalent compounds (e.g., lead and calcium arsenate) have been observed to be carcinogenic, eliciting lung cancer, lymphatic cancer, and skin cancer. While little is known about the relative carcinogenic activity of the two valence states of arsenic in the various inorganic compounds, there is no apparent evidence supporting a distinction between the various inorganic arsenic compounds (OSHA, 1975). The OSHA (1975) recently proposed a permissible exposure limit of 0.004 mg/m^3 As with an active level of 0.002 mg/m^3 and a ceiling limit of 0.01 mg/m^3 over any 15-min period.

It is important to note additional environmental levels of arsenic. For example, background arsenic levels of 10–40 μg/m^3 of air in New York City have been reported (Satterlee, 1956). The presence of arsenic at a concentration of 10–70 ppm has been detected in several common presoaks and household detergents in the United States (Angino et al., 1970). Arsenic levels of 2–8 ppb have been measured in U.S. rivers.

Kroes et al. (1974) reported no evidence of carcinogenicity of sodium arsenate and equivocal evidence of carcinogenicity of lead arsenate in a lifetime (29-month) study in Wistar rats.

Teratogenicity of sodium arsenate in the golden hamster (Ferm and Carpenter, 1968; Ferm et al., 1971), mouse (Hood and Bishop, 1972), and Wistar rat (Beaudoin, 1974) has been demonstrated.

Mutagenicity of arsenic derivatives has been sparsely reported. Paton and Allison (1972) reported chromosome damage in human cell cultures induced by a variety of metal and metalloid derivatives including arsenic. Nishioka (1975) recently reported the mutagenic activity of sodium arsenite (NaAsO$_2$) in the rec-assay using *Bacillus subtilis* strains H17 (*rec*$^+$, *arg*$^-$, and *trp*$^-$) and M45 (*rec*$^-$, *arg*$^-$, and *trp*$^-$) according to the technique of Kada et al. (1972). It was also shown that arsenic compounds such as AsCl$_3$ and NaAsO$_2$, having a valence of -3, seem to be more mutagenic than Na$_2$HAsO$_4$, which has a valence of $+5$, when tested as above. Sodium arsenite was also tested for the induction of tryptophan reversions of *E. coli* strains of WP$_2$ (μvrA^+, *recA*$^+$), WP$_2$ μvr(μvrA^-, *recA*$^+$), and CM571 (μvrA^+, *recA*$^-$). The strain CM571 carrying *recA*$^-$ was hardly mutable by NaAsO$_2$ [as well as K$_2$Cr$_2$O$_7$ and (NH$_4$)$_6$Mo$_7$O$_{24}$], suggesting that the DNA lesions produced in the rec-assay in *B. subtilis* may be repaired through recombination mechanisms and that the *recA* allele may be required for metal mutagenesis.

SUMMARY

Comparative data have been presented (wherever available) on the relative amounts, residues, and transport in the environment of a spectrum of primarily synthetic mutagenic and potentially mutagenic agents representative of diverse categories, including metals in industrial and pesticidal use categories and their degradation products.

The mutagens and potential mutagens surveyed include industrial mutagens (primarily the halogenated hydrocarbons, vinyl chloride, vinylidene chloride, trichloroethylene, tetrachloroethylene, chloroprene, carbon tetrachloride, fluorocarbons, polychlorinated biphenyls, chlorodioxins, haloethers, chlorine, bromoalkanes, and fluorine), phthalate esters, pesticides (DDT, dichlorvos, formaldehyde, and ethylene oxide), and metals and metalloids (lead, mercury, and arsenic).

Information is sparse, as well as lacking in many regards, concerning the environmental reactions and interactions (e.g., in the atmosphere, soil, and water) of many of these mutagens, as well as aspects of their transport, residence times, and stability. Knowledge of the fate of many of these agents (particularly the many halogenated hydrocarbons) in the atmosphere is largely speculative at this time.

It must also be acknowledged that in the vast majority of cases, environmental chemical agents (both naturally occurring and synthetic) have not been extensively and/or adequately tested to permit an evaluation of their relative mutagenic hazard to humans.

REFERENCES

Abbott, D. C., Harrison, R. B., Tatton, J. O. G. and Thompson, J. 1966. Organochlorine pesticides in the atmosphere. *Nature (Lond.)* 211:259–261.

Abernethy, R. C. and Gibson, F. H. 1963. Rare elements in coal. *U.S. Bur. Mines Rep. IC-8163*, p. 21.

Abernethy, R. F. and Gibson, F. H. 1967. Method for determination of fluorine in coal. *U.S. Bur. Mines Rep. RI-7054*, p. 13.

Ahlberg, J., Ramel, C. and Wachtmeister, C. A. 1972. Organo lead compounds shown to be genetically active. *Ambio* 1:29–31.

Albert, R. E., Train, R. E. and Anderson, E. 1977. Rationale developed by the Environmental Protection Agency for the assessment of carcinogenic risks. *J. Natl. Cancer Inst.* 58:1537–1541.

Alderson, T. 1960. Mechanism of formaldehyde-induced mutagenesis. The uniqueness of adenylic acid in the mediation of the mutagenic activity of formaldehyde. *Nature (Lond.)* 187:486–489.

Allison, A. C. and Paton, G. R. 1965. Chromosome damage in human diploid cells following activation by lysosomal enzymes. *Nature (Lond.)* 207:1170–1173.

Altshuller, A. P., Cohen, I. R., Meyer, M.E. and Wartburg, A. F., Jr. 1961. Analysis of aliphatic aldehydes in source effluents in the atmosphere. *Anal. Chem. Acta.* 25:101–117.

American Chemical Society. 1973. *Chemistry in the environment.* Washington, D.C.: American Chemical Society.

Ames, B. N., Durston, W. E., Yamasaki, E. and Lee, F. D. 1973. Carcinogens are mutagens: A simple test system combining liver homogenates for activation and bacteria for detection. *Proc. Natl. Acad. Sci. U.S.A.* 8:2281–2285.

Angino, E. E., Magnuson, L. M., Wauga, T. C., Galle, O. K. and Bredfelt, J. 1970. Arsenic in detergents: Possible danger and pollution hazard. *Science* 168:389–390.

Arata, A. L. and Quispe, P. L. 1969. Concentration de arsenico en tabacosy cigarillos Peruanes. *Rev. Fac. Quim.* 17:15–22.

Auerbach, C., Robson, J. M. and Carr, J. G. 1947. The chemical production of mutations. *Science* 105:243–247.

Autian, J. 1973. Toxicity and health threats of phthalate esters: A review of the literature. *Environ. Health Perspect.* 1:3–26.

Aviado, D. M. 1975a. Toxicity of aerosol propellants in the respiratory and circulatory systems, IX. Summary of the most toxic: Trichlorofluoro-methane (FC-11). *Toxicology* 3:311–319.

Aviado, D. M. 1975b. Toxicity of aerosols. *J. Clin. Pharmacol.* 15:86–104.

Bagchi, K. W., Ganguly, J. D. and Sirdar, J. N. 1940. Lead in food. *Indian J. Med. Res.* 28:441–450.

Bakir, F., Damluji, S. F., Smin-Zaki, M., Mustadita, M., Khalidi, A., Al-Rawi, N. Y., Tikriti, S., Dhahir, H. I., Clarkson, T. W., Smith, J. C. and Doherty, R. A. 1973. Mercury poisoning in Iraq. *Science* 181:230–241.

Barltrop, D. 1969. Environmental lead and its pediatric significance. *Postgrad. Med. J.* 45:129–134.

Barthelmess, A. 1956. Mutagenic drugs. *Arzneim. Forsch.* 6:157–168.

Barthelmess, A. 1970. Mutagenic substances in the human environment. In *Chemical mutagenesis in mammals and man*, eds. F. Vogel and G. Rohrborn, pp. 69–147. Heidelberg: Springer-Verlag.

Bartonicek, V. and Soucek, B. 1959. Der Metabolismus des Trichloräthylen beim Kaninchen. *Arch. Gewerbepathol. Gewerbehyg. 17:283.*

Bartsch, H., Malaveille, C. and Montesano, R. 1975a. Human, rat and mouse liver mediated mutagenicity of vinyl chloride in *S. typhimurium* strains. *Int. J. Cancer* 15:429–437.

Bartsch, H., Malaveille, C., Montesano, R. and Tomatis, L. 1975b. Tissue mediated mutagenicity of vinylidene chloride and 2-chlorobutadiene in *Salmonella typhimurium. Nature (Lond.)* 255:641

Bauchinger, M. and Schmid, E. 1972. Chromosome Analysen in Zellkulturen des Chinesischen Hamsters nach Applikation von Blei Acetat. *Mutat. Res.* 14:95–100.

Bauer, H., Schulz, K. H. and Spiegelberg, U. 1940. Berufliche Vergiftungen bei der Herstellung von Chlorophenol-Verbindungen. *Arch. Gewerbepathol. Gewerbehyg.* 18:538–555.

Beaudoin, A. 1974. Teratogenicity of sodium arsenate in rats. *Teratology* 10:153–158.

Bedford, C. T. and Robinson, J. 1972. The alkylating properties of organo-phosphates. *Xenobiotica* 2:307–337.

Belej, J. A. and Aviado, D. M. 1975. Cardiopulmonary toxicity of propellants for aerosols. *J. Clin. Pharmacol.* 15:105–115.

Bender, M. A. and Gooch, P. C. 1966. Somatic chromosome aberrations induced by human whole body irradiation: The "recuplex" criticality accident. *Radiat. Res.* 29:568–582.

Bengtson, S. A. and Sodergren, A. 1974. DDT and PCB residues in airborne fallout and animals in Iceland. *Ambio* 8:84–86.

Berck, B. 1966. Investigations on fumigants. I. Nature and properties of fumigants. *Occup. Health Rev.* 18:16–26.

Berck, B. 1974. Fumigant residues of carbon tetrachloride and ethylene dibromide in wheat, flour, bran, middlings, and bread. *J. Agric. Food Chem.* 22:977–984.

Bertilsson, L. and Neujahr, H. Y. 1971. Methylation of mercury compounds by methyl cobalamin. *Biochemistry* 10:2805–2808.

Billings, C. E. and Matson, W. R. 1972. Mercury emissions from coal combustion. *Science* 176:1232.

Bird, M. J. 1952. Chemical production of mutations in *Drosophila,* comparison of techniques. *J. Genet.* 50:480–485.

Blake, D. A. and Mergner, G. W. 1974. Inhalation studies on the biotransformation and elimination of [^{14}C]-trichlorofluoromethane and [^{14}C]-dichlorofluoromethane in beagles. *Toxicol. Appl. Pharmacol.* 30:396–407.

Bower, R. K., Haberman, S. and Minton, P. D. 1970. Teratogenic effects in the chick embryo caused by esters of phthalic acid. *J. Pharmacol. Exp. Ther.* 171:314–324.

Boyland, E. 1969. The correlation of experimental carcinogenesis and cancer in man. *Progr. Exp. Tumor Res.* 11:222–234.

Braun, R. and Schoneich, J. 1975. The influence of ethanol and carbon tetrachloride on the mutagenic effectivity of cyclophosphamide in the host-mediated assay with *Salmonella typhimurium. Mutat. Res.* 31:191–194.

Brem, H., Stein, A. B. and Rosenkranz, H. S. 1974. The mutagenicity and DNA modifying effects of haloalkanes. *Cancer Res.* 34:2576–2579.

Bridges, B. A., Mottershead, R. P., Green, M. H. L. and Gray, W. J. H. 1973. The mutagenicity of dichlorovos and methyl methane sulphonate for *E. coli* WP2 and some derivatives deficient in DNA repair. *Mutat. Res.* 19:295–303.

Brown, G., Corbett, D. C. M., Hide, G. A. and Webb, R. M. 1974. Bromine residues in potato and wheat crops grown in soil fumigated with methyl bromide. *Pestic. Sci.* 5:25–29.

Bruhin, A. 1955. Uber die polyploidisierende Wirkung eines Samenbeizmittels. *Phytopathol. Z.* 23:381–394.

Brunelle, M. F., Dickinson, J. E. and Hamming, H. J. 1966. *Effectiveness of organic solvents in photochemical smog formation.* Los Angeles: Air Pollution Control District.

Buchanan, W. D. 1962. *Toxicity of arsenic compounds.* Princeton, N. J.: Van Nostrand.

Buselmaier, W., Rohrborn, G. and Propping, P. 1973. Comparative investigations on the mutagenicity of pesticides in mammalian test systems. *Mutat. Res.* 21:25A.

Butler, T. C. 1961. Reduction of carbon tetrachloride *in vivo* and reduction of carbon tetrachloride and chloroform *in vitro* by tissues and tissue constituents. *J. Pharmacol. Exp. Ther.* 134:311.

Caputo, A., Viola, P. L. and Bigotti, A. 1974. Oncogenicity of vinyl chloride at low concentrations in rats and rabbits. *IRCS Libr. Compend.* 2:1582.

Carlson, G. P. 1974. Enhancement of the hepatotoxicity of trichloroethylene by inducers of drug metabolism. *Res. Commun. Chem. Pathol. Pharmacol.* 7:637–640.

Carlson, R. M., Carlson, R. E., Kipperman, H. L. and Caple, R. 1975. Facile incorporation of chlorine into aromatic systems during aqueous chlorination processes. *Environ. Sci. Technol.* 9:674–675.

Carr, D. H. 1967. Chromosomes after oral contraceptives. *Lancet* 2:830–831.

Carr, D. H. 1970. Chromosome studies in selected spontaneous abortions: I. Conception after oral contraceptives. *Can. Med. Assoc. J.* 103:343–348.

Carter, C. E., Kimbrough, R. D., Liddle, J. A., Cline, R. E., Zack, M. M., Jr., Barthel, W. F., Koehler, R. E. and Phillips, P. E. 1975. Tetrachlorodibenzodioxin: An accidental poisoning episode in horse arenas. *Science* 188:738–740.

Chemical & Engineering News. 1972. Phthalate effect on health still not clear. 50:14–15.

Chemical & Engineering News. 1974. Environmentalists seek fluorocarbon ban. 52:14.

Chemical & Engineering News. 1975a. Federal task force probes ozone issue. 53:17.

Chemical & Engineering News. 1975b. Industry's problems with cancer aired. 53:4.

Chemical & Engineering News. 1975c. Conference explored occupational cancer. 53:16.

Chemical & Engineering News. 1975d. Chloroprene is latest cancer scare. 53:4.

Chemistry and Industry. 1973. Plastics heading for a boom. 13:597.

Chow, T. S. 1973. Our daily lead. *Chem. Br.* 9:258–263.

Chow, T. S. and Johnstone, M. C. 1965. Lead isotopes in gasoline and aerosols of Los Angeles Basin, California. *Science* 147:502–503.

Chrisholm, J. J. and Harrison, H. E. 1956. The exposure of chidren to lead. *Pediatrics* 18:943–958.

Christofferson, D. W. 1961. Coatings for steel water storage tanks. *J. Am. Water Works Assoc.* 53:725–736.

Cicerone, R. J., Stolarski, R. S. and Walters, S. 1975. Stratospheric ozone destruction by manmade chlorofluoromethanes. *Science* 185:1165–1167.

Clark, J. M. 1974. Mutagenicity of DDT. in mice, *Drosophila melanogaster* and *Neurospora crassa. Aust. J. Biol. Sci.* 27:427–440.

Clayton, J. W. 1967. Fluorocarbon toxicity and biological action. *Fluorine Chem. Rev.* 1:197–252.

Cohen, J. M. and Pinkerton, C. 1966. Organic pesticides in the environment. *Adv. Chem. Ser.* 60:163.

Cohen, M. M. 1972. Two human X-autosome translocations identified by autoradiography and fluorescence. *Am. J. Hum. Genet.* 24:583–597.

Collier, L. 1972. Determination of bis-chloromethyl ether at the ppb level in air samples by high-resolution mass spectroscopy. *Environ. Sci. Technol.* 6:930.

Collins, C. J. and Guild, W. R. 1964. Irreversible effects of formaldehyde on DNA. *Biochim. Biophys. Acta.* 157:107–113.

Committee 17. 1974. Environmental mutagenic hazards. *Nature (Lond.)* 187:503–514.

Cook, R. W. 1966. Air pollution by the Florida citrus industry, its causes and prevention. *Proc. Fla. State Hortic. Soc.* 78:260.

Cook, W. A., Giever, P. M., Dinman, B. D. and Magnuson, H. J. 1971. Occupational acroosteolysis, II. An industrial hygiene study. *Arch. Environ. Health* 22:74–82.

Corcoran, E. F. 1973. Gas chromatographic detection of phthalic acid esters. *Environ. Health Perspect.* 3:13–15.

Cory, L., Fjeld, P. and Serat, W. 1971. Environmental DDT and the genetics of natural populations. *Nature (Lond.)* 229:128.

Council on Environmental Quality 1971. *Toxic substances.* Washington, D.C.: Government Printing Office.

County of Los Angeles. 1971. *Profile of air pollution control.* Los Angeles: Air Pollution Control District.

Cramer, J. 1973. Model of the circulation of DDT on earth. *Atmos. Environ.* 7:241–256.

Creech, J. L. and Johnson, M. N. 1974. Angiosarcoma of liver in the manufacture of polyvinyl chloride. *J. Occup. Med.* 16:150–151.

Crosby, D. G. 1973. The fate of pesticides in the environment. *Annu. Rev. Plant Physiol.* 24:467–492.

Crutzen, P. U. 1974a. Estimates of possible variations in total ozone due to natural causes and human activities. *Ambio* 3:201–210.

Crutzen, P. 1974b. A review of upper atmospheric photochemistry. *Can. J. Chem.* 52:1569–1581.

Daniel, J. 1963. Metabolism of ^{36}Cl-labelled trichlorethylene and tetrachloroethylene in the rat. *Biochem. Pharmacol.* 12:795–802.

Dean, B. J. 1972a. The mutagenic effects of organophosphorus pesticides on microorganisms. *Arch. Toxikol.* 30:67–74.

Dean,B. J. 1972a. The effects of dichlorvos on cultured human lymphocytes. *Arch. Toxikol.* 30:75–85.

Dean, B. J. and Thorpe, E. 1972a. Studies with dichlorvos vapor in dominant lethal mutation tests on mice. *Arch. Toxikol.* 30:51–59.

Dean, B. J. and Thorpe, E. 1972b. Cytogenic studies of dichlorvos in mice and Chinese hamsters. *Arch. Toxikol.* 30:75–85.

Dean, B. J., Doak, S. M. A. and Funnell, J. 1972. Genetic studies with dichlorvos in the host-mediated assay and in liquid medium using *Saccharomyces cerevisiae. Arch. Toxikol.* 30:61–66.

Decker, G. C., Bruce, W. N. and Bigger, J. H. 1965. Accumulation or dissipation of residues resulting from the use of aldrin soils. *J. Econ. Entomol.* 58:266–270.

Deknudt, G., Leonard, A. and Ivanov, B. 1973. Chromosome aberrations observed in male workers occupationally exposed to lead. *Environ. Physiol. Biochem.* 3:132.

DeLaMare, P. B. D. and Ridd, J. H. 1959. *Aromatic substitution, nitration and halogenation.* New York: Academic Press.

De Serres, F. J. and Malling, H. V. 1969. Genetic analysis of ad-3 mutants of *Neurospora crassa* induced by ethylene dibromide. a commonly used pesticide with high mutagenic activity. *Genetics* 61:39.

Dinman, B. D., Cook, W. A., Whitehouse, W. M., Mannuson, H. J. and Ditcheck, T. 1971. Occupational acroosteolysis. I. An epidemiological study. *Arch. Environ. Health* 22:74–80.

D'Itri, F. M. 1972. The environmental mercury problem. In *Environmental mercury contamination*, eds. R. Hargung and B. D. Dinman, p. 5. Ann Arbor, Mich.: Ann Arbor Science.

Dobzhansky, T. 1958. Genetics of natural populations, XXVII. The genetic changes in populations of *Drosophila pseudoobscura* in the American Southwest. Evolution 12:385–401.

Dobzhansky, T., Anderson, W. W., Pavlovsky, O., Spassky, S. and Bandwills, C. J. 1964. Genetics of natural populations, XXV. A progress report of genetic changes in populations of *Drosophilia pseudoobscura* in the American Southwest. *Evolution* 18:164–176.

Dobzhansky, T., Anderson, W. W. and Pavlovsky, O. 1966. Genetics of natural populations, XXXVIII. Continuity and change in populations of *Drosophila pseudoobscura* in the western United States. *Evolution* 20:418–427.

Ducatman, A., Hirschhorn, K. and Selikoff, I. J. 1975. Vinyl chloride exposure and human chromosome aberrations. *Mutat. Res.* 31:163–168.

Duce, R. A., Quinn, J. G. and Olney, C. E. 1972. Enrichment of heavy metals and organic compounds in the surface microlayer of Narragansett Bay, Rhode Island. *Science* 176:161.

Dumas, T. 1973. Inorganic and organic bromine residues in foodstuffs fumigated with methyl bromide and ethylene dibromide at low temperature. *J. Agric. Food Chem.* 21:433–436.

Dumas, T. and Bond, E. J. 1975. Bromide residues in apples fumigated with ethylene dibromide. *J. Agric. Food Chem.* 23:95–98.

Durum, W. H. and Haffty, J. 1961. Occurrence of minor elements in water. *U.S. Geol. Surv. Circ.* 445:11.

Dyachuk, I. A. 1970. Hygienic assessment of polyvinyl chloride tiles for covering floors in apartments. *Gig. Sanit.* 35:91.

Dyer, K. F. and Hanna, P. J. 1972. Comparative mutagenic activity and toxicity of triethylphosphate and dichlorvos in bacteria and *Drosophila*. *Mutat. Res.* 21:175–177.

Edwards, C. A. 1966. Insecticide residues in soils. *Residue Rev.* 13:83–132.

Edwards, C. A. 1970. *Persistent pesticides in the environment*. Cleveland, Ohio: Chemical Rubber Co.

Ehrenberg, L., Gustafsson, A. and Lundquist. U. 1956. Chemically induced mutation and sterility in barley. *Acta Chem. Scand.* 10:492–494.

Ehrenberg, L., Hiesche, K. D., Osterman-Golkar, S. and Wennberg, I. 1974. Evaluation of genetic risks of alkylating agents: Tissue doses in the mouse from air contaminated with ethylene oxide. *Mutat. Res.* 24:83–103.

Elgar, K. E., Mathews, B. L. and Bosio, P. 1972. Vapona strips in shops—Residues in foodstuffs. In *Environmental quality and safety*, eds. F. Coulston and F. Korte, vol. 1, pp. 217–221. Stuttgart: Thieme.

Engel, R. E., Hammer, D. I., Horton, R. J. M., Lane, N. M. and Plumlee, L. A., 1971. Environmental and health aspects of lead. *EPA Publ. 3*, Washington, D.C.

Environmental Protection Agency. 1975. Environmental aspects of vinyl/polyvinyl chloride. Research Triangle Park, N.C.: Environmental Protection Agency.

Environmental Science and Technology. 1974. Emerging technology of chlorinolysis. 8:18–19.

Epstein, S. S. 1969. Trimethyl phosphate. *Environ. Mutagen Soc. Newslett.* 2:33.

Epstein, S. S. and Legator, M. S. 1971. *The mutagenicity of pesticides*, p. 30. Cambridge, Mass.: MIT Press.

Epstein, S. S. and Shafner, H. 1971. Chemical mutagens in the human environment. *Nature (Lond.)* 230:259–260.

Epstein, S. S., Joshi, S., Andrea, J., Clapp, P., Falk, H. and Mantel, N. 1967. Synergistic toxicity and carcinogenicity of "Freons" and piperonyl butoxide. *Nature (Lond.)* 214:526.

Epstein, S. S., Bass, W., Arnold, E. and Bishop, Y. 1970. The mutagenicity of trimethyl phosphate in mice. *Science* 168:584–586.

Eshleman, A., Siegel, S. M. and Siegel, B. Z. 1971. Is mercury from Hawaiian volcanoes a natural source of pollution? *Nature (Lond.)* 233:471.

Ettinger, M. B. 1966. Lead in drinking water. *U.S. Public Health Serv. Publ.* 1440:21–27.

European Chemical News. 1974. C. A. argues case against zero VCM exposure limits. May 24, p. 24.

Faberge, A. C. 1955. Types of chromosome aberrations induced by ethylene oxide in maize. *Genetics* 40:571.

Fabre, R. and Truhaut, R. 1952. Contribution de l'etude de la toxicologie du trichloroethylene. *Br. J. Ind. Med.* 9:39.

Fahrig, R. 1973. Nachweis einer genetischem Wirkung von Organophosphor-insektiziden. *Naturwissenschaften* 60:50–51.

Fahrig, R. 1974. Comparative mutagenicity studies with pesticides M161–181. *IARC Monogr. 10.*

Fassett, D. W. 1963. β-Propiolactone. In *Industrial hygiene and toxicology,* ed. F. A. Patty, vol. 2, pp. 1823–1826. New York: Interscience.

Federal Register. 1974. Vinyl chloride, emergency suspension order concerning registrations for certain products and intent to cancel registrations. 30 (82):14573–14574.

Ferm, V. H. and Carpenter, S. J. 1968. Malformations induced by sodium arsenate. *J. Reprod. Fertil.* 17:199–201.

Ferm, V. H., Saxon, A. and Smith, B. M. 1971. The teratogenic profile of sodium arsenate in the golden hamster. *Arch. Environ. Health* 22:557–560.

Figuerova, W. G., Reszkowski, R. and Weiss, W. 1973. Lung cancer in chloromethyl methyl ether workers. *N. Engl. J. Med.* 288:1096–1097.

Filatova, V. S. and Gronsberg, E. S. 1957. Sanitary hygienic conditions of work in the production of polycholorvinyl tar and measures of improvement. *Gig. Sanit.* 22:38–42.

Fimreite, N. 1970. Mercury uses in Canada and their possible hazards as sources of mercury contamination. *Environ. Pollut.* 1:119–131.

Fishbein, G. W. 1972. *Occup. Safety Health Lett.* 2 (6 March): 22.

Fishbein, L. 1969. Degradation and residues of alkylating agents. *Ann. N.Y. Acad. Sci.* 163:869–893.

Fishbein, L. 1972. Natural non-nutrient substances in the food chain. *Sci. Total Environ* 1:211–244.

Fishbein, L. 1973. Mutagens and potential mutagens in the biosphere, I. DDT and its metabolites, polychlorinated biphenyls, chlorodioxins, polycyclic aromatic hydrocarbons, haloethers. *Sci. Total Environ.* 4:305–340.

Fishbein, L. 1974. Toxicity of chlorinated biphenyls. *Annu. Rev. Pharmacol.* 14:139–156.

Fishbein, L. 1974. Mutagens and potential mutagens in the biosphere, II. Metals—mercury, lead, cadmium and tin. *Sci. Total Environ.* 2:341–371.

Fishbein, L., Flamm, W. G. and Falk, H. L. 1970. *Chemical mutagens,* pp. 198–203. New York: Academic Press.

Fiskesjo, G. 1969. Some results from allium tests with organic mercury halogenides. *Hereditas* 62:314–322.

Fiskesjo, G. 1970. The effect of two organic mercury compounds on human leukocytes *in vitro. Hereditas* 64:142–146.

Foltz, V. C. and Fuerst, R. 1974. Mutation studies with *Drosophila melanogaster* exposed to four fluorinated hydrocarbon gases. *Environ. Res.* 7:275–285.

Food and Cosmetics Toxicology. 1970. The air we breathe. 8:212–222.

Foote, R. J. 1972. Mercury vapor concentrations inside buildings. *Science* 177:513–514.

Forni, A. and Secchi, G. 1971. Chromosome changes in preclinical and clinical lead poisoning and correlation with biochemical findings. Presented at the International Symposium on the Environmental Health Aspects of Lead, Amsterdam, October 1–6.

Fowler, S. S. L. 1968. A new metabolite of carbon tetrachloride. *Br. J. Pharmacol.* 36:181.

Friberg, L. and Vostal, J., eds. *Mercury in the environment.* Cleveland, Ohio: CRC Press.

Funes-Cravioto, F., Lambert, B., Lindsten, J., Ehrenberg, L., Natarajan, A. T. and Osterman-Golkar, S. 1975. Chromosome aberrations in workers exposed to vinyl chloride. *Lancet* 1:459.

Gaffney, D. E. 1974. PCB's: Another source. *Science* 183:367–368.

Gage, J. C. 1970. The subacute inhalation toxicity of 109 industrial chemicals. *Br. J. Ind. Med.* 27:1–18.

Gargus, J. L., Reese, W. H., Jr. and Rutter, H. A. 1969. Induction of lung adenomas in new born mice by bis(chloromethyl) ether. *Toxicol. Appl. Pharmacol.* 15:92–96.

Garrett, S. and Fuerst, R. 1974. Sex-linked mutations in *Drosophila* after exposures to various mixtures of gas atmospheres. *Environ. Res.* 7:286–293.

Garrigues, M. R. 1940. Action de la colchicine et dichloral sur la racine de *Vicia faba. Rev. Cytochim. Cytophysiol. Veg.* 4:261.

Gerhardt, P. O. and Witt, J. M. 1965. *Proc. 12th Int. Congr. Entomol. London,* p. 565.

Gillett, J. W. , Harr, J. R., Linstrom, F. T., Mount, D. A., St. Clair, A. D. and Weber, L. J. 1972. Evaluation of human health hazards of dichlorvos (DDVP) especially on resin strips. *Residue Rev.* 44:115–154.

Glass, W. I. 1961. A survey of trichloroethylene degreasing baths in Auckland 1961. *Occup. Health Bull.* 7:15–17.

Goldwater, L. G. 1971. Mercury in the environment. *Sci. Am.* 224:15.

Goodman, G. T. 1974. How do chemical substances affect the environment? *Proc. R. Soc. London Ser. B.* 185:127–148.

Gothe, R., Calleman, C. J., Ehrenberg, L. and Wachtmeister, C. A. 1974. Trapping with 3,4-dichlorobenzenethiol of reactive metabolites formed *in vitro* from the carcinogen, vinyl chloride. *Ambio* 3:234–236.

Graham, P. R. 1973. Phthalate ester plasticizers—why and how they are used. *Environ. Health Perspect.* 3:3–12.

Gray, R. H. 1970. Ultrastructural abnormalities in rat liver after exposure to DDT. *J. Cell Biol.* 47:78A.

Green, A. A., Kane, J. and Gradidge, J. M. G. 1966. The control of *Ephestia elutella* using dichlorvos vapor. *J. Stored Prod. Res.* 2:147–157.

Green, M. H. L., Medcalf, A. S. C., Arlett, C. F., Harcourt, S. A. and Lehmann, A. R. 1974. DNA strand breakage caused by dichlorvos, methyl methane sulphonate. *Mutat. Res.* 24:365–378.

Green, S., Palmer, K. A. and Oswald, E. J. 1973. Cytogenetic effects of the polychlorinated biphenyls (Aroclor 1242) on rat bone marrow and spermatogonial cells. Presented at the 12th annual meeting of the Society of Toxicology, New York, March 18–22.

Guess, W. C., Haberman, S., Rowan, D. F., Bower, R. E. and Autian, J. 1967. Characterization of subtle toxicity of certain plastic compounds used in manufacturing of the polyvinyls. *Am. J. Hosp. Pharm.* 24:494–501.

Haberman, S., Guess, W. C., Rowan, D., Bowman, R. O. and Bower, R. K. 1968. Effects of plastics and their additives on human serum proteins, antibodies and developing chick embryos. *SPE (Soc. Plastics Eng.) J.* 24:62–69.

Haley, T. J. 1975. Vinyl chloride, how many unknown problems? *J. Toxicol. Environ. Health* 1:47.

Hall, S. K. 1972. Pollution and Poisoning. *Environ. Sci. Technol.* 6:31–35.

Hamerton, J. L. 1971. *Human cytogenetics,* vol. 2, p. 345. New York: Academic Press.

Hamming, W. J. 1967. Survey of data relating to the hydrocarbons and oxides of nitrogen relations in photochemical smog. Presented at the aeronautic and space engineering and manufacturing meeting, Society of Automotive Engineers, Los Angeles, Calif., October 2–6.

Hammond, A. L. 1972. Chemical pollution: Polychlorinated biphenyls. *Science* 185:175.

Hammond, A. L. 1975. Ozone destruction: Problem's scope grows, its urgency recedes. *Science* 187:1181–1183.

Hammond, P. B. 1969. Lead poisoning. An old problem with a new dimension. *Essays Toxicol.* 1:115–155.

Hanslian, L. and Pleichingerova, O. 1966. Hygienic aspects of the welding process with basic electrodes. *Cesk. Hyg.* 11:96–104.

Harada, Y. 1968. Congenital (or fetal) Minamata disease. In *Minamata disease*, ed. M. Kutsuna,. pp. 93–117. Kumamoto University, Japan: Study Group of Minamata Disease.

Hardy, H. C., Chamberlain, R. I., Maloof, C. C., Boylen, G. W., Jr. and Howell, M. C. 1971. Lead as an environmental poison. *Clin. Pharmacol. Ther.* 12:982–1002.

Harris, D. K. and Adams, H. G. I. 1967. Acro-osteolysis occurring in men engaged in the polymerization of vinyl chloride. *Br. Med. J.* 3:253.

Harris, C. R., Sans, W. W. and Miles, J. R. W. 1966. Exploratory Studies on occurrences of organochlorine insecticide residues in agricultural soil in southwestern Ontario. *J. Agric. Food Chem.* 14:398.

Harrison, H. C., Loucks, O. L. and Mitchell, J. 1970. Systems studies of DDT transport. *Science* 170:503.

Harvey, G. R. and Steinhauer, W. G. 1974. Atmospheric transport of polychlorobiphenyls to the North Atlantic. *Atmos. Environ.* 8:777–782.

Heath, C. W., Jr., Falk, H. and Creech, J. L. 1975. Characteristics of cases of angiosarcoma of the liver among vinyl chloride workers in the United States. *Ann. N.Y. Acad. Sci.*, 246:231–236.

Helling, C. S. Isensee, A. R., Woolson, E. A., Enfor, P. D. J., Jones, G. E., Plimmer, J. R. and Kearney, P. C. 1973. Chlordioxins in pesticides, soils and plants. *J. Environ. Qual.* 2:171–178.

Hicks, R. M. 1972. Airborne lead as an environmental toxin. *Chem. Biol. Interact.* 5:361–390.

Hill, A. B. and Fanning, E. L. 1948. Studies on the incidence of cancer in a factory handling inorganic compounds of arsenic. I. Mortality experience in the factory. *Brit. J. Ind. Med.* 5:1–6.

Hirschler, D. A., Gilbert, L. F., Lamb, F. W. and Neibylsky, L. M. 1957. Lead compounds in automobile exhaust. *Ind. Eng. Chem.* 49:1131–1142.

Hood, R. D. and Bishop, S. C. 1972. Teratogenic effects of sodium arsenate in mice. *Arch. Environ. Health* 24:62–65.

Hoopingarner, R., Samuel, A. and Krause, D. 1972. Polychlorinated biphenyl interactions with tissue culture cells. *Environ. Health Perspect.* 1:155–158.

Huberman, E., Bartsch, H. and Sachs, L. 1975. Mutation induction in Chinese hamster V79 cells by two vinyl chloride metabolites: Chlorethylene oxide and 2-chloroacetaldehyde. *Int. J. Cancer* 15:539.

Huff, L. C. 1952. Abnormal copper, lead, and zinc content of soil near metalliferous veins. *Econ. Geol.* 47:5–7.

Huntzicker, J. J. 1973. Presented at the 166th American Chemical Society meeting, Chicago, Illinois, August 25–29.

Hurst, D. J., Gardner, D. E. and Coffin, D. L. 1970. Effect of ozone on acid hydrolases of pulmonary alveolar macrophages. *J. Reticuloendothel. Soc.* 8:288–300.

Hussain, S. L., Ehrenberg, L., Löfroth, G. and Getvall, T. 1972. Mutagenic effects of TCDD on bacterial systems. *Ambio.* 1:32–33.

Hutson, D. H. and Hoadley, E. C. 1972. The comparative metabolism of ^{14}C-vinyl dichlorvos in animals and man. *Arch. Toxikol.* 30:9–18.

Iliff, N. 1972. Organic chemicals in the environment. *New Sci.* 53:263–265.

Imura, N., Sukegawa, E., Pan, S. K., Wagar, K., Kim, J. Y., Kwan, T. and Ukita, T. 1971. Chemical methylation of inorganic mercury with methylcobalamin, a vitamin B12 analog. *Science* 172:1248–1249.

Innes, J. R., Ulland, B. M., Valerio, M. G., Petrucelli, L., Fishbein, L., Hart, R., Pallotta, A. J., Bates, R. R., Falk, H. L., Gart, J. J., Klein, M., Mitchell, I. and Peters,, J. 1969. Bioassay of pesticides and industrial chemicals for tumorigenicity in mice. A preliminary note. *J. Natl. Cancer Inst.* 42:1101–1114.

International Agency for Research on Cancer. 1972. *Evaluation of carcinogenic risk,* vol. 1, pp. 53–60, 95–124. Lyon: International Agency for Research on Cancer.

International Agency for Research on Cancer. 1974. Some anti-thyroid and related substances, nitrofurans and industrial chemicals. *IARC Monogr. 7.*

International Committee. 1969. Maximum allowable concentrations of mercury compounds. *Arch. Environ. Health* 19:891–905.

Iosaki, H. 1958. Vinyl chloride finding increased use in Japanese aerosols. *Aerosol Age* 3:22.

Irish, D. D. 1974. Vinylidene chloride. In *Industrial hygiene and toxicology,* 2d ed., ed. F. A. Patty, vol. 2, *Toxicology,* pp. 1305–1307. New York: Wiley-Interscience.

Isensee, A. R., Kearney, P. C., Woolson, E. A., Jones, G. E. and Williams, V. P. 1973. Distribution of alkyl arsenicals in model ecosystem. *Environ. Sci. Technol.* 7:841–845.

Jackson, J. O. 1970. Paint and resins for steel tanks. *J. Am. Water Works Assoc.* 52:1370.

Jackson, W. T. 1972. Regulation of mitosis, III. Cytological effects of 2,4,5-trichlorophenoxyacetic acid and of dioxin contaminants in 2,4,5-T formulations. *J. Cell Sci.* 10:15–25.

Jaeger, R. J. and Rubin, R. J. 1970. Plasticizers from plastic devices: Extraction, metabolism and accumulation by biological systems. *Science* 170:460–461.

Jaeger, R. J. and Rubin, R. J. 1972. Migration of a phthalate ester plasticizer from polyvinyl chloride blood bags into stored human blood and its localization into human tissues. *N. Engl. J. Med.* 287:1114–1118.

Jaeger, R. J. and Rubin, R. J. 1973. Di(2-ethylhexyl) phthalate, a plasticizer contaminant of platelet concentrates. *Transfusion* 13:107–108.

Jaeger, R. J., Trabulus, M. J. and Murphy, S. D. 1973. Biochemical effects of 1,1-dichloroethylene in rats: Dissociation of its hepatotoxicity from a lipoperoxidative mechanism. *Toxicol. Appl. Pharmacol.* 25:457–467.

Jaeger, R. J., Reynolds, E. S., Conolly, R. B., Moslen, M. T., Szabo, S. and Murphy, S. D. 1974. Acute hepatic injury by vinyl chloride in rats pretreated with phenobarbital. *Nature (Lond.)* 252:724–726.

Jagiello, G. and Lin, J. S. 1974. Sodium fluoride as potential mutagen in mammalian eggs. *Arch. Environ. Health* 29:230–235.

Jawarowski, Z. 1967. Stable and radioactive lead in the environment and the human body. *Nucl. Energy Inf. Ctr. Rev. Rep. NEIC-RRL9.*

Jegier, Z. 1969. Pesticide residues in the atmosphere. *Ann. N.Y. Acad. Sci.* 160:143.

Jensen, K. A., Kirk, I., Kolmark, G. and Westergaard, M. 1951. Chemically induced mutations in *Neurospora. Cold Spring Harbor Symp. Quant. Biol.* 16:245–261.

Jensen, S. and Jernelov, A. 1969. Biological methylation of mercury in aquatic organisms. *Nature (Lond.)* 223:753–754.

Jensen, S. and Renberg. L. 1972. Contaminants in pentachlorophenol chlorinated dioxins and predioxins. *Ambio.* 1:62–65.

Jensen, S., Johnels, A. G., Ollson, M. and Otterlind, G. 1969. DDT and PCB in marine animals from Swedish waters. *Nature (Lond.)* 224:247.

Jensen, S., Jernelov, A., Lange, R. and Polmark, K. H. 1970. Chlorinated by-products from vinyl chloride production: A new source of marine pollution. In *FAO technical conference on marine pollution and its effects on living resources and fishing, December 9–18, 1970.* Rome FIR:MP/70. Rome: FAO.

Joensuu, O. I. 1971. Fossil fuels as a source of mercury pollution. *Science* 172:1027.

Johnels, A. G. and Westermark, T. 1969. Mercury contamination of the environment in Sweden. In *Chemical fallout*, eds. M. W. Miller and G. G. Berg, p. 10. Springfield, Ill.: Thomas.

Johnels, A. G., Westermark, T., Berg, W., Persson, P. I. and Sjostrand B. 1967. Pike (*Esox lucius* L) and some other aquatic organisms in Sweden as indicators of mercury contamination in the environment. *Oikos* 18:323–333.

Johnson, G. A. and Jalal, S. M. 1973. DDT induced-chromosomal damage in mice. *J. Hered.* 64:7–8.

Jühe, S. and Lange, C. E. 1972. Sklerodermieartige Hautveranderungen Raynaud Syndrom und Akroosteolysen Belarbeitern der PVC-Herstellenden Industrie. *Dtsch. Med. Wochenschr.* 97:1922–1923.

Kada, T., Sadie, Y. and Tutikawa, D. 1972. *In vitro* and host-mediated "rec-assay" procedures for screening chemical mutagens, and phloxine A mutagenic red dye. *Mutat. Res.* 16:165–174.

Kallos, G. J. and Solomon, R. A. 1973. Investigation of the formation of bis(chloromethyl) ether in simulated hydrogen chloride formaldehyde atmospheric environments. *Am. Ind. Hyg. Assoc. J.* 34:469–473.

Katz, A. 1972. Mercury pollution: The making of an environmental crisis. *Crit. Rev. Toxicol.* 2:517–534.

Kehoe, R. A. 1961. The metabolism of lead in man in health and disease. *J. R. Inst. Public. Health* 24:101,129,177.

Kehoe, R. A. 1969. Toxicological appraisal of lead in relation to the tolerable concentration in the ambient air. *J. Air Pollut. Control Assoc.* 19:690–703.

Kelly-Garvert, F. and Legator, M. S. 1973. Cytogenetic and mutagenic effects of DDT and DDE in a Chinese hamster cell line. *Mutat. Res.* 17:223–229.

Keplinger, M. C., Francher, O. E. and Calandra, J. C. 1971. Toxicological studies with polychlorinated biphenyls. Presented at the PCB Conference, National Institute of Environmental Health, Rougemont, North Carolina, December 20–21.

Khera, K. S. 1973. Reproductive capability of male rats and mice treated with methyl mercury. *Toxicol. Appl. Pharmacol.* 24:167–177.

Kimbrough, R. D. 1974. The toxicity of polychlorinated polycyclic compounds and related chemicals. *Crit. Rev. Toxicol.* 2:445.

Kimmerlle, G. and Eben, A. 1973. Metabolism excretion and toxicology of trichloroethylene after inhalation, I. Experimental exposure on rats. *Arch. Toxicol.* 30:115.

Kimming, J. and Schulz, K. H. 1957. Berufliche Akne (sogenanntenchloroakne) durch chlorierte aromatische zyclische Ather. *Dermetologica* 115:540.

Klein, D. H. 1972. Mercury and other metals in urban soils. *Environ. Sci. Technol.* 6:560.

Kleupfer, R. D. and Fairless, B. J. 1972. Characterization of organic components in a municipal water supply. *Environ. Sci. Technol.* 6:1036–1037.

Kolmark, H. G. and Kilbey, B. J. 1968. Kinetic studies of mutation induction by epoxides in *Neurospora crassa. Genetics* 101:89–98.

Kolmark, G. and Westergaard, M. 1953. Further studies on chemically induced reversions at the adenine locus of *Neurospora. Hereditas* 39:202–224.

Kostoff, D. 1939. Effect of the fungicide "granosan" on atypical growth and chromosome doubling in plants. *Nature (Lond.)* 144:334.

Kramer, C. J. and Mutchler, J. E. 1972. The correlation of clinical and environmental measurements for workers exposed to vinyl chloride. *Am. Ind. Hyg. Assoc. J.* 33:19–30.

Krenkel, P. A. 1973. Mercury: Environmental considerations. Part I. *Crit. Rev. Environ. Control.* 3:303–373.

Kroes, R., Van Logten, M. G., Berkvens, J. M., DeVries, T. and Vanesch, G. J. 1974. Study on the carcinogenicity of lead arsenate and sodium arsenate and on the possible synergistic effect of diethyl-nitrosamine. *Food Cosmet. Toxicol.* 12:671–679.

Kuebler, H. 1958. Vinyl chloride as an aerosol propellant. *Aerosol Age* 3:26.

Kurland, L. T., Faro, S. M. and Seidler, H. 1960. Minamata disease. *World Neurol.* 5:370.

Kuschner, M., Laskin, S., Drew, R. T., Capiello, V. and Nelson, N. 1975. Inhalation carcinogenicity of alpha halo ethers. *Arch. Environ. Health* 30:73–77.

Lake, B. G., Gangolli, S. D., Grasso, P. and Lloyd, A. G. 1975. Studies on the hepatic effects of orally administered di-(2-ethylhexyl) phthalate in the rat. *Toxicol. Appl. Pharmacol.* 32:355–367.

Landner, L. 1970. Biochemical model for the biological methylation of mercury suggested from methylation studies *in vivo* with *Neurospora crassa. Nature (Lond.)* 200:173–174, 452–454.

Lange, C. E., Jühe, S., Stein, G. and Veltman, G. 1974. Die sogenannte Vinylchloride-Krankheit—Eine Berufsbeding Systemskierose? *Int. Arch. Arbeitsmed.* 32:1–32.

Laskin, S., Drew, R. T., Cappiello, V., Kuschner, M. and Nelson, N. 1975. Inhalation carcinogenicity of alpha haloethers. *Arch. Environ. Health* 23:125–176.

Lawless, E. W., Von Rumker, R. and Ferguson, T. L. 1972. Pollution material in pesticide manufacturing. *U.S. Natl. Tech. Inf. Serv. P. B. Rep. 213782/3.*

Lawley, P. D., Shah, S. A. and Orr, D. J. 1974. Methylation of nucleic acids by 2,2-dichlorovinyl dimethyl phosphates. *Chem. Biol. Interact.* 7:171–182.

Lee, A. M. and Fraumeni, J. F., Jr. 1969. Arsenic and respiratory cancer in man, an occupational study. *J. Natl. Cancer Inst.* 42:1045–1052.

Lee, B. K. and Murphy, G. 1969. Determination of arsenic content of American cigarettes by neutron activation analysis. *Cancer* 23:1215–1217.

Legator, M. S., Palmer, K. A. and Adler, T. D. 1973. A collaborative study of *in vivo* cytogenetic analysis. *Toxicol. Appl. Pharmacol.* 24:332–337.

Leibman, K. C. and McAllister, W. J., Jr. 1967. Metabolism of trichloroethylene in liver microsomes, III. Induction of the enzymatic activity and its effect on excretion of metabolites. *J. Pharmacol. Exp. Ther.* 157:574–580.

Leonard, A., Linden, G. and Gerber, G. B. 1972. Étude chez la souris des effets génétiques et cytogénétiques d'une contamination par le plomb. Presented at the International Symposium on the Environmental Health Aspects of Lead, Amsterdam, October 2–6.

Leong, B. K., MacFarland, H. N. and Reese, W. H., Jr. 1971. Induction of lung adenomas by chronic inhalation of bis(chloromethyl) ether. *Arch. Environ. Health* 22:663–666.

Lewis, K. H. 1966. The diet as a source of lead pollution. *U.S. Public Health Publ. 1440:* 17–20.

Liberles, A. 1968. *Introduction to theoretical organic chemistry*, chap. 14. New York: Macmillan.

Lichtenstein, E. P. 1972. Environmental factors affecting the fate of pesticides. In *Degradation of synthetic organic molecules in the biosphere*, pp. 190–205. Washington, D.C.: National Academy of Sciences.

Lichtenstein, E. P. and Schull, K. R. 1959. Persistence of some chlorinated hydrocarbon insecticides as influenced by soil types, rate of application and temperature. *J. Econ. Entomol.* 52:124.

Lichtenstein, E. P., Schulz, K. R., Fuhremann, T. W. and Liang, T. T. 1969. Degradation of aldrin and dieldrin in field soils during a ten-year period. Translocation into crops. *J. Econ. Entomol.* 62:761.

Lindsley, D. L. and Grell, E. H. 1968. Genetic variations of *Drosophila melanogaster. Carnegie Inst. Wash. Pub. 627.*

Löfroth, G. 1970a. Alkylation of DNA by dichlorvos. *Naturwissenschaften* 8:393.

Löfroth, G. 1970b. Methyl mercury, a review of health hazards and side effects associated with the emission of mercury compounds into natural systems. *Ecol. Res. Commun. Swed. Natl. Sci. Res. Counc. Bull.* 2.

Löfroth, G., Kim, C. and Hussain, S. 1969. Alkylating property of 2,2-dichlorovinyl dimethyl phosphate: A disregarded hazard. *EMS Newslett.* 2:21–27.

Loprieno, N., Barale, R., Baroncelli, S., Bauer, C., Bronzetti, G., Cammellini, A., Cercignani, G., Corsi, C., Bervasi, G., Leporini, C., Nieri, R., Rossi, A. M., Stretti, G. and Turci, G. 1975. Evaluation of the genetic effects by vinyl chloride monomer (VCM) under the influence of liver microsomes. *Mutat. Res.* 40:85–96.

Loveless, A. 1953. Chemical and biological problems arising from the study of chromosome breakage by alkylating agents and heterocyclic compounds. *Heredity Suppl.* 6:293–298.

Lovelock, J. C., Maggs, R. J. and Wade, R. J. 1973. Halogenated hydrocarbons in and over the Atlantic. *Nature (Lond.)* 241:194.

Luers, H. 1953. Untersuchungen zur Frage der Mutagenitat des Kontakt Insektizides DDT an *Drosophila melanogaster. Naturwissenschaften* 40:293-294.

Lyon, M. F. and Meredith, R. 1966. Autosomal translocations causing male sterility and viable aneuploidy in the mouse. *Cytogenetics* 5:335-341.

Malaveille, C., Bartsch, H., Barbin, A., Camus, A.M., Montesano, R., Croisy, A. and Jacquignon, P. 1975. Mutagenicity of vinyl chloride, chloroethylene oxide, chloroacetaldehyde, and chloroethanol. *Biochem. Biophys. Res. Commun.* 63:363-370.

Maltoni, C. 1975. The value of predictive experimental bioassays in occupational and environmental carcinogenesis. *Ambio* 4:16-21.

Maltoni, C. and Lefemine, G. 1974. Carcinogenicity bioassays of vinyl chloride 1. Research plan and early results. *Environ. Res.* 7:387-405.

March, E. H. 1965. Residues and some effects of chlorinated hydrocarbon insecticides in biological material. *Residue Rev.* 9:1.

Markaryan, D. W. 1966. The cytogenetic effect of some organochlorine insecticides on the medullary cell nuclei of mice. *Genetika* 2:132-137.

Martin, A. E. 1970. Measurement of fluorides. In *Fluorides and human health. WHO Monogr. 50*, p. 311.

Mathur, S. P. 1974. Phthalate esters in the environment: Pollutants or natural products. *J. Environ. Qual.* 3:189-197.

Maugh, T. H. 1973. DDT: An unrecognized source of polychlorinated biphenyls. *Science* 180:578-579.

Mahley, C. H. 1937. Notes from the reports of public analysts: City of Leeds, annual report of the city analyst for 1936. *Analyst* 62:544.

May, G. 1973. Chloracne from the accidental poisoning of tetrachlordibenzodioxin. *Br. J. Ind. Med.* 30:276-283.

Mayer, F. L., Jr. and Sanders, H. O. 1973. Toxicology of phthalic acid esters in aquatic organisms. *Environ. Health Perspect.* 3:153-158.

Mayer, F. L., Jr., Stalling, D. L. and Johnson, J. L. 1972. Phthalate esters as environmental contaminants. *Nature (Lond.).* 238:411-413.

McBride, B. C. and Wolfe, R. S. 1971. Biosynthesis of dimethyl arsine by *Methanobacterium. Biochemistry* 10:4312-4315.

McConnell, G., Ferguson, D. M. and Pearson, C. R. 1975. Chlorinated hydrocarbons in the environment. *Endeavour* 34:13-27.

McElroy, M. B., Wofsy, S.C., Penner, J. E. and McConnell, J. C. 1974. Atmospheric ozone: Possible impact of stratospheric aviation. *J. Atmos. Sci.* 31:287.

Menz, M., Leutkemeier, H. and Sachsse, K. 1974. Long-term exposure of factory workers to dichlorovos (DDVP) insecticide. *Arch. Environ. Health* 28:72-76.

Metcalf, R. L., Booth, G. M., Schuth, C. K., Hansen, D. J. and Lu, P. Y. 1973. Uptake and fate of di-2-ethylhexyl phthalate in aquatic organisms and in a model ecosystem. *Environ. Health Perspect.* 4:27-34.

Michalek, J. M. and Brockman, H. E. 1969. A test of mutagenicity of Shell "No-Pest Strip Insecticide." *Neurospora Newslett.* 14:8.

Mickey, G. H. and Holden, H., Jr. 1971. Chromosomal effects of chlorine on mammalian cells *in vitro. EMS Newslett.* 4:39-41.

Milgrom, J. 1973. Identifying the nuisance plastics. *New Sci.* 57:184-186.

Miller, E. C. and Miller, J. A. 1971. The mutagenicity of chemical carcinogens: Correlations, problems and interpretations. In *Chemical mutagens: Principles and methods for their detection*, ed. A. Hollaender, pp. 83–119. New York: Plenum.

Miller, M. W. and Berg, G. G., eds. 1969. *Chemical fallout*. Springfield, Ill.: Thomas.

Milnes, M. H. 1971. Formation of 2,3,7,8-tetrachlorodibenzodioxin by thermal decomposition of sodium 2,4,5-trichlorophenate. *Nature* (*Lond.*) 232:395–396.

Mitchell, B. and Gerdes, R. A. 1973. Mutagenic effects of sodium and stannous fluoride upon *Drosophila melanogaster*. *Fluoride* 6:113–117.

Mohamed, A. H. 1968. Cytogenetic effects of hydrogen fluoride treatment in tomato plants. *J. Air Pollut. Control Assoc.* 18:395–398.

Mohamed, A. H. 1969. Cytogenetic effects of hydrogen fluoride upon plants. *Fluoride* 2:76–84.

Mohamed, A. H., Applegate, H. G. and Smith, G. D. 1966a. Cytological reactions induced by sodium fluoride in *Allium cepa* root tip chromosomes. *Can. J. Genet. Cytol.* 8:241–244.

Mohamed, A. H., Smith, J. D. and Applegate, H. G. 1966b. Cytological effects of hydrogen fluoride on tomato chromosomes. *Can. J. Genet. Cytol.* 8:575.

Mohn, G. 1973. 5-Methyl tryptophan resistance mutations in *Escherichia coli* K12, mutagenic activity of monofunctional alkylating agents including organophosphorus insecticides. *Mutat. Res.* 20:7–15.

Moilanen, K. W. and Crosby, D. G. 1973. Vapor phase photodecomposition of p,p'-DDT and its relatives. Presented at the 165th American Chemical Society meeting, Dallas, Texas, April 8–13.

Molina, M. J. and Rowland, F. S. 1974. Stratospheric sink for chlorofluoromethanes: chlorine atom catalysed destruction of ozone. *Nature* (*Lond.*) 249:810–812.

Monsanto Industrial Chemicals. 1971. Public Relations Department news release, November 30.

Moutschen-Dahmen, J., Moutschen-Dahmen, M. and Ehrenberg, L. 1968. Chromosome breaking activity of ethylene oxide and ethylenimine. *Hereditas* 60:267.

Mrak, E. M. 1969. *Report of the Secretary's Commission on Pesticides and Their Relationship to Environmental Health*, parts 1 and 2. Washington, D.C.: Department of Health, Education, and Welfare.

Muro, L. A. and Goyer, J. R. A. 1969. Chromosome damage in experimental lead poisoning. *Arch. Pathol.* 86:660–663.

Murozumi, M. 1967. A new type of mercury chlorine cell (Asahi horizontal rotating cathode cell). *Electrochem. Technol.* 5:236–239.

Nash, R. G. and Woolson, E. A. 1967. Persistence of chlorinated insecticides in soils. *Science* 157:924.

National Academy of Sciences. 1971a. *Biological effects of atmospheric pollutants–fluorides*. Washington, D.C.: National Academy of Sciences.

National Academy of Sciences. 1971b. *Chlorinated hydrocarbons in the marine environment*. Washington, D.C.: National Academy of Sciences.

National Academy of Sciences. 1972. *Report of the Committee on Biological Effects of Atmospheric Pollutants*, p. 131. Washington, D.C.: National Academy of Sciences.

National Academy of Sciences. 1975. *Principles for evaluating chemicals in the environment*, pp. 352–411. Washington, D.C.: National Academy of Sciences.

National Institute of Occupational Safety and Health. 1973. *Occupational exposure to inorganic arsenical,* p. 16. Washington, D.C.: Department of Health, Education and Welfare, Public Health Service.

National Resources Defense Council. 1975. Petition of concern to the Consumer Product Safety Commission. *Chem. Technol.,* pp. 22–27.

Nazir, D. J., Alcaraz, A. P., Bierl, B. A., Beroza, M. and Nair, P. P. 1971. Isolation, identification and specific localization of di-(2-ethylhexyl) phthalate bovine heart muscle mitochondria. *Biochemistry* 10:4228–4232.

Nelson, N., Byerly, T. C., Kolbye, A. C., Jr., Kurland, L. T., Shapiro, R. E., Shibko, S. I., Stickel, W. H., Thompson, J. E., Van Den Berg, L. A. and Weissler, A. 1971. Hazards of mercury. *Environ. Res.* 4:1.

Newsome, J. R., Norman, V. and Keith, C. H. 1965. Vapor-phase analysis of tobacco smoke. *Tob. Sci.* 9:102–110.

Nikonorow, M., Mazur, H. and Piekacz, H. 1973. Effect of orally administered plasticizers and polyvinyl chloride stabilizers in the rat. *Toxicol. Appl. Pharmacol.* 26:253–259.

Nisbet, I. C. T. and Sarafin, A. F. 1972. Rates and routes of transport of PCB's in the environment. *Environ. Health Perspect.* 1:21–38.

Nishioka, H. 1973. Lethal and mutagenic action of formaldehyde in HCR+ and HCR− strains of *Escherichia coli. Mutat. Res.* 17:261–275.

Nishioka, H. 1975. Mutagenic activities of metal compounds in bacteria. *Mutat. Res.* 31:185–189.

Obe, G. and Sperling, K. 1970. Chromosome aberrations in human leucocytes treated with lead *in vitro.* In *Arbeitsgruppe Blei.* Berlin: Kommission fur Umwelt Gefahren, Bundesgesundheitsamt.

Occupational Safety and Health Administration. 1974. Occupational safety and health standards: Part 2. *Fed. Regist.* 39: 23554–23556.

Occupational Safety and Health Administration. 1975. Inorganic arsenic, proposed exposure standard. *Fed. Regist.* 40:3392–3404.

Ogner, G. and Schnitzer, M. 1970. Humic substances: Fulvic acid-dialkyl phthalate complexes and their role in pollution. *Science* 170:317–318.

Olson, W. A., Habermann, R. T., Weisburger, E. K., Ward, J. M. and Weisburger, J H. 1973. Induction of stomach cancer in rats and mice by halogenated aliphatic fumigants. *J. Natl. Cancer Inst.* 51:1993–1995.

Ott, M. G., Holder, B. B. and Gordon, H. L. 1974. Respiratory cancer and occupational exposure to arsenicals. *Arch. Environ. Health* 29:250–254.

Palmer, K. A., Green, S. and Legator, M. S. 1972. Cytogenic effects of DDT and derivatives of DDT in a cultured mammalian cell line. *Toxicol. Appl. Pharmacol.* 22:355–364.

Palmer, K. A., Green, S. and Legator, M. S. 1973. Dominant lethal study of p,p'-DDT in rats. *Food Cosmet. Toxicol.* 11:53–62.

Paton, F. R. and Allison, A. C. 1972. Chromosome damage in human cell cultures induced by metal salts. *Mutat. Res.* 16:332–336.

Peakall, D. B., Lincer, J. L. and Bloom, P. E. 1972. Embryonic mortality and chromosomal alterations caused by Aroclor 1254 in ring doves. *Environ. Health Perspect.* 1:103–104.

Peterle, T. J. 1969. DDT in Antarctic snow. *Nature (Lond.)* 224:620.

Piecuch, P. J. 1974. The chlorination controversy. *J. Water Pollut. Control* 46:2637.

Polani, P. E. 1961. Turner's syndrome and allied conditions. *Br. Med. Bull.* 17:200–205.

Poverenny, A.M., Siomin, Y. A., Saenko, A. S. and Sinzinis, B. I. 1975.

Possible mechanisms of lethal and mutagenic action of formaldehyde. *Mutat. Res.* 27: 123–126.

Powell, J. F. 1945. Oxide formation for trichloroethylene. *Br. J. Ind. Med.* 2:142.

Prendergast, J. A., Jones, R. A., Jenkins, J. and Siegel, J. 1967. Effects on experimental animals of long-term inhalation of trichloroethylene carbon tetrachloride, 1,1,1-trichloroethane, dichlorodifluoromethane, and 1,1-dichloroethylene. *Toxicol. Appl. Pharmacol.* 10:270–289.

Ragelis, E. P., Fisher, B. S., Klimeck, B. A. and Johnson, C. 1968. Isolation and determination of chlorohydrins in foods fumigated with ethylene oxide or with propylene oxide. *J. Assoc. Off. Anal. Chem.* 51:709–715.

Ramel, C. 1967. Genetic effects of organo mercury compounds. *Hereditas* 57:448.

Ramel, C. 1969. Genetic effects of organic mercury compounds, I. Cytological investigations on allium roots. *Hereditas* 61:208–230.

Ramel, C. 1972. Genetic effects. In *Mercury in the Environment*, eds. L. Friberg and J. Vostal, pp. 169–181. Cleveland, Ohio: CRC Press.

Ramel, C. and Magnusson, J. 1969. Genetic effects of organic mercury compounds II. Chromosome segregation in *Drosophila melanogaster. Hereditas* 61:231–254.

Rannug, U., Johansson, A., Ramel, C. and Wachtmeister, C. A. 1974. The mutagenicity of vinyl chloride after metabolic activation. *Ambio* 3:194–197.

Rapoport, I. A. 1948. Action of ethylene oxide glycides and glycols on genetic mutations. *Dokl. Akad. Nauk SSSR* 60:469–472.

Rechnagel, R. O. 1967. Carbon tetrachloride hepatotoxicity. *Pharmacol. Rev.* 19:145.

Reichle, A. and Tengler, H. 1968. Methods for the determination of plasticizer migration from synthetic materials into food. IV. Migration of bis(2-ethylhexyl) phthalate and masamoll from synthetic rubber into milk. *Dtsch. Lebensm. Rundsch.* 64:142–145.

Reinhardt, C. F., Azar, A., Maxfield, M. E., Smith, P. E., Jr. and Mullin, L. S. 1971. Cardiac arrhythmias and aerosol "sniffing". *Arch. Environ. Health* 22:265.

Risebrough, R. W. and DeLappe, B. 1972. Accumulation of polychlorinated biphenyls in ecosystems. *Environ. Health Perspect.* 1:29–45.

Risebrough, R. W., Huggett, R. J., Griffin, J. J. and Goldberg, E. D. 1968a. Pesticides: Transatlantic movements in the northeast trades. *Science* 159:1233–1235.

Risebrough, R. W., Reiche, P., Peakall, D. B., Herman, S. G. and Kirven, M. N. 1968b. Polychlorinated biphenyls in the global ecosystem. *Nature (Lond.)* 220:1098–1101.

Robson, A. O. and Jelliffe, A. M. 1963. Medicinal arsenic poisoning and lung cancer. *Br. Med. J.* 1:207–209.

Rohm & Haas Co. 1972. News release: Reaction of formaldehyde and HCl forms bis CME, December 27.

Roll, R. 1971. Untersuchung uber die Teratogene Wirkung von 2,4,5-T bei Mausen. *Food Cosmet. Toxicol.* 9:671–676.

Rook, H. I., LaFleur, P. D. and Gills, T. E. 1971. Mercury in coal: A new standard reference material. *Environ. Lett.* 2:195–204.

Rosen, A. A., Skeel, R. T. and Ettinger, M. B. 1963. Relationship of river water odor to specific organic contaminants. *J. Water Pollut. Control Fed.* 35:777–782.

Rosenkranz, H. D. (1973). Sodium hypochlorite and sodium perborate: Preferential inhibitors of DNA polymerase-deficient bacteria. *Mutat. Res.* 21:171–174.

Rosenkranz, H. S. and Wlodkowski, T. J. 1974. Mutagenicity of ethylene chlorohydrin. A degradation product present in foodstuffs exposed to ethylene oxide. *J. Agric. Food Chem.* 22:407–409.

Rosenkranz, S., Carr, A. S. and Rosenkranz, H. S. 1974. 2-Haloethanols: Mutagenicity and reactivity with DNA. *Mutat. Res.* 26:367–370.

Roth, F. 1957. The sequelae of chronic arsenic poisoning in Moselle vintagers. *Ger. Med. Mon.* 2:172–175.

Roth, F. 1958. Bronchial cancer of arsenic-poisoned vintagers. *Virchows Arch.* [*Pathol. Anat.*] 331:119–137.

Rowland, M. S. and Molina, M. J. 1974. Chlorofluoromethanes in the environment. *AEC Rep. 1974-1.*

Rubin, E. and Popper, H. 1967. The evolution of human cirrhosis deduced from observations in experimental animals. *Medicine (Baltimore)* 46:163–183.

Ruhling, G. A. and Tyler, G. 1968. An ecological approach to the lead problem. *Bot. Not.* 121:321.

Saha, J. G. 1972. Significance of mercury in the environment. *Residue Rev.* 42:103.

Sakabe, H. 1973. Lung cancer due to exposure to bis(chloromethyl) ether. *Ind. Health* 11:145–148.

Sangioyanni, M. 1974. 1973 Aerosol product survey. *Drug Cosmet. Ind.* June: 43.

Satterlee, H. S. 1956. The problem of arsenic in American cigarette tobacco. *N. Engl. J. Med.* 254:1149–1154.

Scansetti, G. G., Rubino, G. F. and Trompeo, G. 1959. Chronic trichloroethylene poisoning III. Metabolism of trichlorethylene. *Med. Lav.* 50:743–753.

Schmid, E., Bauchiner, M., Pietruck, S. and Hall, G. 1972. Die cytogenetische Wirkung von Blei in menschlichen peripheren Lympocyten *in vitro* und *in vivo. Mutat. Res.* 16:401–406.

Schneider, W. 1968. Daueruntersuchungen zum Fluor Problem in einem industriellen Ballungsgebiet. *Staub* 28:13–18.

Schroeder, H. A. and Tipton, I. H. 1968. The human body burden of lead. *Arch. Environ. Health* 17:965.

Schubert, J. 1973. The chemical environment, presence and fate of chemicals outside the human body. *Ambio. Spec. Rep.* 3:9–11.

Schull, J. 1960. *Mutations*, p. 172. Ann Arbor: Univ. of Michigan Press.

Schulten, G. G. M. and Kuyken, W. 1966. Determination of DDVP in air from vapona strips. *Int. Pest. Control* May/June:18.

Schulz, K. H. 1968. Zur Klinic und Atiologie der Chlorakne. *Arbeitsmed. Soc. Med. Arbeitshyg.* 2:25–29.

Schwanitz, G., Lehnert, G. and Gebhart, E. 1970. Chromosome damage after occupational exposure to lead. Dtsch. Med. *Wochenschr.* 95:1636–1641.

Selikoff, I. 1974. Stillbirths and miscarriages in wives of vinyl chloride workers studied. *Environ. Newslett.* 13:17–19.

Seltzer, R. J. 1975. Reactions grow to trichloroethylene alert. *Chem. Eng. News* 53:41.

Semrau, K. T. 1957. Emission of fluorides from industrial processes. *J. Air Pollut. Control Assoc.* 11:342.

Simler, M., Maurer, M. and Mandard, J. C. 1964. Cancer du foie sur cirrhose au tetrachlorure de carbone. *Strasbourg Med.* 15:910.

Singh, A. R., Lawrence, W. H. and Autian, J. 1972. Teratogenicity of phthalate esters in rats. *J. Pharm. Sci.* 61:51–55.

Singh, A. R., Lawrence, W. H. and Autian, J. 1974. Mutagenic and antifertility sensitivities of mice to di-2-ethylhexyl phthalate (EHP) and dimethoxyethyl phthalate (DMEP). *Toxicol. Appl. Pharmacol.* 29:35–46.

Skerving, S., Hansson, K., Mangs, C., Lindsten, J. and Ryman, N. 1974. Methyl mercury-induced chromosome damage in man. *Environ. Res.* 7:83–98.

Slater, T. F. 1966. Necrogenic action of carbon tetrachloride in the rat: A speculative mechanism based on activation. *Nature (Lond.)* 209:36.

Sledak, N. I. and Teplyakova, R. V. 1974. Hygiene assessment of artificial leather made of polyvinyl. *Gig. Sanit.* 29:17.

Slonka, M. B. 1970. *Facts about no-pest DDVP strips*, p. 18. Shell Chemical Co., Modesto, Calif.

Smith, D. B. 1972. Behavioural effects of lead and other heavy metal pollutants. *Chem. Br.* 8:240–243.

Sobels, F. H. 1963. Peroxides and the induction of mutations by X-rays, ultraviolet light and formaldehyde. *Radiat. Res. Suppl.* 3:171–183.

Sodergren, A., Vensson, B. S. and Ulfstrand, S. 1972. DDT and PCB in south Swedish streams. *Environ. Pollut.* 3:25–36.

Souček, B. and Vlachova, D. 1960. Excretion of trichloroethylene metabolites in human urine. *Br. J. Ind. Med.* 17:60.

Sparrow, A. H., Schairer, L. A. and Villalobos-Pictrini, R. 1974. Comparison of somatic mutation rates induced in *Tradescantia* by chemical and physical mutagens. *Mutat. Res.* 26:265–276.

Sparschau, G. L., Dunn, F. C. and Rowe, V. H. 1971. Study of the teratogenicity of 2,3,7,8-tetrachlorodibenzo-p-dioxin in the rat. *Food Cosmet. Toxicol.* 9:405–412.

Spencer, W. P. and Stern, C. 1948. Experiments to test the validity of the linear R-dose/mutation frequency relation in *Drosophila* at low dosage. *Genetics* 33:43.

Sperling, K., Weiss, G., Minzen, M. and Obe, G. 1970. Cytogenetic effects of lead in man. In *Arbeitsgruppe Blei.* Berlin: Kommission fur Umwelt Gefahren. Bundesgesundheitsamt.

Srinivasan, V. R. 1972. Biodegradation of waste plastics. *Technol. Rev.* 74:45–47.

Staehelin, M. 1958. Reaction of tobacco mosaic virus nucleic acid with formaldehyde. *Biochim. Biophys. Acta* 29:410–417.

Stalling, D. L., Hogan, J. W. and Johnson, J. L. 1973. Phthalate ester residues—their metabolism and analysis in fish. *Environ. Health Perspect.* 3:159–173.

Stanford Research Institute. 1972. *Chemical economics handbook*, sect. C. Stanford, Calif.: Stanford Research Institute.

Stanley, C. W., Barney, J. E., Helton, M. R. and Yobs, A. R. 1971. Measurement of atmospheric levels of pesticides. *Environ. Sci. Technol.* 5:530–535.

Stenburg, R. L., Hangebrauck, R. P., Von Lehmeden, D. H., and Rose, A. H., Jr. 1961. Effects of high-volatile fuel on incinerator effluents. *J. Air Pollut. Control Assoc.* 10:114–120.

Stoltz, D. R., Poirer, L. A., Irving, C. C., Strich, H. F., Weisburger, J. H. and

Grice, H. C. 1974. Evaluation of short-term tests for carcinogenicity. *Toxicol. Appl. Pharmacol.* 29:157–180.

Stuart, J. M. and Smith, D. A. 1965. Degradation of epoxide resins. *J. Appl. Polym. Sci.* 9:3195–3214.

Summers, L. 1955. The 2-haloalkyl ethers. *Chem. Rev.* 55:301–353.

Swain, C. G. and Crist, D. R. 1972. Mechanisms of chlorination by hypochlorous acid. The last chlorination by chloronium ion, Cl^+. *J. Am. Chem. Soc.* 94:3195–3199.

Tabor, E. C. Contamination of urban air through the use of insecticides. *Trans. N.Y. Acad. Sci.* 28:469–478.

Takeuchi, T. 1970. Presented at the International Conference on Environmental Mercury Contamination, Ann Arbor, Michigan, September 30–October 2.

Tarjan, R. and Kemeny, T. 1969. Multigeneration studies on DDT in mice. *Food Cosmet. Toxicol.* 7:215–222.

Tarrant, K. R. and Tatton, J. G. 1968. Organochlorine pesticides in rainwater in the British Isles. *Nature (Lond.)* 219:725–727.

Tatton, J. O'G. and Ruzicka, J. H. A. 1967. Organochlorine pesticides in Antarctica. *Nature (Lond.)* 215:346–349.

Ter Haar, G. 1970. Air as a source of lead in edible crops. *Environ. Sci. Technol.* 4:226–229.

Terrancini, B., Testa, M. C. and Cabral, J. R. 1973. The effects of long-term feeding of DDT to BALB/c mice. *Int. J. Cancer* 11:747–764.

Tessman, I. 1971. Induction of transfersions and transitions by 1,1-Dibromoethane. *EMS Newslett.* 4:33.

Thomas, G. H. 1973. Quantitative determination and confirmation of identity of trace amounts of dialkyl phthalates in environmental samples. *Environ. Health Perspect.* 3:23–28.

Tomatis, L., Turusov, V. and Day, N. 1972. The effect of long-term exposure to DDT on CF-1 mice. *Int. J. Cancer* 10:489–506.

Tomatis, L., Turusov, V., Charles, R. T., Bolocchi, M. and Gati, E. 1974a. Liver tumours in CF-1 mice exposed for limited periods to technical DDT. *Z. Krebsforsch.* 82:25–35.

Tomatis, L., Turusov, V., Charles, R. T. and Bolocchi, M. 1974b. Effect of long-term exposure to 1,1-dichloro-1,1-bis(p-chlorophenyl) ethylene, to 1,1-Dichloro-2,2-bis(p-chlorophenyl) ethane, and to the two chemicals combined on CF-1 mice. *J. Natl. Cancer Inst.* 52:883–891.

Tou, J. C. and Kallos, G. J. 1974. Study of aqueous HCl and formaldehyde mixtures for formation of bis(chloromethyl) ether. *Am. Ind. Hyg. Assoc. J.* 35:419–422.

Tracey, J. P. and Sherlock, P. 1968. Hepatoma following carbon tetrachloride poisoning. *N.Y. State J. Med.* 68:2202.

Train, R. 1974. *Environ. Sci. Technol.* 8:781.

Turusov, V. S., Day, N. E., Tomatis, L., Gati, E. and Charles, R. T. 1973. Tumors in CF-1 mice exposed for six generations to DDT. *J. Natl. Cancer Inst.* 51:983–997.

Umeda, M., Saito, K., Hiroje, K. and Saito, M. 1969. Cytotoxic effects of inorganic phenyl and alkyl mercuric compounds on HeLa cells. *J. Exp. Med.* 39:47–58.

Urone, P., Lutsep, H., Hoyes, C. M. and Parcher, J. F. 1968. Static studies of sulfur dioxide reactions in air. *Environ. Sci. Technol.* 2:611–618.

U.S. Department of Commerce. 1974. *Tariff Commission Report, 1974.* Washington, D.C.: Department of Commerce.

U.S. Department of Health, Education, and Welfare. 1969. *Air quality criteria for particulate matter, Nat. Air Pollut. Control Admin. Publ. AP-49.*

U.S. Department of Interior. 1970. *Bibliography on mercury contamination in the natural environment.* Washington, D.C.: Department of Interior.

U.S. Department of Interior. 1971. *Minerals year book.* Washington, D.C.: Department of Interior, Bureau of Mines.

U.S. Geological Survey. 1970. *U.S. Geol. Surv. Prof. Pap. 7B.*

Vaarama, A. 1947. Experimental studies on the influence of DDT pesticide upon plant mitosis. *Hereditas* 33:191–219.

Van Duuren, B. J. 1974. Chemical mechanisms of vinyl chloride carcinogenesis. Presented at the National Institute of Environmental Health Sciences Conference on Public Health Implications of Plastic Manufacture, Pinehurst, North Carolina, July 29–31.

Van Duuren, B. J., Goldschmidt, B. M., Langseth, L., Mercado, G. and Sivak, A. 1968. Alpha haloethers: A new type of alkylating carcinogen. *Arch. Environ. Health.* 16:472–476.

Van Duuren, B. L., Sivak, A., Goldschmit, B. M., Katz, C., Langseth, C. and Mercado, G. 1969. Carcinogenicity of haloethers. *J. Natl. Cancer Inst.* 43:481–488.

Van Duuren, B. L., Katz, C., Goldschmidt, B. M., Frenkel, K. and Sivak, A. 1972. Carcinogenicity of haloethers II. Structure activity relationships of analogs of bis(chloromethyl) ether. *J. Natl. Cancer Inst.* 48:1431–1439.

Van Oettingen, W. F., Heuper, W. C. and Dcichman-Gruebler, W. 1936. Chlorobutadiene: Its toxicity, pathology and the mechanism of its action. *J. Ind. Hyg. Toxicol.* 28:240–270.

Verburgt, F. 1975. Cited in Bartsch, H. and Montesano, R. 1975. Mutagenic and carcinogenic effects of vinyl chloride. *Mutat. Res.* 32:93–114.

Villaneuva, E. C., Burse, V. W. and Jennings, R. W. 1973. Chlorodibenzo-*p*-dioxin contamination of two commercially available pentachlorophenols. *J. Agric. Food Chem.* 21:739–740.

Villaneuva, E. C., Jennings, R. W., Burse, V. W. and Kimbrough, R. D. 1974. Evidence of chlorodibenzo-*p*-dioxin and chlorodibenzofuran in hexachlorobenzene. *J. Agric. Food Chem.* 22:916.

Viola, P. L., Bigotti, A. and Caputo, A. 1971. Oncogenic response of rat skin, lungs, and bones to vinyl chloride. *Cancer Res.* 31:516–519.

Vogel, E. 1972. Investigations on the mutagenicity of DDT and the metabolites DDE, DDM, DDOM, DDA in *Drosophila melanogaster. Mutat. Res.* 16:157–164.

Von Thiess, A. M., Hey, W. and Zeller, H. 1973. Zur Toxikologie von Dichlorodimethylether: Verdacht auf kanzerogene Wirkung auch beim Menschen. *Zentralbl. Arbeitsmed.* 23:97–102.

Voogd, C. E. and VanderVet, P. 1969. Mutagenic action of ethylene halogenhydrins. *Experientia* 25:85–86.

Voogd, C. E., Jacobs, J. J. J. A. and Vander Stel, J. J. 1972. On the mutagenic action of dichlorvos. *Mutat. Res.* 16:413–416.

Vos, J. G. and Beems, R. B. 1971. Dermal toxicity studies of technical polychlorinated biphenyls and fractions thereof in rabbits. *Toxicol. Appl. Pharmacol.* 19:612–624.

Vos, J. G. and Koeman, J. H. 1970. Comparative toxicologic study with polychlorinated biphenyls in chickens with special reference to porphyria, edema formation, liver necrosis and tissue residues. *Toxicol. Appl. Pharmacol.* 17:656–668.

Vos, J. G., Koeman, J. H., Vander Mass, H. C., Ten Noever, M. C., Debrauw, M. C. and DeVos, H. R. 1970. Identification and toxicological evaluation of chlorinated dibenzofuran and chlorinated naphthalene in two commercial polychlorinated biphenyls. *Food Cosmet. Toxicol.* 8:625–630.

Wadleigh, C. H. 1968. Wastes in relation to agriculture and forestry. *USDA Misc. Publ. 1065*, p. 112.

Wagoner, J. 1972. Epidemiology program of NIOSH. Presented at the American Public Health Association Annual Meeting, Symposium on Occupational Carcinogenesis, Washington, D.C., November.

Waldbott, G. L. and Oelschlager, W. 1974. Fluoride in the environment. *Fluoride* 7:220–222.

Wallace, M. E. 1971. An unprecedented number of mutants in a colony of wild mice. *Environ. Pollut.* 1:175.

Warwick, G. P. 1971. Metabolism of liver carcinogens and other factors influencing liver cancer induction. In *Liver cancer*, pp. 121–157. Lyon: International Agency for Research on Cancer.

Weiss, H. V., Koide, M. and Goldberg, E. D. 1971. Mercury in the Greenland ice sheet: Evidence of recent impact by man. *Science* 174:692.

Wennerberg, R. and Löfroth, G. 1974. Formation of 7-methylguanine by dichlorovos in bacteria and mice. *Chem. Biol. Interact.* 8:339–348.

Wesley, F., Roarke, B. and Darbishire, O. 1965. The formation of persistent toxic chlorohydrins in foodstuffs by fumigation with ethylene oxide and with propylene oxide. *J. Food Sci.* 30:1037–1042.

Wheatley, G. A. 1973. Pesticides in the atmosphere. *Environmental pollution by pesticides*, ed. C. A. Edwards, vol. 3, pp. 365–408. London: Plenum.

Wheatly, G. A. and Hardman, J. A. 1965. Indications of the presence of organochlorine insecticides in rainwater in central England. *Nature (Lond.)* 207:486–487.

Wheatley, G. A., Wright, D. W. and Hardman, J. A. 1960. The re-treatment of soils with dieldrin for the control of carrot fly. *Plant Pathol.* 9:146.

White, G. C. 1972. *Handbook of chlorination.* New York: Van Nostrand-Reinhold.

Wild, D. 1973. Chemical induction of streptomycin-resistant mutations in *Escherichia coli*—Dose and mutagenic effects of dichlorvos and methyl methane sulphonate. *Mutat. Res.* 19:33–41.

Wilson, K. W. 1960. Fixation of atmospheric carbonyl compounds by sodium bisulfite. *Anal. Chem.* 30:1127–1129.

Wlodkowski, T. J. and Rosenkranz, H. S. 1975. Mutagenicity of sodium hypochlorite for *Salmonella typhimurium*. *Mutat. Res.* 31:39–42.

Wofsy, S. C. and McElroy, M. B. 1974. HO_x, NO_x, and ClO_x: Their role in atmospheric photochemistry. *Can. J. Chem.* 52:1582–1591.

Wofsy, S. C., McElroy, M. B. and Sze, N. D. 1974. Freon consumption: Implications for atmospheric ozone. *Science* 187:535–537.

Wood, J. M., Kennedy, F. S. and Rosen, C. G. 1968. Synthesis of methyl-mercury compounds by extracts of methanogenic bacterium. *Nature (Lond.)* 220:173–174.

Woodhouse, D. L. 1965. Demonstration of interaction products of adenine and adenosine phosphates with formaldehyde. *Nature (Lond.)* 192:336–338.

Woodwell, G. M. and Martin, F. T. 1964. Persistence of DDT in soils of heavily sprayed forest strands. *Science* 145:481–483.

Woodwell, G. M., Wurster, C. M. and Isaacson, P. A. 1956. DDT residues in an East Coast estuary: A case of biological concentration of a persistent residue. *Science* 156:821–824.

Woodwell, G. M., Craig, P. P. and Johnson, H. A. 1971. DDT in the biosphere: Where does it go? *Science* 174:1102.

Woolson, E. A. and Kearney, P. C. 1973. Persistence and reactions of ^{14}C-cacodylic acid in soils. *Environ. Sci. Technol.* 7:47.

Wright, A. S., Potter, D., Wooder, M. F., Donninger, C. and Greenland, R. D. 1972. The effects of dieldrin on the subcellular structure and function of mammalian liver cells. *Food Cosmet. Toxicol.* 10:311–332.

Yllner, S. 1961. Urinary metabolites of ^{14}C-tetrachlorethylene in mice. *Nature* (*Lond.*) 191:820.

Younghans, R. S. and McMullen, T. B. 1970. Fluoride concentrations found in NASN samples of suspended particles. *Fluoride* 3:143–152.

Part 5

INFORMATION SYSTEMS

Chapter 11

SPECIALIZED INFORMATION CENTERS IN TOXICOLOGY
I. ENVIRONMENTAL MUTAGEN INFORMATION CENTER (EMIC)

J. S. Wassom
Environmental Mutagen Information Center
Information Center Complex/Information Division
Oak Ridge National Laboratory
Oak Ridge, Tennessee

H. V. Malling
Laboratory of Environmental Mutagenesis
National Institute of Environmental Health Sciences
Research Triangle Park, North Carolina

INTRODUCTION

The study of any discipline assumes mastery of the literature of the subject.[1]

The acquisition and transfer of information are inseparable parts of research and development (R&D) programs, whether they are in the area of

We thank Ms. Vickie Strevel for typing the manuscript and the Environmental Mutagen Information Center staff for their review and helpful comments. Special thanks is also extended to the ORNL Biology Library for their helpful services and to Ms. Lynn Veach, librarian, for her review of the manuscript.

This work was supported by the National Institute of Environmental Health Sciences under contract 40-247-70 with the Oak Ridge National Laboratory, which is operated by Union Carbide Corporation for the Department of Energy.

By acceptance of this article, the publisher or recipient acknowledges the U.S. Government's right to retain a nonexclusive, royalty-free license in and to any copyright covering the article.

[1] Jameson, 1976.

toxicology or some other scientific field. Because of this, scientists and administrators must ensure that measures are instituted that provide for effective information acquisition and transfer. Government, on the other hand, must accept the major responsibility for financing and instituting information programs just as it now accepts major responsibility for funding the experimental aspects of R&D. The need for government involvement is quite obvious when one equates the vast amount of information produced from federally supported research programs with the costs and benefits inherent in providing proper control and availability of this information. Further, government access and use of information from R&D programs is essential since federal agencies must consider all available information in making logical, consistent, and defensible regulatory policy to meet the requirements of legislative mandates—such as, the Toxic Substances Control Act (Public Law 94-469). To ensure effective information acquisition and transfer, every possible method for control should be explored. This may entail implementing new information programs or giving greater support to programs already in operation. Regardless of whether the information program is newly created or existing, it should undergo periodic evaluations by independent and qualified groups of specialists who can assess the program's organizational philosophy, user needs, productivity, cost, operational effectiveness, and so on. Such a system of checks and balances would ensure that funds diverted for information programs are meeting the needs of the research area served. For example, one possible source of such an evaluative group could be the National Bureau of Standards, which recently completed an exhaustive review of the Environmental Mutagen Information Center (EMIC). Such reviews could augment those already occurring for many programs as a matter of their funding policy.

Of all the available methods, techniques, and systems that have been proposed for information control, we believe the concept of the specialized information center, such as the EMIC, and the centralization of the holdings from such centers into an accessible and comprehensive on-line computer system to be the most appealing. The information available from these central files should be available at both the national and the international level to ensure that all countries have equal access to information for use in R&D programs directed toward protecting human health.

Our objectives in this chapter are twofold. First, we wish to provide some background on the importance of information acquisition and transfer to R&D programs by examining the information problem and the specialized information center concept. Second, we describe the organization and operation of one particular specialized information center, which covers the research area of environmental mutagenesis, in order to illustrate the effective interface between a specialized information center and the research discipline it serves.

PROBLEM OF ACCESSING INFORMATION
FROM SPECIFIC DISCIPLINE-ORIENTED RESEARCH
AND DEVELOPMENT PROGRAMS

The National Academy of Sciences' Committee on Scientific and Technical Communication (1969) stated in a report that:

> The steadily expanding volume of scientific and technical information, the emergence of new disciplines and of new links between existing ones, and the increasing number and diversity of user groups and user needs are three obvious and urgent aspects of the information problem.

This statement can be illustrated by examining the most fundamental question that haunts a researcher when planning or reviewing a project: "Do I have all the information I need?" or "Did I search the literature thoroughly?" Likewise, an administrator responsible for making decisions must ask, "Have I considered all the available information?" In most cases, the answer to these questions will be "no," and there will always be the feeling that something important was missed.

The fault, in most cases, does not rest with the individual but rather with the information collection system; the literature is simply too awesome and diverse to be searched effectively. Hess (1977) has stated that there are not less than 3,000 abstracting and indexing services throughout the world engaged in the surveillance of published literature. Even with all these helpful resources, the task of finding information either in the primary literature or by use of most secondary literature sources, such as the aforementioned abstracting and indexing services, requires the expenditure of too much time. Workers in the information science field have recognized this problem, and many innovative systems, techniques, and types of equipment have been developed to make the collection and dissemination of information easier, but these have not been adequately applied to the problem of keeping pace with the increase in information in most areas of science. To correct this situation, more emphasis must be placed on the need to provide access to scientific information by the government agencies funding R&D programs. A beginning in solving the information problem would be to renew support for existing specialized information centers or to create new ones. Concurrent with this is the need to make sure that on-line computer systems are available to serve as centralized collection points for the data bases assembled by these centers.

Before going further in our consideration of the specialized information center concept, which will be illustrated by a description of the EMIC, a brief look at how most scientific investigators regard the acquisition and transfer of information will be helpful. No one would disagree with the statement that scientists and health administrators must have information to do their jobs effectively. In the past, and even now, the health administrator has relied on the scientist for advice and to provide the needed information, while the scientist has relied on experience and the knowledge of colleagues for the information to be supplied to the administrator. Although this is an important aspect of information transfer, it is not sufficient because individuals cannot surmount the obstacles presented by the volume of published material. This statement is universal to all research areas and is particularly applicable to toxicology.

Since access to the primary literature of a subject has passed the abilities of individuals, an investigator or administrator is left with essentially four options:

1. Concentrate only on information provided by certain key journals and the counsel of colleagues.

2. Screen one or several of the secondary literature services.

3. Use the specialized information center (if one presently exists in the area of concern) directly.

4. Query centralized on-line collections of the data bases from specialized information centers directly or have others such as response centers, do searches.

Of these options, the ones that give the best assurance that most of the necessary data will be available within a particular discipline are the specialized information center and the centralized collection of data bases from specialized information centers. The advantage of querying (directly or indirectly) a central facility is that it can provide valuable supporting information from related areas in addition to the specific information requested.

Since the information files created by the specialized information center offer the best solution to the information problem in strict scientific disciplines, the next section explores this concept of information control.

SPECIALIZED INFORMATION CENTER CONCEPT

All areas of toxicology are experiencing a phenomenal information increase, which has necessitated the need for strict organization of the data being published. Through such organization, scientists and administrators can work more effectively. The question is, "What is the best method of organizing information?" As the previous section has suggested, the specialized information center offers the best option for information control. This is not a new idea, and the concepts envisioned for the operation of the specialized information center conform for the most part to the following description by the President's Science Advisory Committee (Weinberg et al., 1963):

> An information analysis center is a formally structured organizational unit, specifically (but not necessarily exclusively) established for the purpose of acquiring, selecting, storing, retrieving, evaluating, analyzing, and synthesizing a body of information and/or data in a clearly defined specialized field or pertaining to a specified mission with intent of compiling, digesting, repackaging, or otherwise organizing and presenting pertinent information and/or data in a form most authoritative, timely, and useful to a society of peers and management.
>
> The activities of the most successful (information analysis) centers are an intrinsic part of science and technology. The centers not only disseminate and retrieve information; they create new information. . . . The process of sifting through large masses of data often leads to new generalizations. . . . In short, knowledgeable scientific interpreters who can collect relevant data, review a field, and distill information in a manner that goes to the heart of a technical situation are more help to the overburdened specialist than is a mere pile of relevant documents. Such knowledgeable scientific middlemen 'who themselves contribute to science' are the backbone of the information (analysis) center; they make an information center a technical institute rather than a technical library. The essence of a good technical information center is that it is operated by highly competent working scientists and engineers—people who see in the operation of the center an opportunity to advance and deepen their own personal contact with their science and technology.

In addition to conforming to these criteria, it is also desirable that the specialized toxicology information center be a computerized facility that has been commissioned to collect, organize, and disseminate information in a specific area of toxicology. To facilitate the work of the center, it is important that it be located at a research laboratory where work is under way in the area covered and where excellent library resources are available. It is also desirable that the center be actively supported by a research society from whose membership it can seek advice, counsel, and/or opinions on matters regarding policy. A peer review board could also be obtained from the society's members to assess the technical competence of the center's program in conjunction with other review efforts (see p. 350).

The material selected to become a part of the center's information file must be obtained from the international literature. This will require that the center's staff be versatile in languages and follow a clearly defined format regarding technical scope in their efforts to exhaust every means available for screening the literature from all countries. Once articles are found, it is paramount that the information indexed be accurately recorded. To do this, the center must have a copy of every document selected to go into the system. This necessitates that the center be linked to excellent library facilities. To remove individual biases, no judgment or analysis is made of publications selected to become a part of the center's file to determine the quality of the work reported. All information must be processed in the same manner. The center, for the most part, should leave value judgment and analysis strictly in the hands of the individual receiving the information. This is not to say that the center does not participate in evaluating data. Data evaluation, in our present context, is thought of in two dimensions: (1) reliability and worth of the study under question, and (2) significance of the reported results as they are related to human health.

How is the specialized information center involved in this first dimension of data evaluation? As pointed out earlier, we propose that the specialized information center collect all its data from primary literature sources and that the data selected for entry into the center's system be thoroughly indexed. The subject matter to be included in this indexing regimen should contain the most important data the researcher and administrator require. From this information, it then becomes easier to select only papers that fit specific requirements an individual may have. In other words, since the reliability criteria used to determine the value of a paper differ among individuals, selection of data elements to coincide with these various discretions will be possible. By following a nondiscriminatory selection and indexing scheme, the center is not limiting its capabilities to the opinions of its own staff.

As for the second dimension of data evaluation, the center can be of best service by assisting in the publication of a review journal in its area of interest, if one is already in existence, or by helping to start one. The objective of such a publication would be to provide reviews authored by recognized experts on specific issues of interest to the scientific discipline served by the center. These reviews could either summarize and evaluate important subjects with emphasis on potential hazards to humans or focus on the need for further research in certain areas to aid our understanding. The specialized information center can play a key role in the production of such a journal. For example, in this particular arrangement the editorial board of the review journal would have the primary responsibility for selecting subjects and authors and the specialized information center would supply the resource material. This information source, coupled with the one previously described, provides one of the best mechanisms of assisting and participating in the evaluation process, which emphasizes the assessment of potential hazards or benefits to humans from environmental agents.

The specialized information center can also play a role in helping make it possible to publish results from routine testing programs. For instance, publication of data from these tests could be mediated through a special supplement to a recognized journal in the field or serve as the basis for the establishment of a new journal. It is especially important to make these data available since they are needed in the assessment of potential health risks for the following reasons:

1. Testing data are accumulating rapidly from existing testing programs and will increase even more as new private and government-funded testing programs begin in response to recent legislation in the United States and other countries. Public health-oriented scientists and health administrators must have access to these data.

2. Existing journals may not have the ability or desire to publish the quantity of testing data now being generated or expected.

3. Rapid publication of testing data may prevent unnecessary duplication of research efforts, saving both time and money.

In view of these facts, we believe that researchers will seek ways to publish their experimental results. If there is no mechanism for publication of these data, an important incentive for voluntary toxicological testing of environmental compounds will be drastically diminished; it may also make it difficult for governments and industrial laboratories to obtain capable scientists to carry out testing programs. Most important, however, the information will be lost. As previously mentioned, a solution to the problem of publishing testing data could be a special journal designed specifically to handle only data from standard screening tests. We believe that the only way such a publication could be successful would be to have the active participation of the specialized information center, which could computerize all testing results either before or after publication. To do this, the center and the editorial board of the journal could recommend specific formats to be used in reporting testing results for publication, which then could be used to input directly into the center's computer file. These data then would be made available to testing laboratories for their planning and analysis through (1) journal publication, (2) the specialized information center, or (3) the central on-line computer system, queried directly or through a response center for toxicology information such as the Toxicology Information Response Center (Gerstner et al., 1977).

The following outline summarizes what a specialized information center is:

1. An information-collecting activity in a specifically defined research discipline (e.g., mutagenesis, teratogenesis, and carcinogenesis) with the purpose of acquiring, selecting, storing, retrieving, and analyzing information.

2. An information activity that has the active support and overview of the scientific discipline it serves.

3. An information activity that collects and prepares information for computer storage directly from copies of the published material selected for its data base. This literature is then maintained in a document library.

4. An information activity staffed primarily by individuals with backgrounds and research experience in the field covered.

5. An information activity whose primary function is to provide direct information to researchers and health administrators and/or their scientific advisors.

6. An information activity that attempts to keep its staff oriented to the scientific discipline served by attendance and/or participation in workshops and scientific meetings. Site visits to active research institutes should also be encouraged.

7. An information activity that explores and implements new programs to keep pace with the changing demands presented by the field covered and the user community served.

These are all obvious points, and one might have a tendency to think that they are natural to all information programs and that therefore the statement of such straightforward ideas is naive, but unfortunately they are not standard practice. These ideas, along with a further explanation of the specialized information center concept, are discussed on pp. 359–382.

Even though this section has dealt primarily with the organization and contributions that can be made by specialized toxicological information centers, the ideas can be applied to such centers in other areas of science. The main objective is to keep these facilities directly linked with the scientific discipline served and have the technical staff of the center working in cooperation with scientists actively engaged in experimental work in the field covered under the center's charter. If specialized information centers pursue the objectives outlined in this section, they will become an integral functioning part of R&D programs.

CENTRALIZATION OF DATA BASES
FROM SPECIALIZED TOXICOLOGY INFORMATION CENTERS

Specialized toxicology information centers such as the EMIC have evolved from the large secondary literature sources like *Chemical Abstracts, Biological Abstracts,* and so on (see Table 1). To obtain maximum use of the information files maintained by these centers, they must be brought together into a central system that users can search directly on-line. It is vitally important that these information files be available on a national scale. A program is under way in the United States through the auspices of the

National Library of Medicine to do just this, through their TOXLINE, CHEMLINE, and CANCERLINE systems, as well as other programs (see Table 2).

Centralized information files obtained from specialized information centers should follow the basic format shown in Table 3. As previously stated, the National Library of Medicine is the only organization, to our knowledge, that has a system that follows this concept. If scientific and technical information is to be made available in a usable form, it is best that it come from information files of the specialized information center.

ENVIRONMENTAL MUTAGEN INFORMATION CENTER (EMIC)

The Environmental Mutagen Information Center is a computerized information facility that was organized in 1969 and is located at Oak Ridge National Laboratory (ORNL) (Wassom, 1973; Wassom et al., 1977). The mission of the center is to collect, organize, and disseminate information of relevance to the subject of environmental mutagenesis. The decision to begin such an activity was stimulated by the fact that many geneticists who were concerned about the genetic hazards of environmental chemicals were finding it difficult to keep up with the literature. Because of this concern, the involvement of the research community in EMIC's operation began during the early stages of its development.

Papers selected for entry into the EMIC file contain information that is primarily concerned with the testing of chemicals (or other environmental agents, excluding for the most part papers dealing solely with uv and ionizing radiation) for mutagenicity. Papers are also selected that contain information on peripheral subjects that may be useful in understanding the known or suspected mutagenic activity of environmental agents (see Table 4).

To accomplish its task of data collection, EMIC uses a variety of methods to locate publications of interest. The most productive of these methods is the manual searching of 40 key journals that regularly publish manuscripts on mutagenesis studies (see Table 5). These journals are scanned as soon as they are available in the ORNL Biology Library and yield about 50% of the papers selected. The other 50% are obtained by searching large data bases such as those produced by the Chemical Abstracts Service, the BioSciences Information Service (*Biological Abstracts* and *BioResearch Index*), the Institute for Scientific Information, and the U.S. Department of Agriculture (Agricola). Descriptions of these and other data bases are found in Table 1. These secondary literature resources are searched by computer, using a unique set of terms significant to genetics and mutagenicity. Other secondary sources, such as *Genetics Abstracts, Carcinogenesis Abstracts, Current Contents,* and *Excerpta Medica,* are manually screened, as are books, symposia, and other publications available from the ORNL Biology Library.

TABLE 1A Secondary Literature Sources (Publications) Containing Toxicological Information

Biological Abstracts	BioSciences Information Service, Philadelphia, Pennsylvania	Life sciences	8,000 source publications from 100 countries	1. A subject-oriented, author-indexed collection of abstracts published twice monthly under the title *Biological Abstracts* 2. Computerized searches available either from the producer or from institutions that have purchased these tapes for use in their search services (see section B)
BioResearch Index	BioSciences Information Service, Philadelphia, Pennsylvania	Life sciences	More than 100,000 articles from the following sources are reported annually: institutional reports, bibliographies, letters, notes, preliminary reports, reviews, government reprints, semipopular journals, symposia, trade journals	1. A monthly publication containing bibliographical information and some abstracts 2. Computerized searches available either from the producer or from institutions that have purchased these tapes for use in their search services (see section B)

Name	Producer	Scope	Coverage	Description
Chemical Abstracts	American Chemical Society, Columbus, Ohio	World chemical literature	Approximately 1,000 primary journals	1. A weekly collection of abstracted information that has been indexed according to subject keyword, numerical patent, patent concordance, and author 2. Magnetic tapes available from producer for sale to customers for searching; searches also available from institutions that have purchased these tapes for use in their search services (see section B)
Index Medicus	National Library of Medicine, Washington, D.C.	Biomedical literature	Approximately 2,300 sources of periodical literature	A monthly subject- and author-indexed bibliography; information computerized and searchable via MEDLINE (see section B)
Current Contents	Institute for Scientific Information, Philadelphia, Pennsylvania	Life sciences	Approximately 1,000 journals	1. A weekly collection of the tables of contents of screened journals 2. Computerized searches of tables of contents of key journals by journal name and/or title keywords available; service called ASCA (Automated Science Center Alert)

TABLE 1A Secondary Literature Sources (Publications) Containing Toxicological Information (*Continued*)

Genetics Abstracts	Information Retrieval Limited, London, England	Literature of genetics and related disciplines	3,000 journals	A monthly collection of subject-indexed abstracts
Carcinogenesis Abstracts	National Cancer Institute, Bethesda, Maryland	Literature reporting on carcinogenesis research	Not available	A monthly collection of subject-indexed abstracts
Cancer Chemotherapy Abstracts	National Cancer Institute, Bethesda, Maryland	Literature reporting on carcinogenesis research	Not available	A monthly collection of subject-indexed abstracts
Excerpta Medica	Excerpta Medica Foundation, Amsterdam, Netherlands	World biomedical literature	Approximately 3,400 journals	A monthly collection of subject- and author-indexed abstracts

From all of this one can easily see that neither EMIC, nor any other specialized information center, can do its job without the use and help of special libraries and secondary literature services. EMIC is particularly fortunate to have access to the ORNL Biology Library, which is one of the finest in the world. In addition, geneticists around the world assist EMIC by sending reprints of their work and copies of material from journals and books published in their countries that have a limited geographic distribution. Such cooperation is frequently the only means of obtaining information from some of these foreign sources. Table 4 summarizes EMIC's selection and information processing techniques. Output from EMIC's computerized data base can take the form of publications, specialized indexed bibliographies, computer-readable tapes, or microfiches.

The services and publications of EMIC are available without charge to requesters to whom the EMIC funding agencies have given an exempt status. EMIC's charge policy has been formulated in compliance with a directive issued from the government's Office of Management and Budget. This directive states that all federally supported information activities must initiate a cost recovery policy for their products and services. Such a charge policy was, of course, worked out in conjunction with each federal agency providing financial support. Since EMIC presently has two different funding agencies— the National Institute of Environmental Health Sciences (NIEHS) and the National Cancer Institute (NCI)—its charge policy reflects the administrative and research attitudes of each of these agencies as well as those of ORNL. Basically, individuals and/or government agencies exempt from EMIC's charge policy are comprised of the following:

1. The President and Congress

2. All staff members of either of EMIC's two funding agencies, their contractors, subcontractors, or any individual or institution designated by one or more of these agencies

3. The membership of all Environmental Mutagen Societies belonging to the International Association of Environmental Mutagen Societies

4. All students or individuals not receiving direct support for research projects

5. Collaborators, authors, or institutions providing material and/or significant consulting services to EMIC

The EMIC data base is available for use on two on-line computer systems, TOXLINE and RECON. TOXLINE is a collection of toxicology data files sponsored and maintained by the National Library of Medicine. RECON is an on-line system of data files sponsored by the Department of Energy (DOE) and of interest primarily to DOE-funded researchers. This file is

TABLE 1B Secondary Literature Sources (On-Line Computer Systems[a]) Containing Toxicological Information

Name	File, number of records, and period covered	File description
DIALOG Lockheed Information Systems, Palo Alto, California	AGRICOLA *AGRIC*ultural *On-L*ine *A*ccess 835,000 1970–present	NATIONAL AGRICULTURAL LIBRARY. Worldwide index to the literature of agriculture and allied sciences. Subjects are: agricultural economics, animal industry, entomology, forestry, plant science, pesticides, soils, pollution, etc. Cites journal articles, monographs, government documents, special reports, proceedings, etc. Includes the Agricultural Economics file and the Food and Nutrition File. Corresponds to the *Bibliography of Agriculture* and the *National Agricultural Library Catalog*
	BIOSIS Previews 1,100,000 1969–present	*BIOS*CIENCES *I*NFORMATION *S*ERVICE. Worldwide coverage of research in the life sciences from more than 8,000 journals, as well as monographs, reports, symposia proceedings, etc. Subjects include microbiology, plant and animal science, biochemistry, botany, environmental biology, experimental medicine, genetics, public health, toxicology, virology, and other interdisciplinary areas. Citations from both *Biological Abstracts* and *BioResearch Index*
	CASIA *CA S*ubject *I*ndex *A*lert 1,000,000 1973–present	CHEMICAL ABSTRACTS SERVICE, AMERICAN CHEMICAL SOCIETY. General subject index headings and Chemical Abstracts Service (CAS) registry numbers for documents covered by CA Condensates.
	CHEMCON or CAC *Chem*ical Abstracts *C*ondensates 2,000,000 1968–present	CHEMICAL ABSTRACTS SERVICE, AMERICAN CHEMICAL SOCIETY. Worldwide coverage of literature in chemistry and chemical engineering, including biochemistry, organic chemistry, physical and analytical chemistry, etc. Corresponds to the printed *Chemical Abstracts.* Includes bibliographic citations to journal articles, monographs, patents, government reports, and proceedings of conferences and symposia

Note: See p. 369 for footnote.

CDA
*Comprehensive Dissertation
  Abstracts*
540,000
1961–present

UNIVERSITY MICROFILMS INTERNATIONAL.
Subject, title, and author guide to doctoral dissertations from accredited universities (predominantly U.S.). Based on *Dissertation Abstracts International, American Doctoral Dissertation,* and *Comprehensive Dissertation Index*

NTIS or GRA
*National Technical Information
  Service or Government
  Reports Announcements*
520,000
1964–present

NATIONAL TECHNICAL INFORMATION SERVICE.
A broad interdisciplinary file containing citations and abstracts of government-sponsored R&D reports and other reports prepared by contractors and grantees of the federal government. Some foreign language translations included. Corresponds to *Weekly Government Abstracts* and *Government Reports Announcements*

POLLUTION
Pollution *abstracts*
43,000
1970–present

POLLUTION ABSTRACTS DIVISION, DATA COURIER, INC.
Covers foreign and domestic reports, journals, contracts, symposia, etc. in the areas of pollution, its sources, and its control. Includes air, water, and land pollution, sewage and water treatment, and legal developments. Corresponds to the printed *Pollution Abstracts*

SCISEARCH
Science Citation Index
1,000,000
1974–present

INSTITUTE FOR SCIENTIFIC INFORMATION.
Multidisciplinary index to the literature of science and technology, including animal and plant science, biochemistry, drug research, experimental medicine, and microbiology. Unique feature is indexing cited papers. Corresponds to the printed *Science Citations Index*

ENVIROLINE or ESI
Environment (On-Line) or
Environment Science Index
60,000
1971–present

ENVIRONMENT INFORMATION CENTER.
Covers key environmental journals and reports as well as films and the *Federal Register.* Corresponds to *Environment Abstracts*

TABLE 1B Secondary Literature Sources (On-Line Computer Systems[a]) Containing Toxicological Information (*Continued*)

Name	File, number of records, and period covered	File description
	CEC *Council for Exceptional Children* 2,200 1966–present	COUNCIL FOR EXCEPTIONAL CHILDREN. Literature dealing with education of handicapped and gifted children
	PA *Psychological Abstracts* 240,000 1967–present	AMERICAN PSYCHOLOGICAL ASSOCIATION. Covers the world literature in psychology and other behavioral sciences. Indexes articles from more than 800 journals, as well as books, dissertations, and reports. Corresponds to the printed *Psychological Abstracts*
ORBIT System Development Corporation, Santa Monica, California	AGRICOLA	See entry under Lockheed's DIALOG system
	CHEMCON or CAC	See entry under Lockheed's DIALOG system
	LIBCON/E LIBCON/F LIBCON/S *Library of Congress* 1,000,000+ 1965–present	INFORMATION DYNAMICS CORPORATION. Covers all subject areas in monographic literature and audiovisual materials. Includes MARC records from the Library of Congress as well as many more LC-cataloged items. English (E), non-English (F), and current (S) files
	NTIS or GRA	See entry under Lockheed's DIALOG system

PNI
*Pharmaceutical News
Index*
14,000
1974–present

PHARMACEUTICAL NEWS INDEX, DATA COURIER, INC.
Indexes four weekly publications: *Drug Research Reports, FDC Reports, PMA Newsletter,* and *Washington Drug and Device Letter.* Covers major health bills, FDA recalls, and court actions, legislative actions, etc.

POLLUTION

See entry under Lockheed's DIALOG system

SSIE
*S*mithsonian *S*cience
*I*nformation *E*xchange
130,000
Current research for 3
fiscal yr

SMITHSONIAN SCIENCE INFORMATION EXCHANGE.
Covers ongoing and recently completed research in the life, physical, and social sciences, both basic and applied research projects. Includes federally funded projects (grants, contracts, etc.) and some privately sponsored research. A search retrieves Notices of Research Projects

MEDLINE
National Library
of Medicine,
Bethesda, Maryland

MEDLINE/NLM
MEDLARS On-Line
Current file 652,000
Most recent 2–3 yr
Backfiles 1,644,000
Older material from 1966

NATIONAL LIBRARY OF MEDICINE.
Contains references from more than 3,000 biomedical journals published throughout the world. Monographs and conference proceedings added in 1976. Corresponds to *Index Medicus.* Contains full bibliographic citations and index terms for all records. Some abstracts included. SDILINE, the monthly current awareness service, part of file

TOXLINE
*TOX*icology Information
On-*LINE*
Current file 350,000
1971–present
Backfiles (TOXBACK)
200,000
Older material

NATIONAL LIBRARY OF MEDICINE, TOXICOLOGY INFORMATION PROGRAM.
An extensive collection of toxicology information with references to human and animal toxicity studies, effects of environmental chemicals, pesticides, and pollutants, adverse drug reactions, and analytical methodology. Abstracts and/or indexing terms included in addition to full bibliographic citations. Information derived from five major secondary sources and five special collections of material:

TABLE 1B Secondary Literature Sources (On-Line Computer Systems[a]) Containing Toxicological Information (*Continued*)

Name	File, number of records, and period covered	File description
		1. CBAC (*Chemical-Biological Activities*) from CAS; 1965–present
		2. HEEP (*Health Effects of Environmental Pollutants*) from BIOSIS; 1972–present
		3. IPA (*International Pharmaceutical Abstracts*) from American Society of Hospital Pharmacists; 1970–present
		4. TOXBIB (*Toxicity Bibliography*) from NLM; 1968–present
		5. PESTAB (*Pesticides Abstracts,* formerly HAPAB) from EPA; 1966–present
		6. Hayes file on Pesticides, from EPA; 1940–1966
		7. EMIC (Environmental Mutagen Information Center) from ORNL; 1968–present
		8. TMIC (Toxic Materials Information Center) from ORNL; 1971–1974
		9. ETIC (Environmental Teratology Information Center) from ORNL; 1950–present
		10. TERA (Teratology) from IFI/Plenum Data Corporation; 1950s–1974
	CANCERLINE *Cancer* On-*Line* 37,000 1963–present	NATIONAL CANCER INSTITUTE. Cancer therapy and chemical, physical, and viral carcinogenesis from *Carcinogenesis Abstracts* and *Cancer Therapy Abstracts*
	CANCERPROJ *Cancer Projects* 10,000 Current Research (3 fiscal yr)	NATIONAL CANCER INSTITUTE, CURRENT CANCER RESEARCH PROJECTS ANALYSIS CENTER. Contains summaries of ongoing cancer research projects that have been provided by cancer scientists in many countries

	EPILEPSY *Epilepsy* On-Line 19,000 1945–present	**NATIONAL INSTITUTE OF NEUROLOGICAL DISEASES AND STROKE.** Contains citations and abstracts to literature on epilepsy, including information on the scientific, clinical, and social aspects of the disease. Corresponds to the printed *Epilepsy Abstracts* published by Excerpta Medica

RECON
Oak Ridge National
  Laboratory,
Computer Sciences
  Division,
DOE/RECON
  Project,
Oak Ridge,
  Tennessee
	EMIC
	*Environmental Mutagen
	Information Center*
	17,500
	1968–present
		NATIONAL INSTITUTE OF ENVIRONMENTAL HEALTH SCIENCES AND NATIONAL CANCER INSTITUTE, OAK RIDGE NATIONAL LABORATORY.
		Indexes worldwide journal and report literature on genetic effects of environmental agents, excluding radiation. CAS registry numbers included for all chemical agents. Full document file maintained for all material indexed

	ETIC *Environmental Teratology Information Center*	**NATIONAL INSTITUTE OF ENVIRONMENTAL HEALTH SCIENCES.** Indexes worldwide journal and report literature on the evaluation of agents for teratogenic activity in warm-blooded animals. CAS registry numbers included for all chemical agents. Full document file maintained for all material indexed
	NSA *Nuclear Science Abstracts* 550,000 1967–1976 (June)	**DEPARTMENT OF ENERGY, TECHNICAL INFORMATION CENTER**, Oak Ridge. Comprehensive coverage of international nuclear science literature. Includes reports as well as books, journals, conference proceedings, etc. Corresponds to *Nuclear Science Abstracts*. File closed in June 1976 and the information processed for this data base now included in the Energy Data Base portion of this information system

[a]Material in this section was adapted from a compilation prepared by M. L. Calkins (personal communication).

TABLE 2 Information Files Provided by the National
Library of Medicine of Interest to the Toxicologist[a]

CANCERLINE
CANCERPROJ
CHEMLINE
TOXLINE
    CBAC (*C*hemical-*B*iological *AC*tivities)
    HEEP (*H*ealth *E*ffects of *E*nvironmental *P*ollutants)
    IPA (*I*nternational *P*harmaceutical *A*bstracts)
    TOXBIB (*TOX*icity *BIB*liography)
    PESTAB (*PEST*icides *AB*stracts, formerly HAPAB)
    HAYES (*HAYES* file on pesticides)
    EMIC (*E*nvironmental *M*utagen *I*nformation *C*enter)
    TMIC (*T*oxic *M*aterials *I*nformation *C*enter)
    TERA (*TERA*tology)
    ETIC (*E*nvironmental *T*eratology *I*nformation *C*enter)

[a]See Table 1 for further information.

maintained for the DOE by the ORNL Computer Science Division. More details about each of these systems can be found in Table 1.

As of September 30, 1977, the EMIC data base contained 22,000 papers that cite information on approximately 8,000 different chemicals. EMIC is an example of a successful effort to establish a specialized information center that is closely allied with and supported by the scientific discipline it serves.

Literature of Environmental Mutagenesis[2]

During the last 12 yr, issues regarding the relationship between humans and their environment have become demanding subjects in all sciences, and naturally the threat to human health from environmental agents has become a major concern. It has been established that chemical exposure can lead to cancer and congenital defects. Another hazard to human health is posed by environmental mutagens that have the potential of changing human genetic material by inducing mutations. Problems associated with the elucidation of such a threat to human genetic welfare range from the identification of mutagenic agents to the more difficult problems of evaluating their genetic effects on humans. These problems began to be recognized in the literature during the late 1950s and more so during the 1960s. The environmental influence has created a new climate for research with demands for testing priorities, new assay procedures, and population-monitoring techniques. These areas have added another dimension to the extensive knowledge that has accumulated in this field since the early days, when research efforts were

[2]This section is based primarily on information contained in an article previously published under this section heading by Wassom (1973).

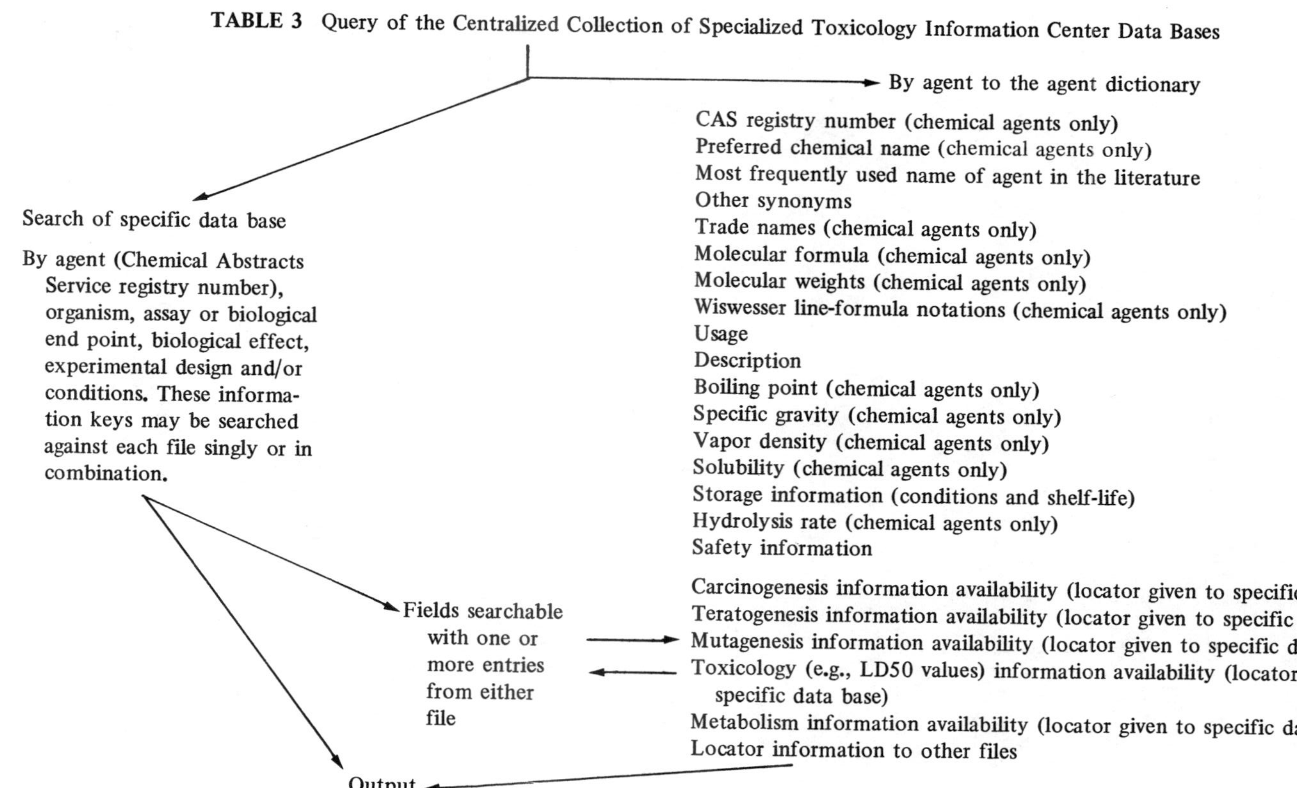

TABLE 3 Query of the Centralized Collection of Specialized Toxicology Information Center Data Bases

TABLE 4 The Processing Format for Chemical Mutagenesis Information
at the Environmental Mutagen Information Center

Information selection and processing techniques

I. *Screening of the international scientific literature*

A. Search methods
 1. Computerized searches of secondary literature sources (see Table 1)
 2. Manual screening of key source journals (Table 5)
 3. Correspondents[a]

B. Selection criteria
 Articles are selected that report on or review the testing of chemicals and/or
 biologicals on the induction of
 1. Mutations
 2. Chromosomal and chromatid aberrations (breaks, gaps, etc.
  or effects on
 3. DNA (binding, breaks, base modification, repair, etc.)
 4. Mitosis
 5. Meiosis
 6. Oogenesis
 7. Spermatogenesis

II. *Processing of information from copies of all selected papers*

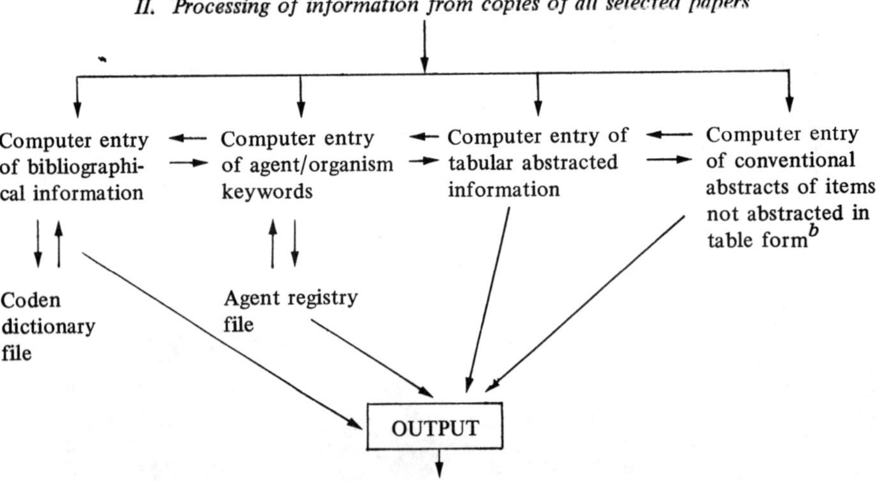

1. Annual surveys of the chemical mutagenesis literature
2. Special subject bibliographies
3. Searches
4. File made available to two on-line computer systems, TOXLINE and RECON

---

[a]Individuals located in various countries throughout the world who screen the
literature of their respective countries for material to be considered for the EMIC data
file.

[b]These aspects of EMIC's information processing program are not fully operational
at this writing.

TABLE 5 Key Journal Sources Used by the Environmental
Mutagen Information Center

1. *Mutation Research*	22. *Comptes Rendus Hebdomadaires des Seances de l'Academie des Sciences, Serie D: Sciences Naturelles*
2. *Soviet Genetics* (USSR)—English translation of *Genetika*	
3. *Cancer Research*	23. *Radiation Research*
4. *Genetics*	24. *Journal of the National Cancer Institute*
5. *Nature (London)*	
6. *Journal of Bacteriology*	25. *Toxicology and Applied Pharmacology*
7. *Molecular and General Genetics*	26. *Canadian Journal of Genetics and Cytology*
8. *Biochimica et Biophysica Acta*	
9. *Proceedings of the National Academy of Sciences U.S.A.*	27. *Biochemical Pharmacology*
10. *Experimental Cell Research*	28. *Doklady Biological Sciences*
11. *Chemico-Biological Interactions*	29. *Cytologia*
12. *Cytology and Genetics* (USSR) and its Russian original *Tsitologiya i Genetika*	30. *Bulletin of Experimental Biology and Medicine (USSR)*
13. *Experientia*	31. *Virology*
14. *Hereditas*	32. *Journal of Virology*
15. *Biochemical and Biophysical Research Communications*	33. *Lancet*
	34. *Indian Journal of Radiation Biology*
16. *Tsitologiya* (Russian)	35. *Biochemical Journal*
17. *Science* (Washington)	36. *Journal of Reproduction and Fertility*
18. *Journal of Cell Biology*	
19. *Human Genetics*	37. *Chromosoma*
20. *Japanese Journal of Genetics*	38. *Nucleus (Calcutta)*
21. *Journal of Molecular Biology*	39. *Biochemistry*
	40. *Journal of General Microbiology*

dominated by pure rather than applied research. Today, efforts to understand the nature of induced mutations and to evaluate their effect on humans demand that concerned researchers, administrators, and government officials have access to all available information related to environmental mutagenesis. This has contributed significantly to the enormous growth of the literature in this area, as can be seen by a review of the number of publications produced over a period of recent years. For instance, from nominal yearly increases prior to 1960, the rate of papers being published increased almost twofold during the decade of the 1960s compared with that of the late 1940s and 1950s. From 1968 to 1973 published material grew at a rate of 200–700 articles per year (Table 6).

There was a drop in papers published during 1974, 1975, and 1976, which is somewhat surprising. On analysis it seems that the decline in papers offered for publication during these years was probably a result of the following factors:

1. Articles overwhelmed the journals publishing manuscripts containing mutagenicity information.

2. Stricter editorial policy made data from straight mutagenicity testing more difficult to publish.

3. Negative results were being considered nonpublishable.

4. Many tests were done under contracts and the results were proprietary and therefore never published.

5. Results from most government-funded research projects were published as government reports, whose public availability is minimal.

Future publication trends will be influenced by the level of experimentation and interest this field attains in the years ahead and the availability of publication outlets. An increase in the publication of negative data and data from routine testing, which heretofore have not been published with any regularity, promises to be a factor contributing to the growth expectancy of this literature field.

Primary Literature Sources and Article Types Comprising the Mutagenesis Literature

Documents that are indexed in the EMIC file are of several different types, such as review articles, symposium proceedings, and conference abstracts, but the majority are journal articles that give detailed descriptions of results from original research. To illustrate this point, the forms in which the 22,000 records in the EMIC file were published are shown in Table 7. There is a wide range of sources to which an author may submit writings for

TABLE 6 Yearly Publication Frequencies
of the Mutagenesis Literature

Year of publication	Number of documents collected
pre-1968	2,723
1968	922
1969	1,360
1970	1,918
1971	2,336
1972	2,476
1973	2,611
1974	2,096
1975	2,153
1976	1,805
1977	1,600
Total –	~ 22,000[a]

[a]Number of documents in the EMIC information file as of September 30, 1977.

publication. As science has expanded in scope, certain publication sources have evolved that accept and publish articles along strict disciplinary lines. Most of the information on environmental mutagenesis is now found in sources publishing on genetic, carcinogenic or biochemical subjects. There is, however, a trend developing for specific journals that publish only papers relevant to mutagenesis. For example, the international journal *Mutation Research* and its three supplements—*Environmental Mutagenesis and Related Subjects, Reviews in Genetic Toxicology*, and *Genetic Toxicology Testing*—have come into existence within the last few years and carry 10% of all the papers published in this field. The records at EMIC show that writings in all forms about environmental mutagens are now found in approximately 2,000 different publications (see Table 2).

After a prospective record has been selected and a hard copy of the article obtained, the index terms describing the biographical data, agent/ organism keywords, and Chemical Abstracts Service (CAS) registry numbers are recorded and sent to the computer. Table 8 shows an example of these types of entries.

Further processing of a document depends on the type of literature at hand. For instance, all items in which experimental results of original work are published as journal articles are subject to additional indexing in a form called tabular abstracts or extracts. Conventional written abstracts are prepared for documents not indexed in tabular form, such as review articles, meeting abstracts, and editorial comments.

All these methods of information processing except tabular abstracting, or data extraction, as it is also called, are used quite commonly today and are relatively self-explanatory. The idea of tabular abstracts, however, is a relatively new approach in the computer manipulation of data from mutagenicity research. This indexing technique makes it possible to segregate essential data under different column headings, thus providing a means by which key information from a citation may be summarized for the user. The type of information indexed by this method and the format used to process it

TABLE 7 Types of Published Work in the Data Base
of the Environmental Mutagen Information Center

1. Original data	15,649
2. Abstracts	3,390
3. Reviews	1,398
4. Symposia	554
5. Reports and notes	387
6. Letters to editors	91
8. Hypotheses or theory papers	134
9. Miscellaneous (books, book chapters, etc.)	397
Total	22,000[a]

[a]Number of documents in the EMIC information file as of September 30, 1977.

TABLE 8 Example of the Entry of Bibliographic and Agent/Organism Data
at the Environmental Mutagen Information Center

Accession number	10549
Literature type	Journal article with original data
Publication date	1971
Author(s)	Lieberman, Michael W.; Baney, Richard N.; Lee, Robert E.; Sell, Stewart; Farber, Emmanuel
Title	Studies on DNA repair in human lymphocytes treated with proximate carcinogens and alkylating agents
Publication source	*Cancer Research* 31:1297–1306
Selection source	Key journal screening
Test object, common classification	Mammal, human cell culture
Test object, specific classification	*Homo sapiens*
Agent(s) tested/Chemical Abstract Service registry numbers	EMS(62-50-0); MMS(66-27-3); *N*-acetoxy-2-acetylaminofluorene(6098-44-8); beta-propiolactone(57-57-8); nitrogen mustard (51-75-2); DMN(62-75-9); 3-methyl-4-dimethylaminoazobenzene(55-80-1); 2-acetylaminofluorene(53-96-3); iodoacetamide (144-48-9)

for the computer are illustrated in Table 9. Data extracted in this manner can be associated by the computer in a variety of ways, such as by compound or organism, and printed in tabular form. Entries within such a table can be queried individually or in combination with data contained under other headings, which makes it a very powerful tool, particularly in document selection.

To supplement its search methods, EMIC is constructing a computerized agent registry. Table 10 shows an entry that is included in this file. This registry makes it possible to locate and associate synonyms for chemical agents through their unique CAS registry numbers. These numbers are then used in lieu of chemical names to search the EMIC master file. This feature lends an important dimension to the retrieval of information. Instead of searching the data base with each of a compound's synonyms, its CAS registry number is used. This unique number collates all the synonyms and all the available information in the data base. In addition, these unique numbers are used as the primary means of providing links to other information files or reference documents, such as the NCI publication entitled *Survey of Com-*

pounds Which Have Been Tested for Carcinogenic Activity (PHS 149), the monographs of the International Agency for Research on Cancer (IARC), and the Agent Registry of the Environmental Teratology Information Center (see Table 11).

Also included in this registry is a substructural search program that makes it possible to draw correlations between chemically active groups and mutagenic activity, a capability that could have some prognostic value concerning the mutagenic activity of new chemicals. Also, this substructural search program makes it possible to identify and list compounds with similar structural characteristics.

EMIC has also adopted a chemical classification scheme for use in assigning classes to the 8,000 chemicals presently in its agent registry. In devising this classification system, consideration was given to the major reactions between chemicals and DNA, such as alkylation, arylation, and intercalation, as well as to chemical structures and/or functional groups. The classification scheme follows, with few exceptions, the system used by the DHEW subcommittee on environmental mutagenesis and its committee on testing procedures.

The system is composed of 16 primary chemical groups and, in some instances, several subgroups denoting particular functional moieties. These groups were selected after examining several thousand of the chemicals in the EMIC registry file and are shown in Table 12.

These chemical classes will be used as a mechanism for searching the EMIC file for information on general groups of compounds and drawing parallels between the types and numbers of compounds tested in various assay

TABLE 9　Tabular Abstracting Format of the Environmental
Mutagen Information Center

EMIC accession number	10549
Agent	Dimethylnitrosamine (CAS No. 62-75-9)
Test object	Cultured human lymphocytes
Assay	Unscheduled DNA synthesis
Treatment conditions	Chemical added to culture for 1 hr; cells cultured 12 additional hr in media with tritiated thymidine
Agent concentrations tested	0.0001–10.0 mM
Method of detection	TCA-precipitable activity in cells measured by liquid scintillation counting
Reported biological effect	All exposures produced negative results
Comment	Negative results were presumably found because no activation system was present

TABLE 10 Environmental Mutagen Information Center Agent Registry

EMIC name	Ethylene dibromide
CAS registry number	106-93-4
Preferred name	Ethane, 1,2-dibromo
Synonyms	Bromofume; sym-dibromoethane; Dowfume, W 8; Dowfume MC-2; EDB; Glycol dibromide; Iscobrome D; Soilfume; Aadibroom; Dowfume W 85; Nefis; Sanhyuum; ethylene dibromide; ethylene bromide; dibromoethane.
Molecular formula	C2-H4-Br2
Wiswesser linear notation	E2E
Usage	Pesticide (fumigant); gasoline additive.
Description	Heavy colorless to light brown nonflammable liquid. Has a pungent chloroform-like odor.
Boiling point	131°C
Specific gravity	$2.180\,\frac{20}{4}$
Vapor density	6.5
Solubility	Soluble in about 250 parts H_2O; completely soluble in alcohol, acetone, benzene, dimethyl formamide, and dimethyl sulfoxide.
Storage	Compound is light-sensitive and should therefore be stored in an airtight amber container located in a refrigerated (4°C) storage cabinet.
Hydrolysis rate	—
Toxicity	Acute oral LD50 (male rat), 146 mg/kg; acute vapor toxicity, 200 ppm; signs and symptoms of intoxication in humans include headache, prolonged vomiting, sometimes diarrhea, weak and rapid pulse, tinnitus. Brief exposures may produce conjunctival and respiratory irritation, anorexia, headache. Skin contact may result (depending on exposure) in burning pain, erythema, inflammation, blisters. Sensitization (on repeated skin contact) is reported.
Metabolism	Compound metabolized to *S*-(hydroxyethyl)cysteine-*S*-(2-hydroxyethyl)cysteine-*N*-acetate after oral administration to rats and mice; ip injections yielded only *S*-(hydroxyethyl) cysteine. REF: EMIC No. 7931.
Safety	The greatest potential danger from EDB comes from handling. This compound is highly penetrating and most commonly used lab safety materials or equipment offer only token protection. For example, this chemical penetrates most varieties of rubber gloves, which makes them unsatisfactory for use during handling operations. Nylon-neoprene has been

TABLE 10 Environmental Mutagen Information Center Agent Registry (*Continued*)

	found to offer the best protection for use in handling operations. Hands should, in any case, be washed thoroughly with soap and water after all experiments. Experimental work areas should be well ventilated and all manipulations involving transfers of this chemical should be done in a properly functioning hood. (*Encyclopaedia of Occupational Health and Safety*, vol. 1, pp. 384–385, International Labour Office, Geneva 22, Switzerland, 1973).
Carcinogenic data availability	PHS 149[a], Supplement I, Accession No. 155; *IARC Monograph 12*
Teratogenic data availability	No data available per ETIC[b] (5/1/77)
Sources	Aldrich Chemical Co.; Dow Chemical Co.; Excel Industries (India); Great Lakes Chemical Corp.; Kerr-McGee Chemical Co.; Michigan Chemical Corp.
EMIC availability	5480; 6861; 7225; 7931; 8212; 11767; 12223; 13302; 13817; 14101; 15901.

[a]PHS 149 is an acronym for the following publication: *Public Health Serv. Publ. 149, Survey of compounds which have been tested for carcinogenic activity*, prepared for the National Cancer Institute by John I. Thompson and Company, Rockville, Maryland.
[b]Environmental Teratology Information Center.

TABLE 11 Results of Cross-Referencing Agents in the Environmental Mutagen Information Center Registry with Other Toxicological Information Sources

No. of chemicals in EMIC agent registry	No. of chemicals in agent registries cross-referenced to EMIC		No. of chemicals common to both files
8,000	ETIC[a]	2,880	1,177
	PHS 149[b]	3,634	1,180
	IARC Monographs (through vol. 11)[c]	357	232

[a]ETIC, Environmental Teratology Information Center.
[b]PHS 149, *Public Health Serv. Publ. 149, Survey of compounds which have been tested for carcinogenic activity*.
[c]IARC, International Agency for Research on Cancer, Lyon, France.

TABLE 12 Chemical Classification System for Substances
in the Environmental Mutagen Information Center
Agent Registry

I. Alkylating agents
   A. Aziridines
   B. Triazines
   C. Nitrogen, sulfur, and oxide mustards
   D. Phosphoric acid esters, phosphonates, phosphoramides, thio analogues
   E. Epoxides
   F. Lactones
   G. Aldehydes
   H. Alkyl sulfates
   I. Alkylsulfonic acid esters (salts)
   J. Diazoalkanes
   K. Aryl dialkyltriazenes
   L. Alkyl halides
   M. Azoxy and hydrazo alkanes

II. Nitrosamines, nitrosamides, nitrosoureas
   A. Nitrosamines
   B. Nitrosamides and nitrosoimides
   C. Nitrosoureas

III. Organic peroxides

IV. Polynuclear aromatics, NOC[a]
   A. Fluorenes

V. Heterocyclics, NOC
   A. Benzimidazoles
   B. Phenothiazines
   C. Dicarboximides
   D. Thioxanthenes
   E. Acridines
   F. Dibenzo-*p*-dioxins
   G. Furocoumarins

VI. Inorganic derivatives, NOC
   A. Metal and metalloid derivatives
   B. Halogens and derivatives
   C. Sulfur and nitrogen oxides and derivatives
   D. Ozone

VI. Natural products, NOC
   A. Mycotoxins
   B. Pyrrolizidine alkaloids
   C. Antibiotics
   D. Xanthines
   E. Steroids

VIII. Halogenated ethers, halohydrins, and cyanohydrins

TABLE 12 Chemical Classification System for Substances
in the Environmental Mutagen Information Center
Agent Registry (*Continued*)

IX. Halogenated hydrocarbons and related derivatives
    A. Vinyl and vinylidene derivatives
    B. Halogenated aromatics and alicyclics
    C. Fluorocarbons
    D. Cyclodienes

X. Six-membered diazine derivatives (purines, pyrimidines, and pteridines)

XI. Hydrazines, hydroxylamines, carbamates, hydrazides, ureas, thioureas, and their
    cyclic analogues
    A. Hydrazines
    B. Hydroxylamines
    C. Carbamates
    D. Hydrazides
    E. Ureas
    F. Thioureas
    G. Guanidines
    H. Aliphatic amines and nitriles
    I. Thiocyanates
    J. Sulfamates

XII. Aromatic amines and phenolics (not part of heterocyclic)

XIII. Nitro derivatives, NOC
    A. Nitroquinolines and derivatives
    B. Nitrofurans
    C. Nitroimidazoles

XIV. Organometallics, NOC
    A. Organolead derivatives
    B. Organomercury derivatives

XV. Amino acid analogues

XVI. Other, NOC
    A. Intercalating agents
    B. Azo compounds
    C. Esters and anhydrides
    D. Quaternary ammonium compounds (and partially substituted ammonium
        compounds)
    E. Quinones
    F. N-Oxides
    G. Sulfites
    H. Sultones

[a]NOC, Not otherwise classified.

systems. For example, the system would tell how many aldehydes had been tested in a particular mutagenicity assay such as the sex-linked recessive lethal test in *Drosophila*.

The guiding principle used in devising this scheme has been to classify materials tested for mutagenic activity in large, well-defined chemical groups; other coding techniques such as Wiswesser line notation and the Environmental Protection Agency's substructure search system (Heller et al., 1977) are to be used for examining chemicals on the basis of more detailed structural features or combinations of features.

EVALUATION OF PUBLISHED DATA
FROM MUTAGENICITY TESTS

Extreme care is taken to ensure that the information selected to become a part of the EMIC data file is accurately recorded. No judgment or analysis is made to determine the quality of the work reported, as all information that conforms to the scope of the center is processed in the same manner. The center, for the most part, leaves value judgment and analysis strictly in the hands of the individual receiving the information. This is not to say that EMIC does not participate in evaluating data, for it does. As already stated (p. 354), data evaluation is thought of in two dimensions: (1) the reliability of the study in question, and (2) the significance of the reported results to humans. EMIC is involved in the first dimension of data evaluation by collecting all data that are indexed, as shown in Tables 8 and 9. This makes it possible to select only papers that fit specific requirements an individual may have when making reliability estimates. Since reliability criteria differ from one individual to another, information can be selected to meet these various discretions. By entering all papers within the scope of the center, the chance of personal biases influencing the content of the data base is eliminated.

As for the second dimension of data evaluation, EMIC assists the new supplement to *Mutation Research* entitled *Reviews in Genetic Toxicology*. The objective of this new publication is to provide reviews authored by recognized experts on the genetic effects of chemicals or other environmental mutagens and the potential genetic hazards of such compounds to humans. Articles may also point out the need for further research in order to provide relevant data in this general area.

Topics to be reviewed and prospective authors are selected by the editorial board, EMIC, and the NIEHS Laboratory of Environmental Mutagenesis. Also, along the same lines, EMIC assists the IARC in the preparation of the mutagenicity section of their monograph series *Evaluation of Carcinogenic Risks of Chemicals to Man*. In this case, EMIC provides information to experts selected by the IARC. This procedure also involves two of EMIC's primary funding agencies, NIEHS and NCI. EMIC is thus involved in data evaluation, but in a manner that we believe is most suitable for information centers.

F. H. Sobels, managing editor of *Mutation Research*, and several of his coeditors wrote an editorial pointing out the need for a special publication to handle results from standard mutagenicity tests (Sobels et al., 1976). EMIC and the NIEHS Laboratory of Environmental Mutagenesis drafted a suggested format for articles to be submitted to such a journal (see Table 13). The

TABLE 13 Suggested Format for Articles Submitted
to *Genetic Toxicology Testing*

Title of paper
Author(s)
Address(es)

  I.   Summary

  II.   Introduction

  III. Materials and methods
     A. Test agents
       1. Pure chemicals
       2. Commercial mixtures
       3. Waste products and chemically contaminated samples from
          the environment
       4. Comments
     B. Biological test material
       1. Specific or taxonomic name of test organism, to include all
          strain designations
         a. Cells (virus, bacteria, conidia, mammalian
           cells, etc.)
         b. Animals
         c. Plants
     C. Description of the method
       1. Test system
       2. Preparation of the test solution
       3. Treatment conditions

  IV. Results
     A. Requirements for reporting experimental data
       1. Controls
         a. Positive controls
         b. Negative controls
       2. Test results
       3. Statistical evaluation
       4. Results obtained for agents that did not show an increase
          in the mutation frequency
       5. Presentation of data

  V.   Discussion

  VI. References

Elsevier Scientific Publishing Company, which publishes *Mutation Research* and two special sections on environmental subjects and reviews, agreed to publish a third section. The first issue of this new section appeared in January, 1976, under the title supplement of *Genetic Toxicology Testing.*

There is much more to be said about this topic, but because of the considerable amount of material already discussed in this chapter it will not be possible to cover every aspect of the EMIC program. Further details of the information presented here, as well as the other facets of the operation of EMIC, can be obtained by writing the Environmental Mutagen Information Center, Oak Ridge National Laboratory, P.O. Box Y, Building 9224, Oak Ridge, Tennessee 37830.

CONCLUSION

The eminent risk to human health resulting from exposure to environmental agents adds urgency to the task of providing access to toxicology information. Specialized information centers in the research area of toxicology are therefore needed. The government must support these information centers as R&D programs in their own right to ensure that information generated by toxicological research will be available for use in the assessment of health problems.

EMIC is an example of such a specialized information center. As of September 30, 1977, 22,000 documents were indexed and on file, which contained information on approximately 8,000 different compounds, many of which are pollutants of air, land, and water. The resources of EMIC provide, in our opinion, the best means available for reviewing the voluminous literature from this specific area of toxicology (mutagenesis).

We believe that the specialized information center concept, as described in this chapter, offers the best solution to the problem of keeping up with and making the best use of the information provided by R&D programs in any area of science.

REFERENCES

Gerstner, H. B., Huff, J. E. and Ulrikson, G. U. 1977. *Am. Lab.* 9:41.
Heller, S. R., Milne, G. W. A. and Feldmann, R. J. 1977. *Science* 195:253.
Hess, E. L. 1977. *Fed. Proc.* 36:1.
Jameson, D. L. 1976. In *Benchmark papers in genetics,* eds. J. W. Drake and R. E. Koch, vol. 4, p. vii. Stroudsburg, Pa.: Dowden, Hutchinson and Ross.
Sobels, F. H., de Serres, F. J., Malling, H. V., Vogel, E. and Wassom, J. S. 1976. *Mutat. Res.* 40:1.
Wassom, J. S. 1973. In *Chemical mutagens. Principles and methods for their detection,* A. Hollaender, vol. 3, pp. 271–287. New York: Plenum.

Wassom, J. S., Shelby, M. D. and Von Halle, E. S. 1977. *Proc. Symp. Toxicology Information Subcommittee DHEW to Coordinate Toxicology and Related Programs, 1976.* National Institutes of Health. In press.
Weinberg, A. M., Baker, W. O., Cohen, K., Crawford, H. H. Jr., Hammett, L. P., Kalitinsky, A., King, G. W., Knox, W. T., Lederberg, J., Lee, M. O., Tukey, J. W., Wigner, E. P. and Kelley, J. H. 1963. In *Science, government, and information. A report of the President's Science Advisory Committee.* Washington, D.C.: Government Printing Office.

INDEX